D1609464

The Ruminants

Color Atlas of
Veterinary Anatomy

The Ruminants

Raymond R. Ashdown PhD, BVSc, MRCVS
Emeritus Reader in Veterinary Anatomy, University of London

Stanley Done BA, BVet, PhD, MRCVS
Formerly Lecturer in Veterinary Anatomy, University of London

Photography by
Stephen W. Barnett BA, MIST
Formerly Chief Technician at the
Royal Veterinary College, London

University Park Press · Baltimore
Gower Medical Publishing · London · New York

Color Atlas of Veterinary Anatomy. The Ruminants

Distributed in the United States of America and Canada by:
University Park Press
300 North Charles St.
Baltimore
Maryland 21201

Distributed in Japan by:
Nishimura Co. Ltd.
1-754-39, Asahimachi-dori
Niigata-Shi 951
Japan

Distributed in all countries except the United States of America and
Canada by:
Baillière Tindall
1 St. Anne's Road
Eastbourne
BN21 3UN
England

ISBN 0-8391-1760-4 (University Park Press)
ISBN 0-906923-04-2 (Gower Medical Publishing)

Library of Congress Catalog #: 82-50120

Slide Atlas of Ruminant Anatomy
The slide atlas, which is based on the material in this book, has been
specially designed to provide a high quality, practical aid to teachers. It is
presented as a number of volumes in which printed material, containing
color photographs and labelled and captioned drawings, is bound
together with wallets holding 35mm slides of all the illustrations in the
book.

The 'Slide Atlas of Ruminant Anatomy' is available from:

Gower Medical Publishing
101 5th Avenue, New York, New York 10003 USA

Project Editor Marinella Nicolson
    Designer Phil Jones
    Illustrator Jeremy J.D. Cort
Printed in Hong Kong by Mandarin Offset Ltd.

Author's preface

This book is intended for veterinary students and practising veterinary surgeons. Important features of topographical anatomy are presented in a series of full-color photographs of detailed dissections. The structures are identified in accompanying colored line drawings, and the nomenclature is based on that of the Nomina Anatomica Veterinaria (1973); latin terms are used for muscles, arteries, veins, lymphatics and nerves, but anglicized terms are used for all other structures. When necessary, information needed for interpretation of the photographs is given in the captions. Each section begins with photographs of regional surface features taken before dissection, and complementary photographs of an articulated bovine skeleton illustrate the important palpable bony features of these regions. All dissections and photographs have been specially prepared for this book.

The cattle (two cows and four calves) were all Jerseys and the three goats were of the British Saanen breed. The specimens were embalmed, for the most part, in the standing position using methods routinely employed in the Department of Anatomy at the Royal Veterinary College. Every effort was made to ensure that the final position corresponded to that of normal level standing. In most cases red neoprene latex was injected into the arteries. The dissections follow the pattern of prosections that have been used for teaching at the Royal Veterinary College for the past ten years.

The aim of these dissections and photographs is to reveal the topography of the animal as it would be presented to the veterinary surgeon during a routine clinical examination. Therefore, lateral views predominate and we have, as far as possible, avoided photographs of parts removed from the body or the use of views from unusual angles, or of unusual bodily positions. It is our earnest hope that this book will enable students and veterinary surgeons to see, beneath the outer surface of the animals entrusted to their care, the muscles, bones, vessels, nerves and viscera that go to make up each region of the body and each organ system.

Author's acknowledgements

The dissections and photography for this book were carried out at the Royal Veterinary College, University of London. We are grateful to the Department of Anatomy for the provision of specialised facilities, without which this work could not have been possible. In particular we would like to thank Susan Evans, M.I.S.T., Chief Technician in Anatomy, for advice and assistance with the dissections and photography. The task of preparing and caring for the specimens before and during dissection was undertaken by Douglas Hopkins and Andrew Crook, both of whom also assisted with the dissections.

The programme of prosections of the cow used in this book has been based on that developed over several years in this Department of Anatomy, by Harry Merlen, M.R.C.V.S.; he also prepared the dissections of the abdomen of the goat.

The idea of producing an atlas of ruminant anatomy based on our yearly teaching programme of prosection of cow and calf, resulted from discussions within Gower Medical Publishing. We are very grateful to the project editor, designer and illustrators for their hard work and for sustaining us with their optimism and enthusiasm.

Our wives have been somewhat neglected at times during the past three years while we picked at the carcases and puzzled over transparencies. We would like to thank them for their forbearance and understanding.

RRA
SD

Numerous original papers have been consulted during this work but our studies have mainly been supported by a range of anatomical textbooks. We would especially acknowledge our debt to the following, which have been our constant companions throughout the preparation of the specimens and the text:-

Berg, R. (1973) Angewandte und topographische Anatomie der Haustiere. Jena; Fischer.

Bressou, C. (1978) Les ruminants. Anatomie régionale des animaux domestiques Vol. II (Montané, L., Bourdelle, E. & Bressou, C. editors). 2nd edition. Paris; Baillière.

Butterfield, R.M. & May, N.D.S. (1966) Muscles of the ox. St. Lucia; Univ. of Queensland.

Dyce, K.M. & Wensing, C.J.G. (1971) Essentials of bovine anatomy. Amsterdam, Utrecht; de Bussy, Oosthoek.

Ellenberger, W. & Baum, H. (1943) Handbuch der vergleichenden Anatomie der Haustiere. (Zietzschmann, O., Ackernecht, E. & Grau, H. editors) 18th edition. Berlin: Springer.

Field, E.J. & Harrison, R.J. (1968) Anatomical terms. Their origin and derivation. 3rd edition. Cambridge; Heffer.

Ghoshal, N.G., Koch, T. & Popesko, P. (1981) The venous drainage of the domestic animals. Philadelphia; Saunders.

Greenhough, P.R., MacCallum, F.J. & Weaver, A.D. (1981) Lameness in cattle. (Weaver, A.D., editor) 2nd edition. Bristol; Wright.

Habel, R.E. (1970) Guide to the dissection of domestic ruminants. 2nd edition. Ithaca; Habel.

Habel, R.E. (1973) Applied veterinary anatomy. Ithaca; Habel.

Hecker, J.F. (1974) Experimental surgery of small ruminants. London; Butterworth.

McFadyean's osteology and arthrology of the domesticated animals. 4th edition. (Hughes, H.V. & Dransfield, J.W. editors) London; Ballière, Tindall, Cox.

Martin, P. & Schauder, W. (1938) Lehrbuch der Anatomie der Haustiere Bd.III Anatomie der Hauswiederkäuer. 3rd edition. Stuttgart; Schickhardt, Ebner.

Nickel, R., Schummer, A. & Seiferle, E. (1968) Lehrbuch der Anatomie der Haustiere Bd.I Bewegungsapparat. 3rd edition. Berlin, Hamburg; Parey.

Nickel, R., Schummer, A. & Seiferle, E. (1973) The viscera of the domestic animals. Translated and revised by Sack, W.O., Berlin, Hamburg; Parey.

Nickel, R. Schummer, A. & Seiferle, E. (1981) The anatomy of the domestic animals Vol. 3. The circulatory system, the skin, and the cutaneous organs of the domestic mammals. Schummer, A., Wilkins, H., Vollmerhaus, B.K., Habermehl, K.H. Translated by Siller, W.G. & Wight, P.A.L. Berlin, Hamburg; Parey.

Nickel, R., Schummer, A., & Seiferle, E. (1975) Lehrbuch der Anatomie der Haustiere Bd. IV. Nervensystem, Sinnesorgane, Endokrine Drüsen. Seiferle, E., Berlin, Hamburg; Parey.

Nomina Anatomica Veterinaria (1973) 2nd edition, published by the International Committee on Veterinary Anatomical Nomenclature, World Association of Veterinary Anatomists; Vienna.

Popesko, P. (n.d.) Atlas of topographical anatomy of the domestic animals. Vols I-III. Translated by Getty, R. & Brown, J. Philadelphia; Saunders.

Raghavan, D. & Kachroo, P. (1964) Anatomy of the ox. New Delhi; Indian council of agricultural research.

Rosenberger, G., Dirksen, G., Grunder, H.D., Grunert, E., Krause, D. & Stober, M. (1979) Clinical examination of cattle. Translated by Mack, R., Berlin, Hamburg; Parey.

Sisson, S. & Grossman, J.D. (1953) The anatomy of the domestic animals. 4th. edition, revised. Philadelphia; Saunders.

Sisson & Grossman's The anatomy of the domestic animals. Vol. I (1975). (Getty, R. editor) 5th edition. Philadelphia; Saunders.

Taylor, J.A. (1955-1970) Regional and applied anatomy of the domestic animals. Parts I-III. Edinburgh; Oliver, Boyd.

Vollmerhaus, B. & Habermehl, K.H. (n.d.) Topographical anatomical diagrams of injection technique in horses, cattle, dogs and cats. Marburg, Lahn; Hoechst, Behringwerke A.G.

Contents

Introduction

The range of the Veterinary Curriculum is continually expanding, and in many subjects its depth is continually increasing, yet the overall length of the course remains constant. As a result, there is pressure to allocate less and less time to some subjects, of which Anatomy is a notable example. Furthermore, within departments of Anatomy the desire to give greater emphasis to functional and applied aspects of the discipline, to radiological anatomy, and to teratology makes it increasingly difficult to allocate adequate time to personal dissection of each species by each student. An obvious solution to this problem is to rely more and more upon prepared dissections for the teaching of topographical anatomy. This saves much student time, but has several major disadvantages. Firstly the student loses the chance to gain manipulative skills, and is unable to see and feel the structures as they are progressively revealed by scalpel and scissors. Secondly, it means that the student must rapidly and in quick succession master complexities that were more surely understood by the leisurely methods of thirty years ago. Nothing can fully compensate for the lack of personal dissection by the skilled dissector supplemented by the intelligent use of graphic methods to record the work as it progresses. However, our experience at the Royal Veterinary College over the past fifteen years has convinced us that the work of the skillful prosector, carefully studied, recorded and annotated, can be more useful than personal dissections of large animals carried out hurriedly by a group of inexpert students. One problem in the teaching of topographical anatomy from prepared specimens has been the difficulty of providing students with enough good preparations of a full range of dissection stages of specific regions. It is our sincere hope that this photographic atlas of dissections will help to compensate for this deficiency in prepared specimens. For those students who are able to carry out their own detailed dissections, this atlas will provide a permanent reminder of what they saw, or should have seen, during each stage (often transitory) of the dissection.

The sequence of dissections presented in this volume is an expanded version of that used by us for a series of twelve three-hour sessions on the topographical anatomy of ruminants. Each stage of the work has been photographed in order to show many more stages of each major dissection than can be shown in our practical demonstration classes. We hope that this will compensate for the loss of the third dimension that is inevitable in photographs of dissections. We have tried to present the progression of required dissections as they occurred. Where the specimen was "unusual" or where we were not completely successful in demonstrating all of the structures as planned, we have not substituted a different specimen in the sequence; this would have broken the thread of the narrative. Occasionally, for the sake of clarity, we have reversed photographs of dissections made on one side, so that they fit more readily into the major sequence, but when this has been done it is clearly indicated in the legends. In every dissection room it is, from time to time, advantageous to mount "extra" demonstrations. For some regions we also have done this to show a different dissection procedure or a different specimen. Students should beware of treating these "extras" as optional or unnecessary complications – often they are of considerable importance.

A comment is needed on the technique of dissection shown in these photographs. In many instances we have not cleaned away all of the connective tissue from the structures being displayed. In "complete" dissections it is often impossible to preserve accurately the original topographical relationships of vessels and nerves. Also, such dissections encourage the student to think that textbook drawings are "real" and that adipose, fascial and areolar tissues should not exist. We have tried to make the photographs represent the structures as they really appear during the course of an actual dissection.

It is no part of our plan as teachers of veterinary anatomy to entice the students out of the dissection room, away from the specimens, and into the comfort of armchairs for their study of practical topographical anatomy. Rather, we have attempted to provide an atlas with which they can extend their own personal study of dissections of ruminants at times when the dissections are no longer readily available.

This is not an atlas of applied Veterinary Anatomy, but it is intended for veterinary students; considerable emphasis is given to those regions and structures that seem important for the veterinarian in practice. As far as possible, the photographs have been taken to provide information about the animal as it is seen during a routine clinical examination – other views have been avoided, even though they are sometimes more informative from a strictly anatomical standpoint. It is hoped that the clinical student and the practicing veterinarian may find this approach of value in examination, diagnosis and treatment of the standing animal. The experimentalist may also find that some of his problems of topographical anatomy are illuminated by these photographs of dissections. We realize that his requirements are diverse and unpredictable and have made our labelling of the various series of dissections as complete as possible with this in mind.

R.R.A.
S.D.

1 The Head

Fig. 1.1 Palpable surface features of the bovine head, in left lateral view.

The hair covering the palpable surface features was shaved off before embalming commenced.

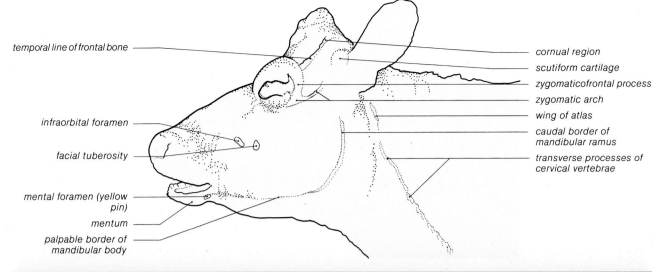

temporal line of frontal bone
infraorbital foramen
facial tuberosity
mental foramen (yellow pin)
mentum
palpable border of mandibular body

cornual region
scutiform cartilage
zygomaticofrontal process
zygomatic arch
wing of atlas
caudal border of mandibular ramus
transverse processes of cervical vertebrae

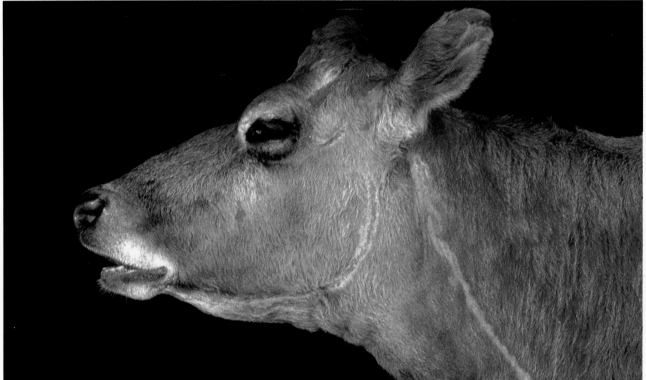

Fig. 1.2 The skull and first five cervical vertebrae.

Palpable features shown in fig. 1.1 are coloured red.

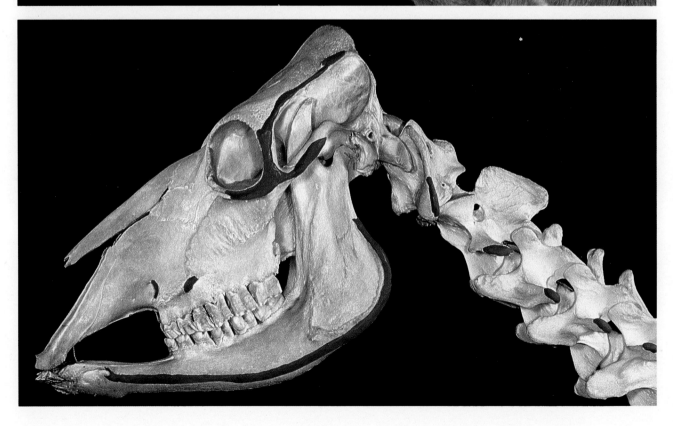

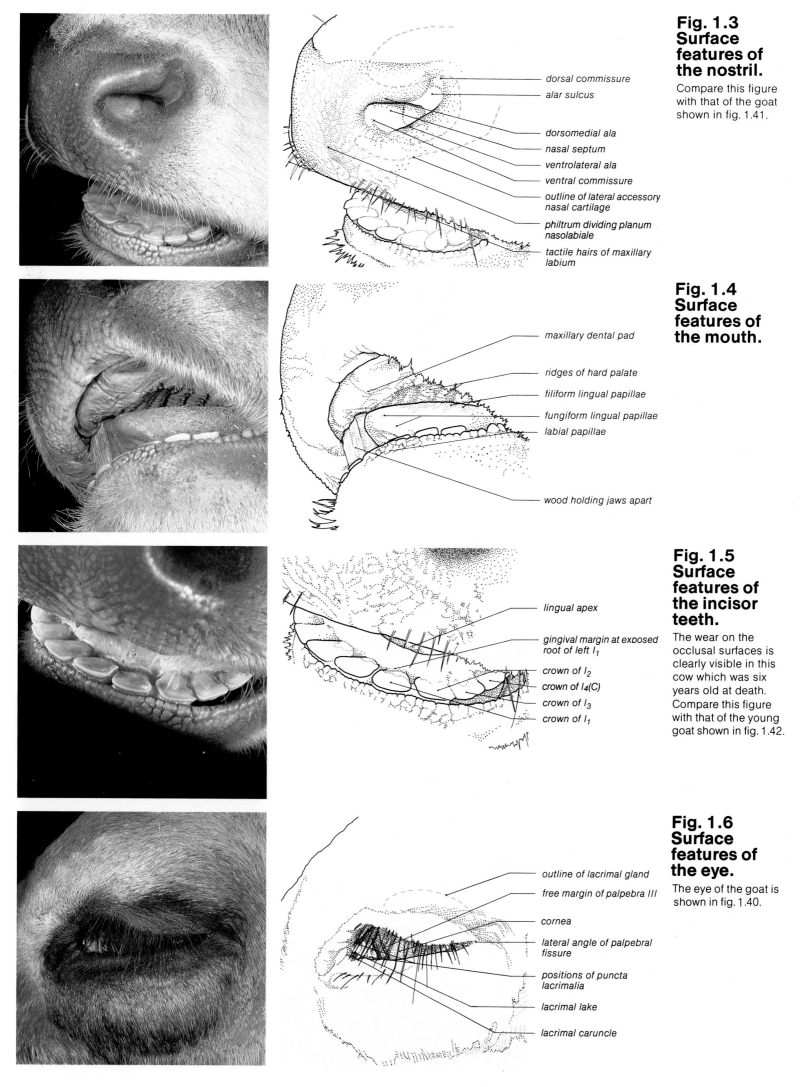

**Fig. 1.3
Surface features of the nostril.**
Compare this figure with that of the goat shown in fig. 1.41.

- dorsal commissure
- alar sulcus
- dorsomedial ala
- nasal septum
- ventrolateral ala
- ventral commissure
- outline of lateral accessory nasal cartilage
- philtrum dividing planum nasolabiale
- tactile hairs of maxillary labium

**Fig. 1.4
Surface features of the mouth.**

- maxillary dental pad
- ridges of hard palate
- filiform lingual papillae
- fungiform lingual papillae
- labial papillae
- wood holding jaws apart

**Fig. 1.5
Surface features of the incisor teeth.**
The wear on the occlusal surfaces is clearly visible in this cow which was six years old at death. Compare this figure with that of the young goat shown in fig. 1.42.

- lingual apex
- gingival margin at exposed root of left I_1
- crown of I_2
- crown of $I_4(C)$
- crown of I_3
- crown of I_1

**Fig. 1.6
Surface features of the eye.**
The eye of the goat is shown in fig. 1.40.

- outline of lacrimal gland
- free margin of palpebra III
- cornea
- lateral angle of palpebral fissure
- positions of puncta lacrimalia
- lacrimal lake
- lacrimal caruncle

1.3

Fig. 1.7 Superficial structures of the head, in left lateral view.

Further details of selected areas are given in figs. 1.8, 1.9 and 1.10. The vascular notch in the ventral border of the body of the mandible in the sheep and goat contains only the facial vein. In these species the transverse facial artery is large and the parotid duct crosses the surface of the masseter muscle as illustrated by the broken blue line. The dotted lines highlight the palpable bony prominences.

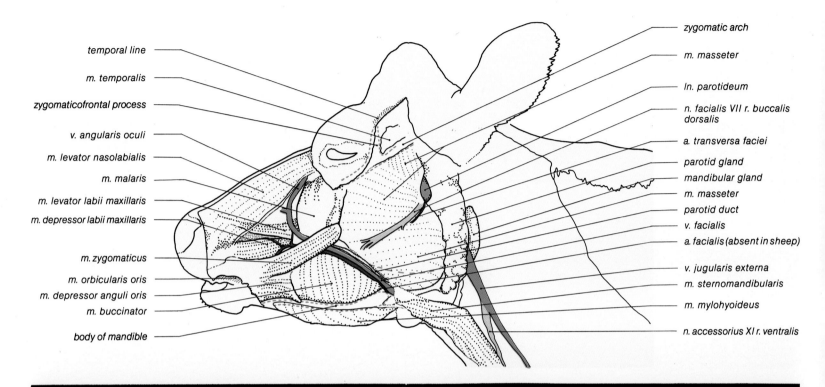

temporal line
m. temporalis
zygomaticofrontal process
v. angularis oculi
m. levator nasolabialis
m. malaris
m. levator labii maxillaris
m. depressor labii maxillaris
m. zygomaticus
m. orbicularis oris
m. depressor anguli oris
m. buccinator
body of mandible

zygomatic arch
m. masseter
ln. parotideum
n. facialis VII r. buccalis dorsalis
a. transversa faciei
parotid gland
mandibular gland
m. masseter
parotid duct
v. facialis
a. facialis (absent in sheep)
v. jugularis externa
m. sternomandibularis
m. mylohyoideus
n. accessorius XI r. ventralis

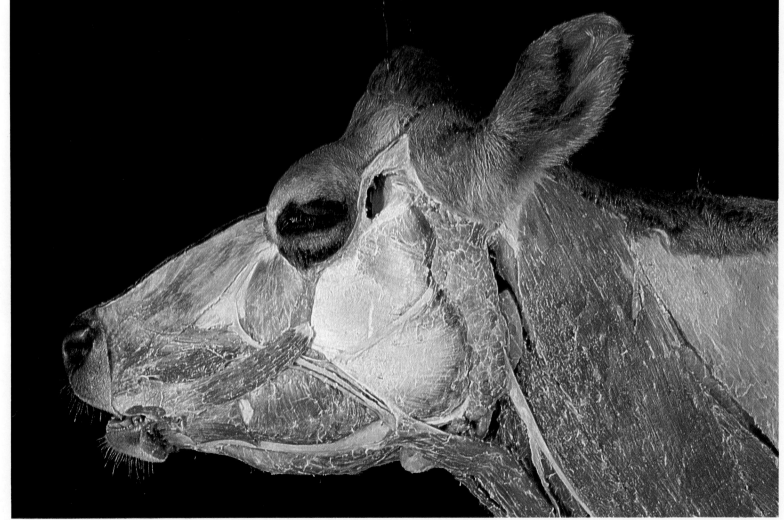

Fig. 1.8 Superficial structures of the head – relationships of the infraorbital foramen.

The levator labii maxillaris muscle has been slightly depressed to reveal the infraorbital foramen.

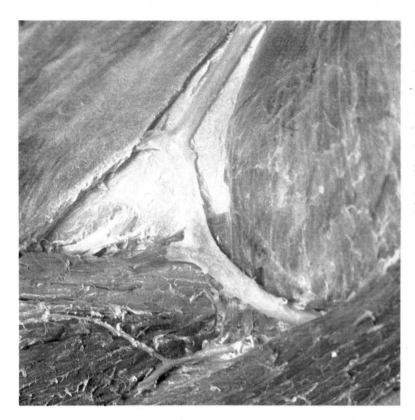

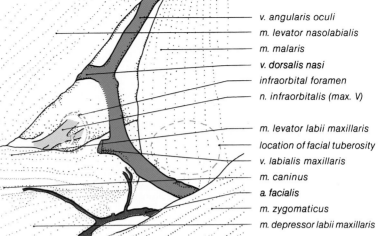

- v. angularis oculi
- m. levator nasolabialis
- m. malaris
- v. dorsalis nasi
- infraorbital foramen
- n. infraorbitalis (max. V)
- m. levator labii maxillaris
- location of facial tuberosity
- v. labialis maxillaris
- m. caninus
- a. facialis
- m. zygomaticus
- m. depressor labii maxillaris

Fig. 1.9 Superficial structures of the head – relationships of the mental foramen.

An oval hole has been cut in the depressor labii mandibularis muscle to reveal the mental foramen.

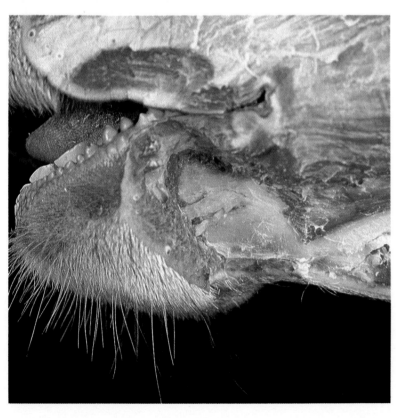

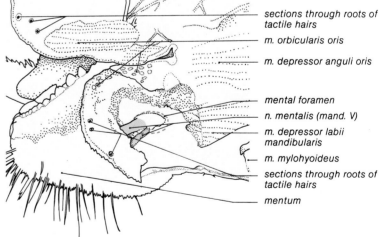

- sections through roots of tactile hairs
- m. orbicularis oris
- m. depressor anguli oris
- mental foramen
- n. mentalis (mand. V)
- m. depressor labii mandibularis
- m. mylohyoideus
- sections through roots of tactile hairs
- mentum

Fig. 1.10 Superficial structures of the parotid region.

The auriculotemporal (mand. V) and auriculopalpebral (VII) nerves are not shown, but they are both present in fig. 1.32.

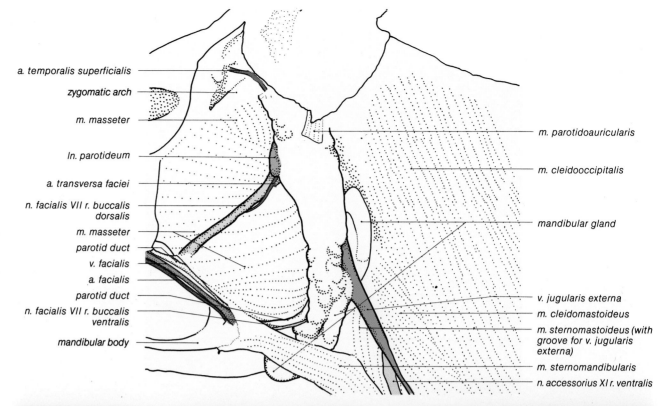

a. temporalis superficialis
zygomatic arch
m. masseter
ln. parotideum
a. transversa faciei
n. facialis VII r. buccalis dorsalis
m. masseter
parotid duct
v. facialis
a. facialis
parotid duct
n. facialis VII r. buccalis ventralis
mandibular body

m. parotidoauricularis
m. cleidooccipitalis
mandibular gland
v. jugularis externa
m. cleidomastoideus
m. sternomastoideus (with groove for v. jugularis externa)
m. sternomandibularis
n. accessorius XI r. ventralis

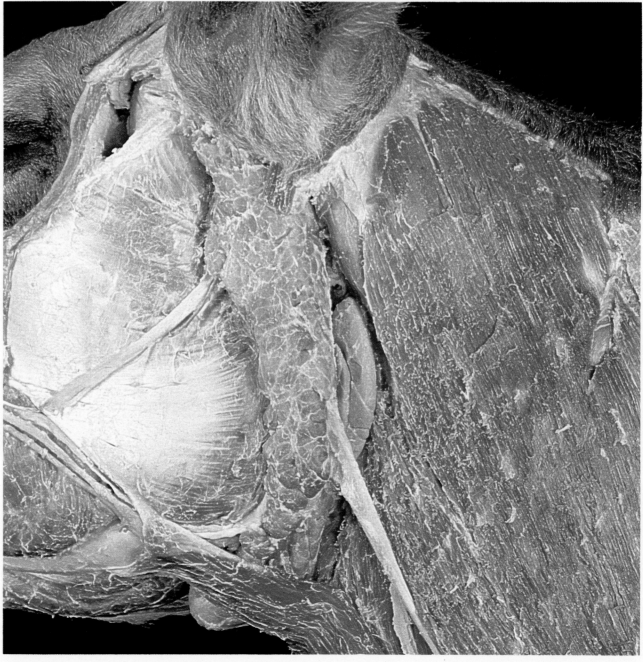

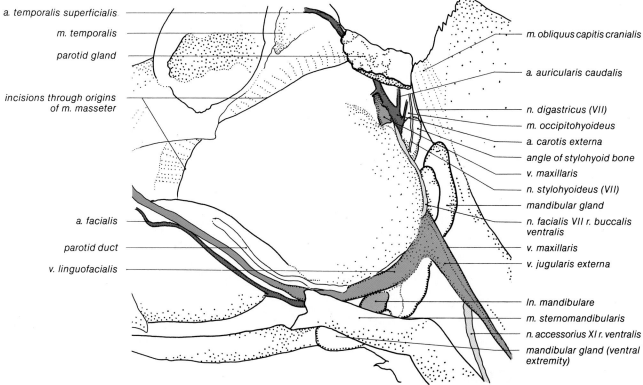

a. temporalis superficialis

m. temporalis

parotid gland

incisions through origins of m. masseter

a. facialis

parotid duct

v. linguofacialis

m. obliquus capitis cranialis

a. auricularis caudalis

n. digastricus (VII)

m. occipitohyoideus

a. carotis externa

angle of stylohyoid bone

v. maxillaris

n. stylohyoideus (VII)

mandibular gland

n. facialis VII r. buccalis ventralis

v. maxillaris

v. jugularis externa

ln. mandibulare

m. sternomandibularis

n. accessorius XI r. ventralis

mandibular gland (ventral extremity)

Fig. 1.11 The structures lying deep to the parotid gland.

The lateral retropharyngeal lymph node lies too far rostral in this specimen to be visible at this stage of the dissection. It often protrudes from the caudal edge of the mandibular gland (see figs. 1.15 and 1.32).

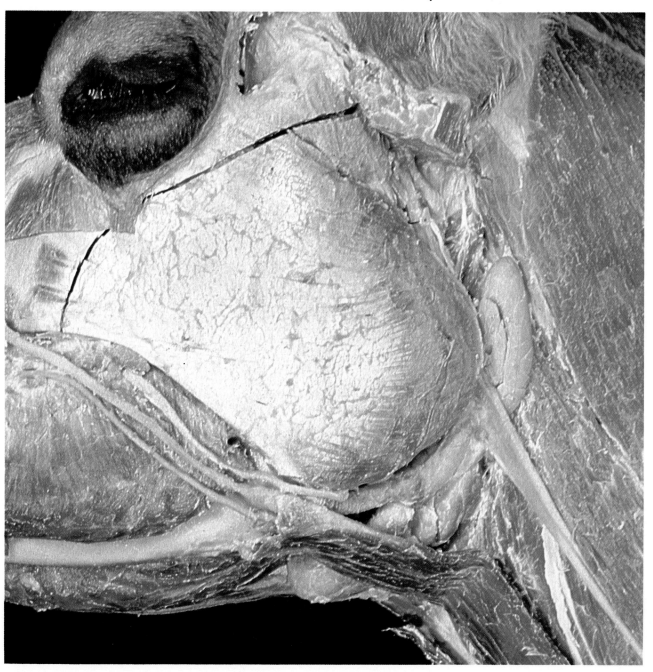

Fig. 1.12 The mandible and caudal buccal wall.

The facial vessels and parotid duct occupy a distinct notch in the ventral border of the mandible. The mandible has been sawn ready for removal as shown in fig. 1.13.

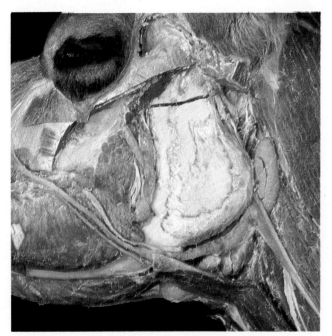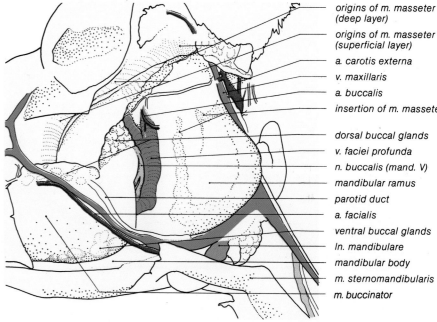

origins of m. masseter (deep layer)
origins of m. masseter (superficial layer)
a. carotis externa
v. maxillaris
a. buccalis
insertion of m. masseter
dorsal buccal glands
v. faciei profunda
n. buccalis (mand. V)
mandibular ramus
parotid duct
a. facialis
ventral buccal glands
ln. mandibulare
mandibular body
m. sternomandibularis
m. buccinator

Fig. 1.13 The structures lying medial to the mandible.

The lateral pterygoid muscle covers the lingual nerve (mand. V) and this nerve is therefore not visible (see fig. 1.14).

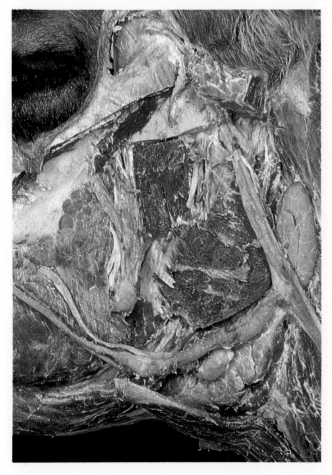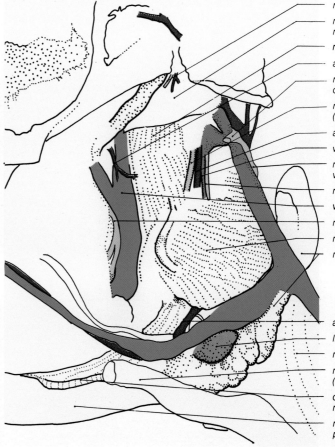

n. massetericus (mand. V)
remains of mandibular ramus
m. pterygoideus lateralis
a. buccalis
n. facialis VII r. buccalis dorsalis
n. alveolaris mandibularis (mand. V)
a. alveolaris mandibularis
v. alveolaris mandibularis
n. facialis VII r. buccalis ventralis
n. mylohyoideus (mand. V)
v. faciei profunda
n. buccalis (mand. V)
m. pterygoideus medialis
mandibular gland
a. facialis
ln. mandibulare
m. sternomastoideus
m. sternomandibularis (cut and displaced)
cut insertion of m. digastricus (rostral part)
m. mylohyoideus (rostral part)

Fig. 1.14 The structures lying deep to the pterygoid muscles.

The sternocephalicus and brachiocephalicus muscles have been entirely cut away to reveal the deeper structures of the neck region. The muscular wall of the pharynx rostral to the stylohyoid bone has been partly removed in order to expose the palatine tonsil.

Fig. 1.15 The lateral and medial retropharyngeal lymph nodes.

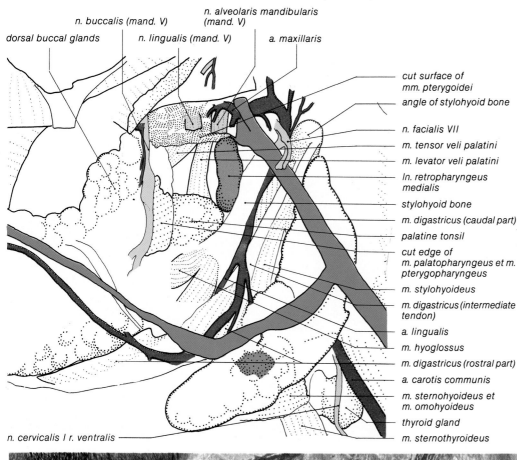

n. buccalis (mand. V)

n. alveolaris mandibularis (mand. V)

dorsal buccal glands

n. lingualis (mand. V)

a. maxillaris

cut surface of mm. pterygoidei

angle of stylohyoid bone

n. facialis VII

m. tensor veli palatini

m. levator veli palatini

ln. retropharyngeus medialis

stylohyoid bone

m. digastricus (caudal part)

palatine tonsil

cut edge of m. palatopharyngeus et m. pterygopharyngeus

m. stylohyoideus

m. digastricus (intermediate tendon)

a. lingualis

m. hyoglossus

m. digastricus (rostral part)

a. carotis communis

m. sternohyoideus et m. omohyoideus

thyroid gland

n. cervicalis I r. ventralis

m. sternothyroideus

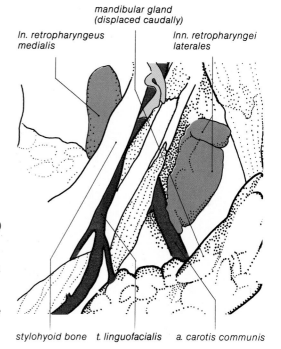

mandibular gland (displaced caudally)

ln. retropharyngeus medialis

lnn. retropharyngei laterales

stylohyoid bone   t. linguofacialis   a. carotis communis

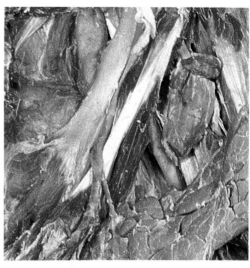

By displacing the mandibular gland, the lateral retropharyngeal lymph nodes are exposed and their position relative to the stylohyoid bone can be compared with that of the medial node.

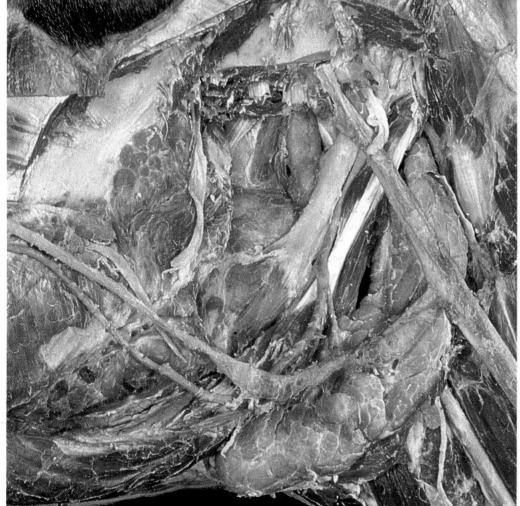

Fig. 1.16 The maxillary cheek teeth and the muscles of the pharynx.

The mandibular gland, ventral neck muscles and buccal wall have been removed. The veins have also been cut away to permit a clearer presentation of additional structures.

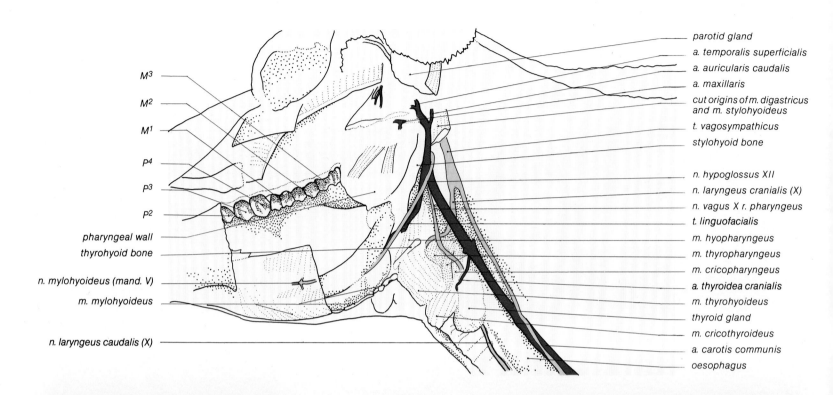

M³
M²
M¹
P⁴
P³
P²
pharyngeal wall
thyrohyoid bone
n. mylohyoideus (mand. V)
m. mylohyoideus
n. laryngeus caudalis (X)

parotid gland
a. temporalis superficialis
a. auricularis caudalis
a. maxillaris
cut origins of m. digastricus and m. stylohyoideus
t. vagosympathicus
stylohyoid bone
n. hypoglossus XII
n. laryngeus cranialis (X)
n. vagus X r. pharyngeus
t. linguofacialis
m. hyopharyngeus
m. thyropharyngeus
m. cricopharyngeus
a. thyroidea cranialis
m. thyrohyoideus
thyroid gland
m. cricothyroideus
a. carotis communis
oesophagus

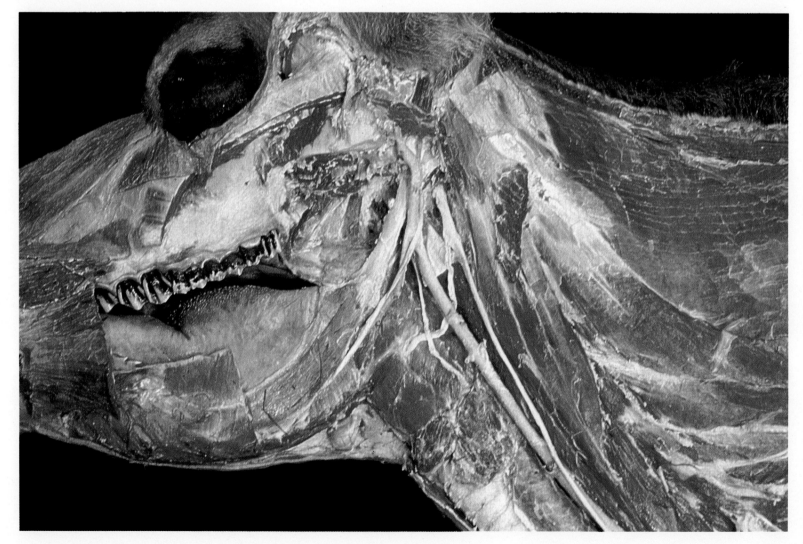

Fig. 1.17 The sublingual salivary gland and the sublingual fold.

The sublingual fold and its papillae mark the line of the orifices of the ducts of the polystomatic part of the sublingual gland. The duct of the monostomatic part, like that of the mandibular gland, opens at the rostral extremity of this fold.

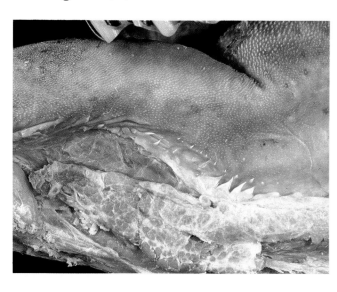

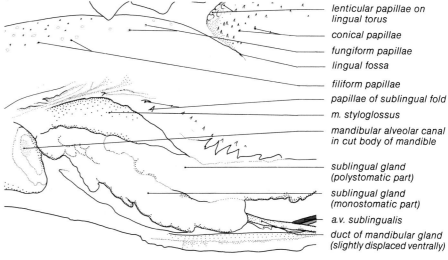

lenticular papillae on lingual torus
conical papillae
fungiform papillae
lingual fossa
filiform papillae
papillae of sublingual fold
m. styloglossus
mandibular alveolar canal in cut body of mandible
sublingual gland (polystomatic part)
sublingual gland (monostomatic part)
a.v. sublingualis
duct of mandibular gland (slightly displaced ventrally)

Fig. 1.18 Surface features and muscles of the tongue.

palatine tonsil
n. hypoglossus XII
lingual torus
vallate papillae
lingual fossa
a. facialis
a. lingualis
m. styloglossus
thyrohyoid bone
m. lingualis proprius
m. hyoglossus
right mandibular gland
a. sublingualis
m. geniohyoideus
cut edge of m. mylohyoideus
m. genioglossus

Fig. 1.19 The muscles of the tongue.

stylohyoid bone
m. hyoglossus
m. styloglossus (cut origin)
a. lingualis
n. hypoglossus XII
m. hyoglossus
n. laryngeus cranialis (X) (reflected ventrally)
m. genioglossus
right mandibular gland
a. sublingualis
m. geniohyoideus

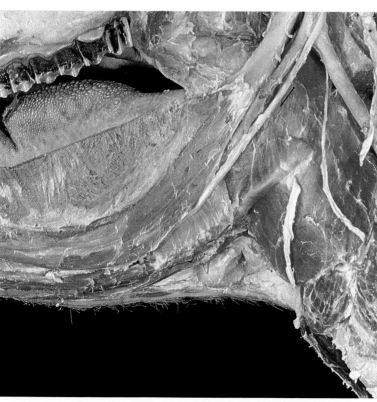

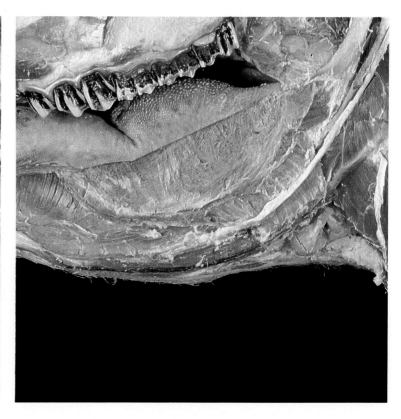

Fig. 1.20 The hyoid apparatus, pharynx and larynx.

The stylohyoid and epihyoid bones have been removed. After reflecting the linguofacial artery, the caudal and middle constrictor muscles of the pharynx and part of the hyoid apparatus have been removed to expose the caudal part of the stylopharyngeal muscle and the dorsal edge of the thyroid cartilage.

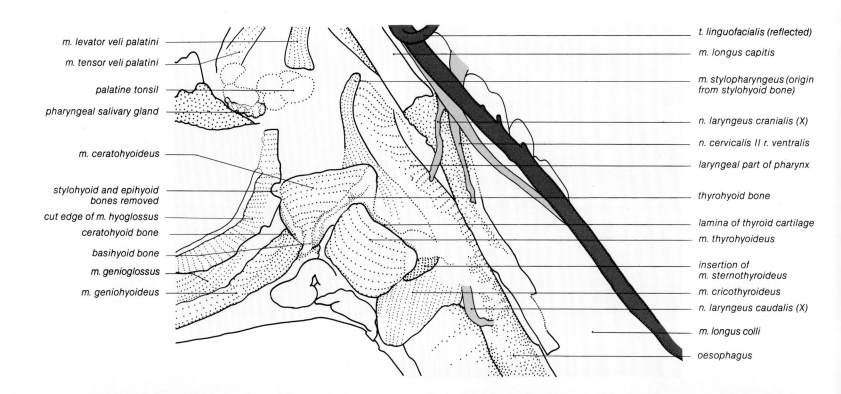

m. levator veli palatini

m. tensor veli palatini

palatine tonsil

pharyngeal salivary gland

m. ceratohyoideus

stylohyoid and epihyoid bones removed

cut edge of m. hyoglossus

ceratohyoid bone

basihyoid bone

m. genioglossus

m. geniohyoideus

t. linguofacialis (reflected)

m. longus capitis

m. stylopharyngeus (origin from stylohyoid bone)

n. laryngeus cranialis (X)

n. cervicalis II r. ventralis

laryngeal part of pharynx

thyrohyoid bone

lamina of thyroid cartilage

m. thyrohyoideus

insertion of m. sternothyroideus

m. cricothyroideus

n. laryngeus caudalis (X)

m. longus colli

oesophagus

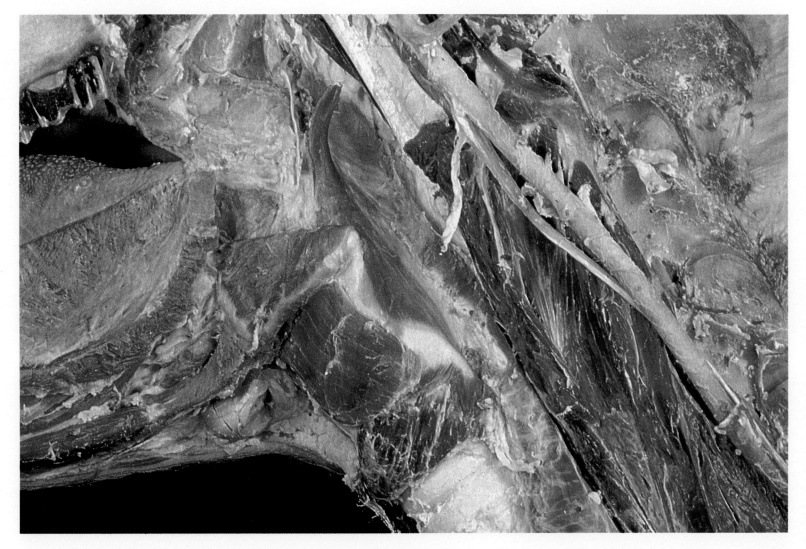

Fig. 1.21 The pharynx and larynx.

The lateral wall of the nasopharynx and laryngeal pharynx has been removed. The corniculate process of the arytenoid cartilage is unusually dark in colour. The border of the mandible is shown by a blue dotted line, but it should be remembered that its relationships are greatly changed in life during flexion and extension of the atlantooccipital articulation.

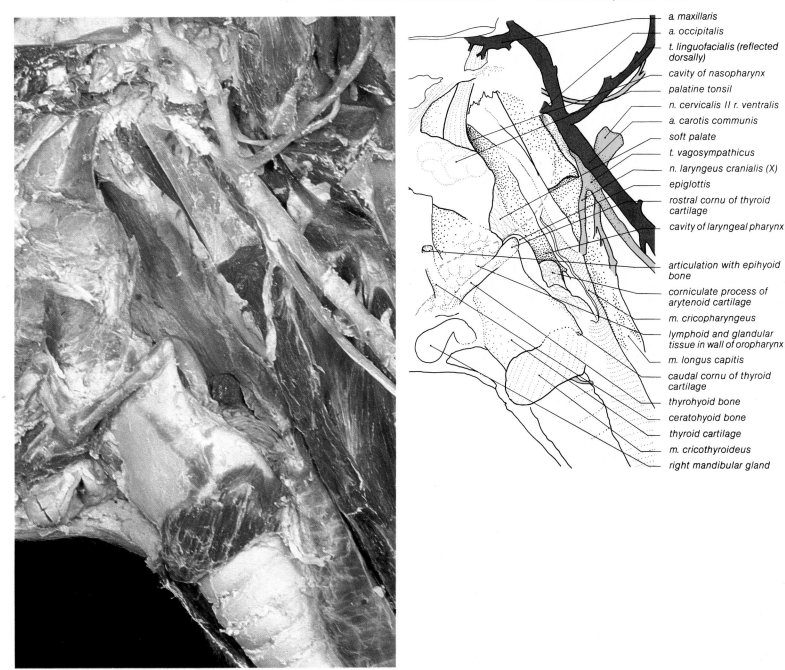

a. maxillaris
a. occipitalis
t. linguofacialis (reflected dorsally)
cavity of nasopharynx
palatine tonsil
n. cervicalis II r. ventralis
a. carotis communis
soft palate
t. vagosympathicus
n. laryngeus cranialis (X)
epiglottis
rostral cornu of thyroid cartilage
cavity of laryngeal pharynx
articulation with epihyoid bone
corniculate process of arytenoid cartilage
m. cricopharyngeus
lymphoid and glandular tissue in wall of oropharynx
m. longus capitis
caudal cornu of thyroid cartilage
thyrohyoid bone
ceratohyoid bone
thyroid cartilage
m. cricothyroideus
right mandibular gland

Fig. 1.22 The oral, nasal and laryngeal parts of the pharynx.

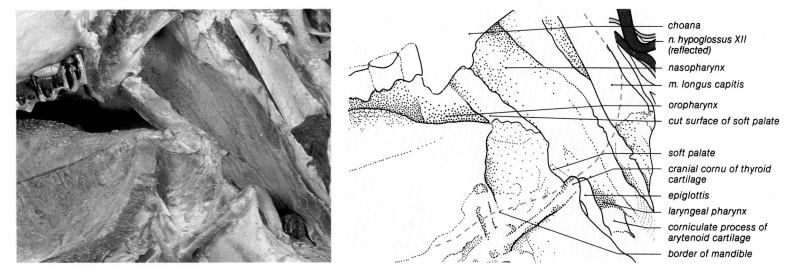

choana
n. hypoglossus XII (reflected)
nasopharynx
m. longus capitis
oropharynx
cut surface of soft palate
soft palate
cranial cornu of thyroid cartilage
epiglottis
laryngeal pharynx
corniculate process of arytenoid cartilage
border of mandible

1.13

Figs. 1.23–1.26 Surface features and bones of the cornual region in a dehorned cow.

temporal line of frontal bone   site of horn (dehorned cow)   intercornual prominence

long hairs on rostral part of auricular helix
dorsal border of orbit
scutiform cartilage

zygomaticofrontal process
lateral angle of palpebral fissure
zygomatic arch, temporal part
zygomatic arch, zygomatic part
wing of atlas
caudal border of mandibular ramus

site of horn (dehorned cow)
scutiform cartilage
temporal line of frontal bone
temporal fossa
supraorbital foramen (also position of a convergent hair vortex)
dorsal border of orbit
zygomatic arch, temporal part
pigmented border of palpebra III
ventral border of orbit
divergent hair vortex
zygomatic arch, zygomatic part
transverse processes of cervical vertebrae
caudal border of mandibular ramus

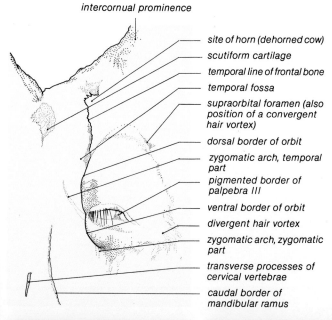

Fig. 1.23 Frontal, temporal, cornual and auricular regions.

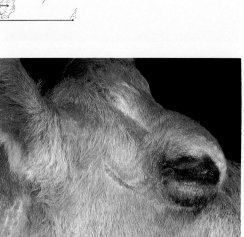

Fig. 1.24 Skull, mandible and cervical vertebrae. Palpable features shown in fig. 1.23 are coloured red.

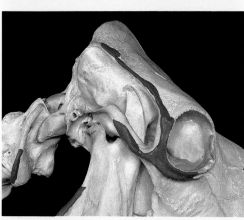

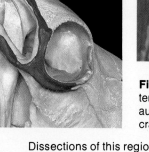

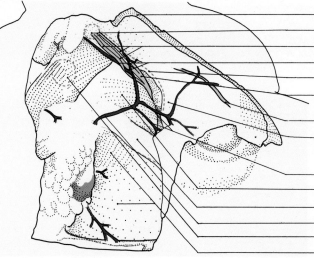

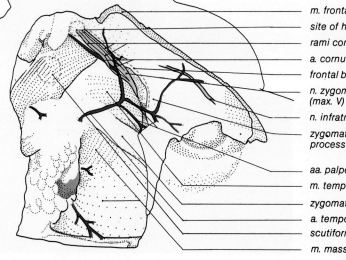

Fig. 1.25 Frontal, temporal, cornual and auricular regions in cranial view.

Fig. 1.26 Skull and cervical vertebrae. Palpable features shown in fig. 1.25 are coloured red.

Fig. 1.27 Nerves and blood vessels of the right cornual region.

Dissections of this region in immature and horned ruminants are shown in figs. 1.33 and 1.43. The cornual artery is relatively larger in horned individuals. The fine branches of the frontal nerve (oph. V) that run parallel and caudal to the infratrochlear nerve, could not be identified, and the auriculopalpebral nerve (VII) is not shown.

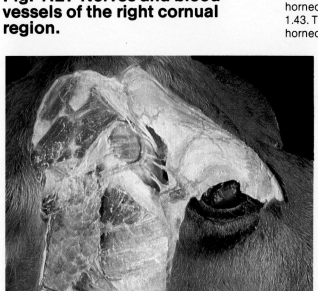

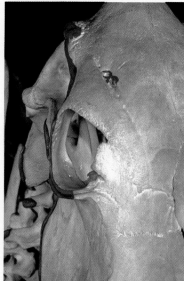

m. frontalis (cut)
site of horn
rami cornuales
a. cornualis
frontal bone, temporal line
n. zygomaticotemporalis (max. V)
n. infratrochlearis (oph. V)
zygomaticofrontal process
aa. palpebrales
m. temporalis
zygomatic arch
a. temporalis superficialis
scutiform cartilage
m. masseter

Fig. 1.28 The frontal and maxillary paranasal sinuses, in right lateral view.

Further details of these sinuses are shown in figs. 1.29, 1.30 and 1.31.

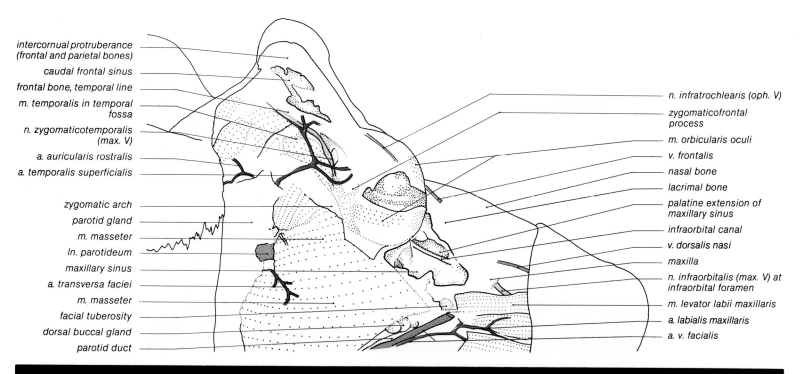

intercornual protruberance (frontal and parietal bones)
caudal frontal sinus
frontal bone, temporal line
m. temporalis in temporal fossa
n. zygomaticotemporalis (max. V)
a. auricularis rostralis
a. temporalis superficialis

zygomatic arch
parotid gland
m. masseter
ln. parotideum
maxillary sinus
a. transversa faciei
m. masseter
facial tuberosity
dorsal buccal gland
parotid duct

n. infratrochlearis (oph. V)
zygomaticofrontal process
m. orbicularis oculi
v. frontalis
nasal bone
lacrimal bone
palatine extension of maxillary sinus
infraorbital canal
v. dorsalis nasi
maxilla
n. infraorbitalis (max. V) at infraorbital foramen
m. levator labii maxillaris
a. labialis maxillaris
a. v. facialis

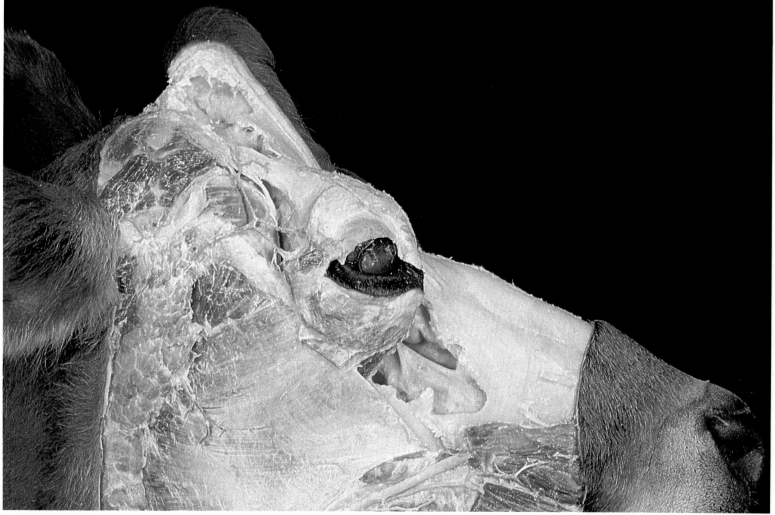

Fig. 1.29 The maxillary paranasal sinus in right craniolateral view.

Part of the lacrimal bone surrounding the nasolacrimal duct has been removed and the position of the duct is shown by a white wire. The palatine extension of the sinus is often considered to be a separate sinus.

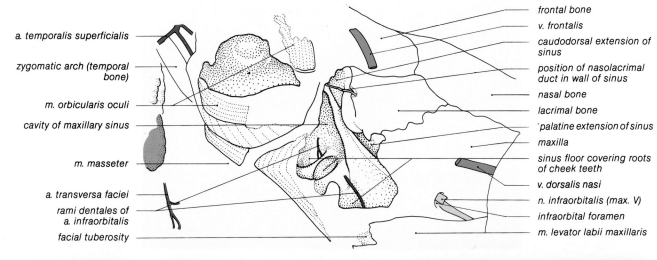

a. temporalis superficialis

zygomatic arch (temporal bone)

m. orbicularis oculi

cavity of maxillary sinus

m. masseter

a. transversa faciei

rami dentales of a. infraorbitalis

facial tuberosity

frontal bone

v. frontalis

caudodorsal extension of sinus

position of nasolacrimal duct in wall of sinus

nasal bone

lacrimal bone

palatine extension of sinus

maxilla

sinus floor covering roots of cheek teeth

v. dorsalis nasi

n. infraorbitalis (max. V)

infraorbital foramen

m. levator labii maxillaris

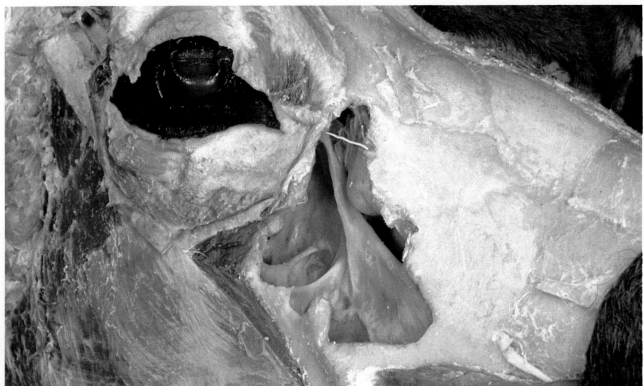

Fig. 1.30 The maxillary paranasal sinus in cranial view.

The sinus extends caudally into the lacrimal bulla to reach the level of the zygomaticofrontal process (see fig 1.39).

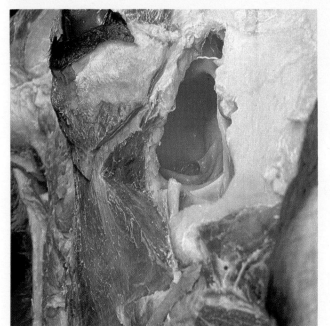

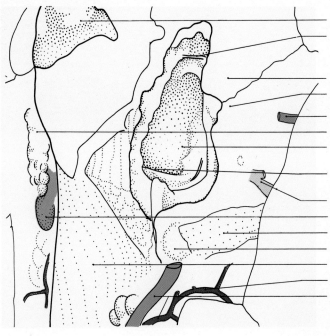

cornea of right eyeball

position of nasolacrimal duct in wall of sinus

lacrimal bone

maxilla

v. nasalis dorsalis

parotid gland

caudal extension of sinus into lacrimal bulla

sinus floor covering roots of cheek teeth

n. infraorbitalis (max.V)

ln. parotideum

m. levator labii maxillaris

facial tuberosity

m. masseter

a. labialis maxillaris

a. v. facialis

Fig. 1.31 The maxillary and frontal paranasal sinuses in cranial view.

The specimen was freeze-dried before being photographed for this figure.

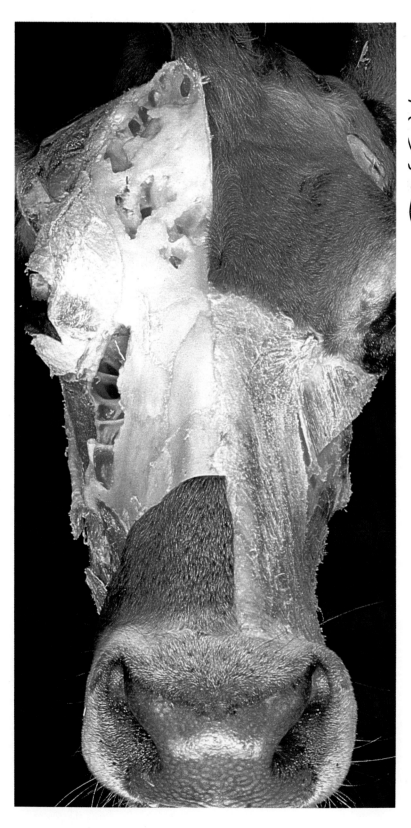

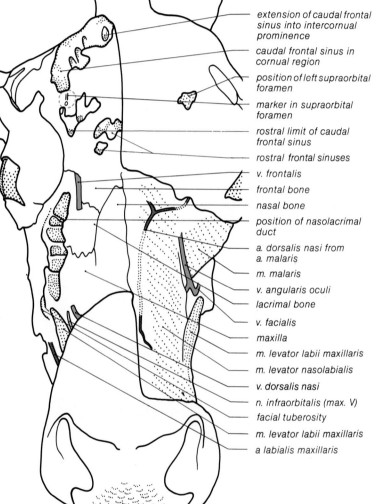

extension of caudal frontal sinus into intercornual prominence

caudal frontal sinus in cornual region

position of left supraorbital foramen

marker in supraorbital foramen

rostral limit of caudal frontal sinus

rostral frontal sinuses

v. frontalis

frontal bone

nasal bone

position of nasolacrimal duct

a. dorsalis nasi from a. malaris

m. malaris

v. angularis oculi

lacrimal bone

v. facialis

maxilla

m. levator labii maxillaris

m. levator nasolabialis

v. dorsalis nasi

n. infraorbitalis (max. V)

facial tuberosity

m. levator labii maxillaris

a labialis maxillaris

Fig. 1.32 Superficial structures of the head in the bull calf – parotid, masseteric and facial regions.

This calf was about one week old.

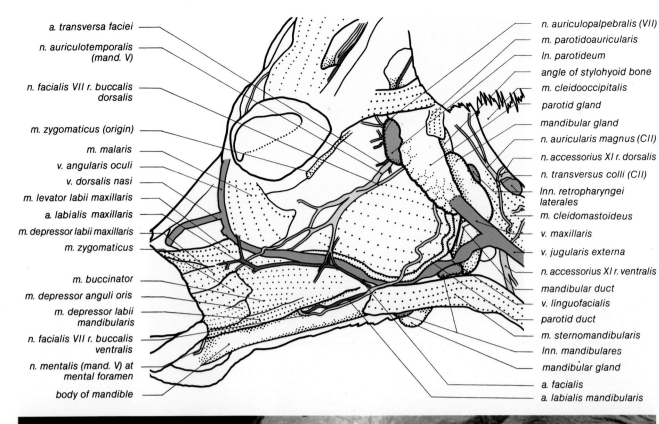

- a. transversa faciei
- n. auriculotemporalis (mand. V)
- n. facialis VII r. buccalis dorsalis
- m. zygomaticus (origin)
- m. malaris
- v. angularis oculi
- v. dorsalis nasi
- m. levator labii maxillaris
- a. labialis maxillaris
- m. depressor labii maxillaris
- m. zygomaticus
- m. buccinator
- m. depressor anguli oris
- m. depressor labii mandibularis
- n. facialis VII r. buccalis ventralis
- n. mentalis (mand. V) at mental foramen
- body of mandible

- n. auriculopalpebralis (VII)
- m. parotidoauricularis
- ln. parotideum
- angle of stylohyoid bone
- m. cleidooccipitalis
- parotid gland
- mandibular gland
- n. auricularis magnus (CII)
- n. accessorius XI r. dorsalis
- n. transversus colli (CII)
- lnn. retropharyngei laterales
- m. cleidomastoideus
- v. maxillaris
- v. jugularis externa
- n. accessorius XI r. ventralis
- mandibular duct
- v. linguofacialis
- parotid duct
- m. sternomandibularis
- lnn. mandibulares
- mandibular gland
- a. facialis
- a. labialis mandibularis

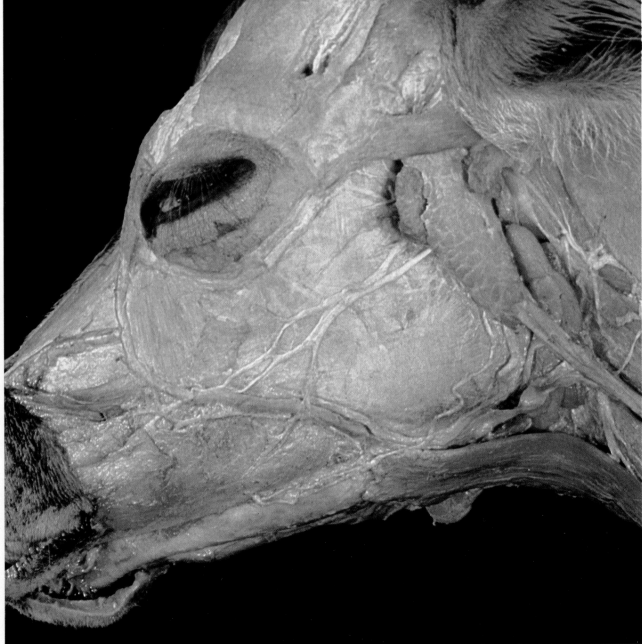

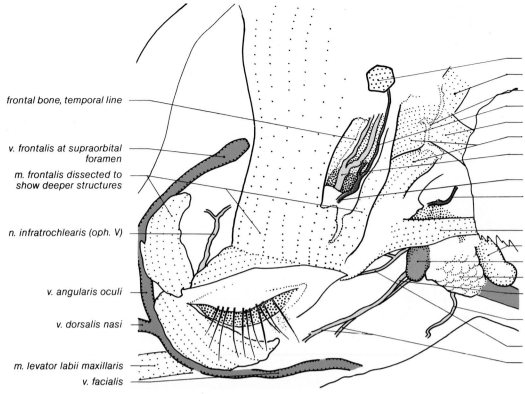

frontal bone, temporal line

v. frontalis at supraorbital foramen

m. frontalis dissected to show deeper structures

n. infratrochlearis (oph. V)

v. angularis oculi

v. dorsalis nasi

m. levator labii maxillaris

v. facialis

skin of horn bud
m. cervicoscutularis
scutiform cartilage
a. cornualis
m. scutuloauricularis
m. frontoscutularis
n. zygomaticotemporalis (max. V)
a. temporalis superficialis
a. auricularis rostralis

m. zygomaticoauricularis
mandibular gland
ln. parotideum
parotid gland
n. auriculotemporalis (mand V)
n. facialis VII r. buccalis ventralis
n. auriculopalpebralis (VII)
n. facialis VII r. buccalis dorsalis

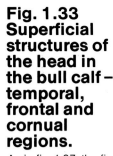

Fig. 1.33 Superficial structures of the head in the bull calf – temporal, frontal and cornual regions.

As in fig. 1.27, the fine branches of the frontal nerve (oph. V) could not be identified.

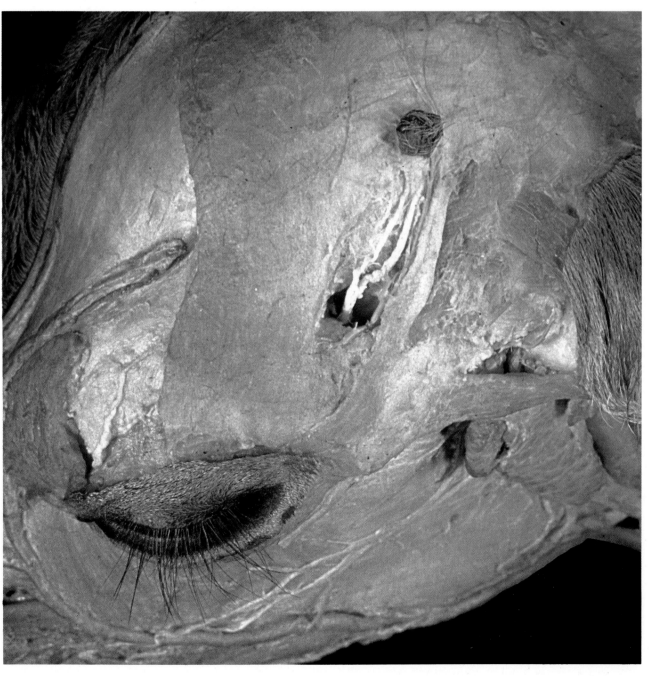

Fig. 1.34 The frontal and maxillary paranasal sinuses of the calf at one week of age: left craniolateral view.

The longitudinal dorsal skin incision has been made just to the right side of the midsagittal plane.

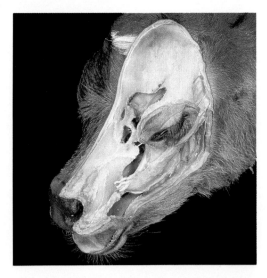

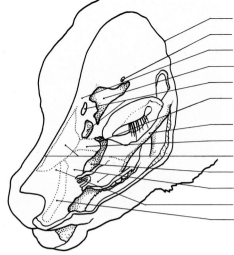

- horn bud
- supraorbital foramen
- frontal bone
- caudal frontal sinus
- rostral frontal sinuses
- marker in nasolacrimal duct
- zygomatic bone
- lacrimal bone
- nasal bones
- maxillary sinus
- maxilla
- nasoincisive notch
- incisive bone

Fig. 1.35 The paranasal sinuses and nasal cavity of the calf: left craniolateral view.

A space labelled "nasal septum" has been excavated within the cartilage of the septum. Lateral to this, the dorsal nasal meatus has been exposed. The cavity of the dorsal nasal concha lies lateral to the meatus and has not been opened.

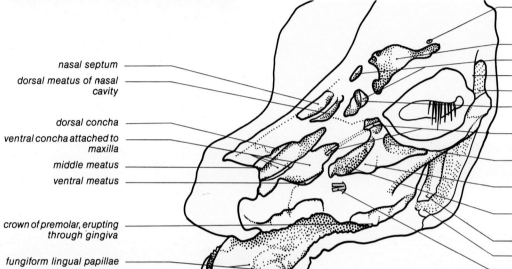

- nasal septum
- dorsal meatus of nasal cavity
- dorsal concha
- ventral concha attached to maxilla
- middle meatus
- ventral meatus
- crown of premolar, erupting through gingiva
- fungiform lingual papillae

- supraorbital foramen (not yet enclosed by the frontal sinus)
- caudal frontal sinus
- rostral frontal sinuses
- frontal bone, temporal line
- m. temporalis
- origin of sinus from ethmoidal meatus
- marker in nasolacrimal duct
- extension of sinus into lacrimal bulla
- infraorbital canal traversing maxillary sinus
- extension of sinus into hard palate ("palatine" sinus)
- ramus of mandible
- m. masseter
- n. infraorbitalis (max. V) at infraorbital foramen

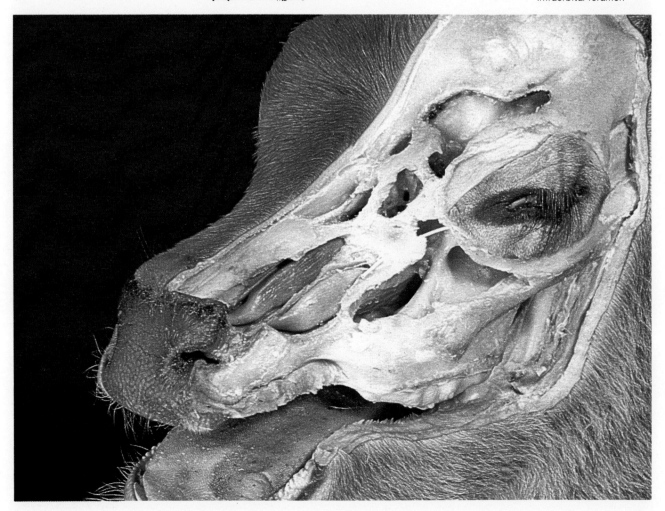

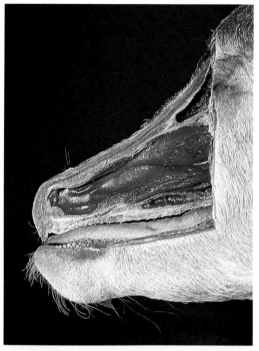

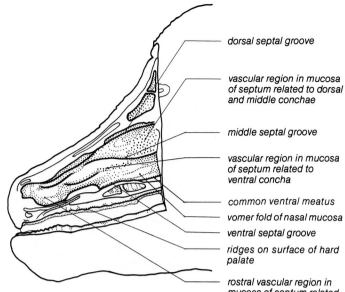

Fig. 1.36 The left mucosal surface of the nasal septum in the calf.

dorsal septal groove

vascular region in mucosa of septum related to dorsal and middle conchae

middle septal groove

vascular region in mucosa of septum related to ventral concha

common ventral meatus

vomer fold of nasal mucosa

ventral septal groove

ridges on surface of hard palate

rostral vascular region in mucosa of septum related to alar and basal folds

The left nasal cavity has been cut away by a paramedian sagittal incision to show that the highly vascular mucosa of the nasal septum conforms closely to the shape of the conchae which are related to it. The vascular enlargements of the septal mucosa are divided by grooves, labelled here as "septal grooves".

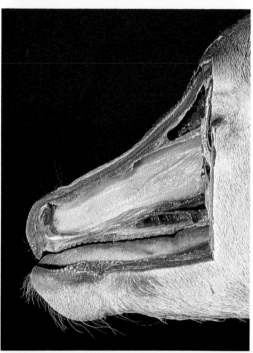

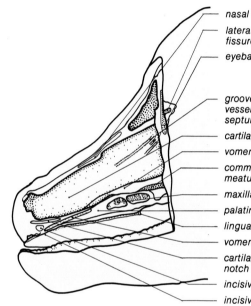

Fig. 1.37 The cartilaginous nasal septum of the calf, in left lateral view.

nasal bone

lateral angle of palpebral fissure

eyeball on cut surface

grooves occupied by vessels and nerves of nasal septum

cartilaginous nasal septum

vomer

common ventral nasal meatus

maxillary paranasal sinus

palatine process of maxilla

lingual fossa

vomeronasal organ

cartilage of interincisive notch

incisive bone

incisive papilla

The mucosa of the nasal septum, shown in fig. 1.36, has been removed to expose the perpendicular septal plate of the ethmoid bone which is entirely cartilaginous in this young calf.

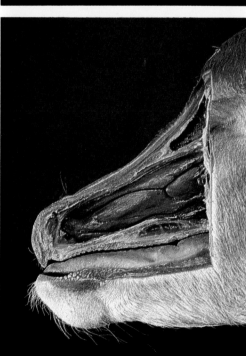

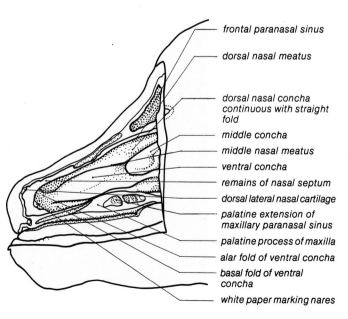

Fig. 1.38 The right nasal conchae in the calf after removal of the nasal septum: left lateral view.

frontal paranasal sinus

dorsal nasal meatus

dorsal nasal concha continuous with straight fold

middle concha

middle nasal meatus

ventral concha

remains of nasal septum

dorsal lateral nasal cartilage

palatine extension of maxillary paranasal sinus

palatine process of maxilla

alar fold of ventral concha

basal fold of ventral concha

white paper marking nares

Comparison of this figure with fig. 1.36 shows the close correspondence between the anatomy of the mucosa of the nasal septum and that of the nasal conchae related to it.

1.21

Fig. 1.39 The nasal cavity and associated structures of the calf, in left craniolateral view.

The specimen is at the same stage of dissection as that shown in fig. 1.38, but is here viewed from a more cranial and dorsal aspect.

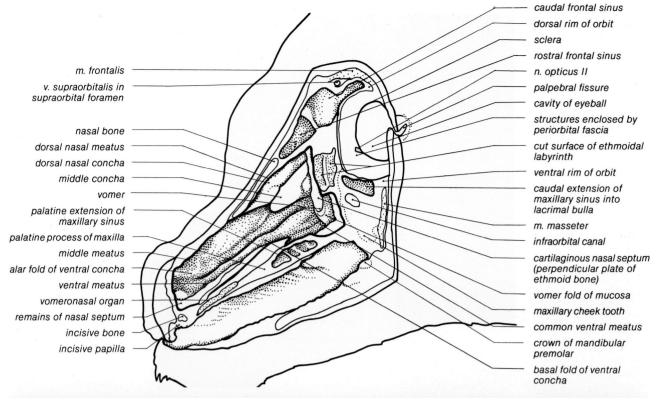

m. frontalis

v. supraorbitalis in supraorbital foramen

nasal bone
dorsal nasal meatus
dorsal nasal concha
middle concha
vomer
palatine extension of maxillary sinus
palatine process of maxilla
middle meatus
alar fold of ventral concha
ventral meatus
vomeronasal organ
remains of nasal septum
incisive bone
incisive papilla

caudal frontal sinus
dorsal rim of orbit
sclera
rostral frontal sinus
n. opticus II
palpebral fissure
cavity of eyeball
structures enclosed by periorbital fascia
cut surface of ethmoidal labyrinth
ventral rim of orbit
caudal extension of maxillary sinus into lacrimal bulla
m. masseter
infraorbital canal
cartilaginous nasal septum (perpendicular plate of ethmoid bone)
vomer fold of mucosa
maxillary cheek tooth
common ventral meatus
crown of mandibular premolar
basal fold of ventral concha

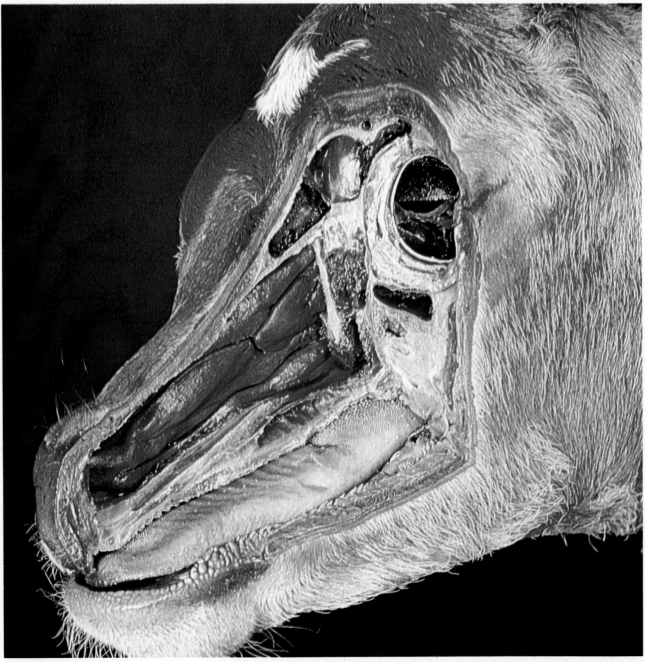

Fig. 1.40 Surface features of the left eye of the goat.

The eye was photographed a few minutes after death.

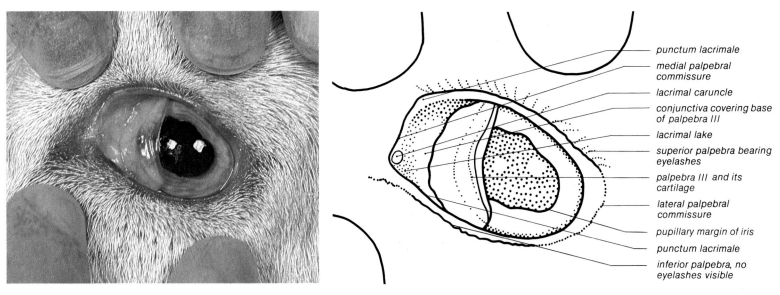

- punctum lacrimale
- medial palpebral commissure
- lacrimal caruncle
- conjunctiva covering base of palpebra III
- lacrimal lake
- superior palpebra bearing eyelashes
- palpebra III and its cartilage
- lateral palpebral commissure
- pupillary margin of iris
- punctum lacrimale
- inferior palpebra, no eyelashes visible

Fig. 1.41 Surface features of the nostrils and mouth of the goat.

The specimen was photographed a few minutes after death. Compare with fig. 1.3.

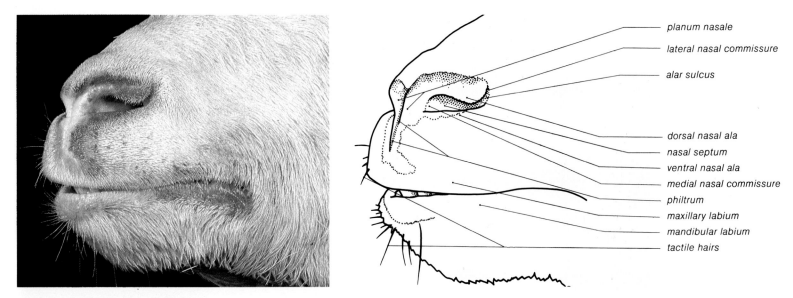

- planum nasale
- lateral nasal commissure
- alar sulcus
- dorsal nasal ala
- nasal septum
- ventral nasal ala
- medial nasal commissure
- philtrum
- maxillary labium
- mandibular labium
- tactile hairs

Fig. 1.42 The deciduous incisor dentition of the young goat (aged 2 years).

The specimen was photographed a few minutes after death. Compare with the permanent bovine incisor dentition shown in fig. 1.5.

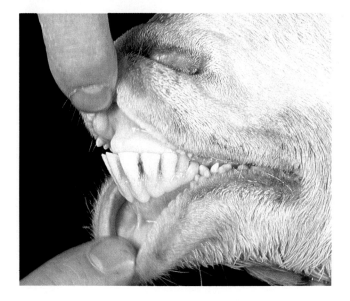
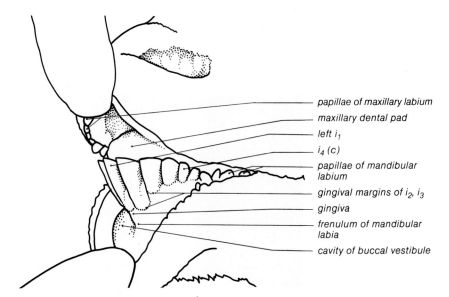

- papillae of maxillary labium
- maxillary dental pad
- left i_1
- i_4 (c)
- papillae of mandibular labium
- gingival margins of i_2, i_3
- gingiva
- frenulum of mandibular labia
- cavity of buccal vestibule

**Fig. 1.43
Nerves and
blood vessels
of the left
cornual
region in the
male goat.**
This figure should be
compared with fig.
1.27 (dehorned cow)
and fig. 1.33 (bull calf).
The fine branches of
the frontal nerve (oph. V)
could not be identified.

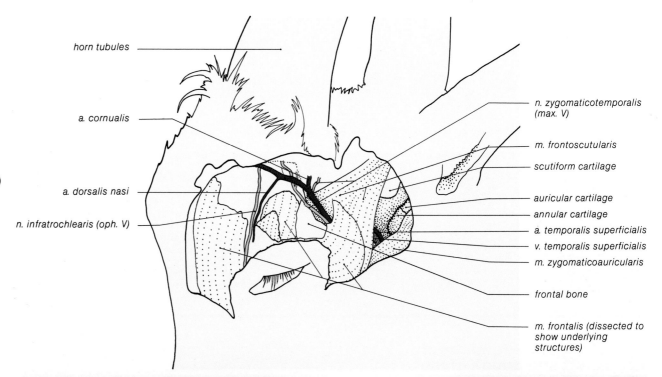

horn tubules

a. cornualis

a. dorsalis nasi

n. infratrochlearis (oph. V)

n. zygomaticotemporalis
(max. V)

m. frontoscutularis

scutiform cartilage

auricular cartilage

annular cartilage

a. temporalis superficialis

v. temporalis superficialis

m. zygomaticoauricularis

frontal bone

m. frontalis (dissected to
show underlying
structures)

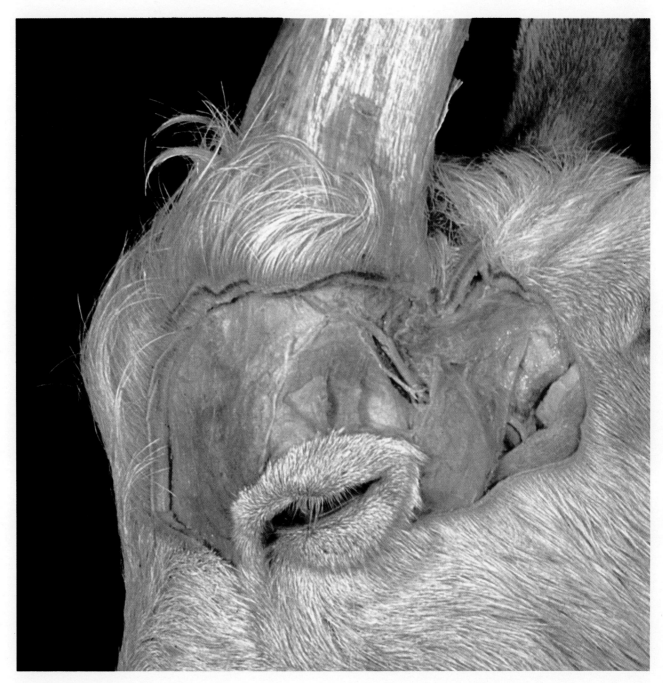

2 The Neck

Fig. 2.1 Surface features of the neck in left lateral view.

The first rib, which demarcates the caudal boundary of the neck, is palpable medial to the major tuberosity of the humerus. The cranial border of the scapula is covered by muscles and is not clearly palpable.

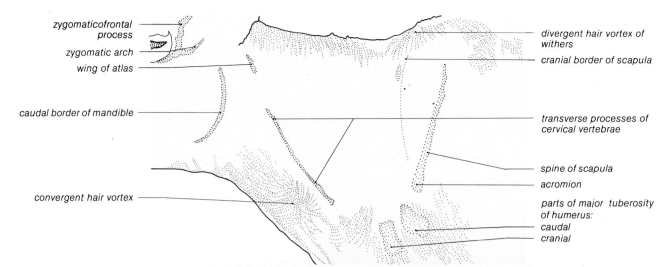

zygomaticofrontal process

zygomatic arch

wing of atlas

caudal border of mandible

convergent hair vortex

divergent hair vortex of withers

cranial border of scapula

transverse processes of cervical vertebrae

spine of scapula

acromion

parts of major tuberosity of humerus:
caudal
cranial

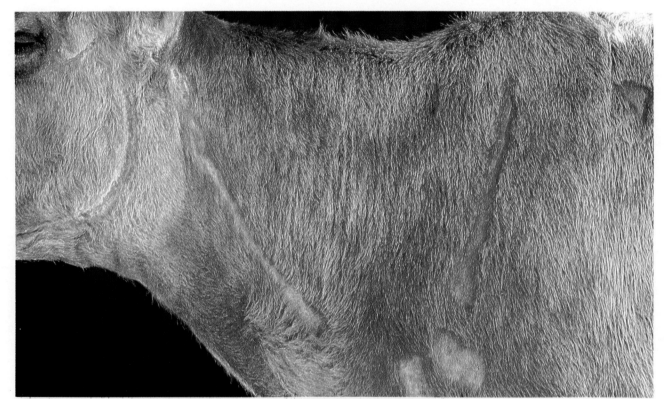

Fig. 2.2 Cervical vertebrae and scapula

The palpable features shown in fig. 2.1 are coloured red.

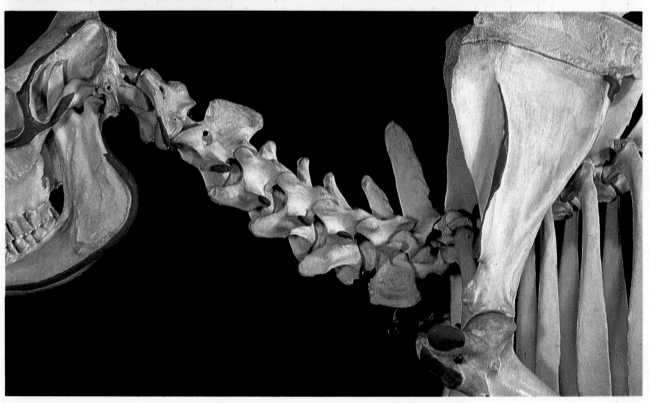

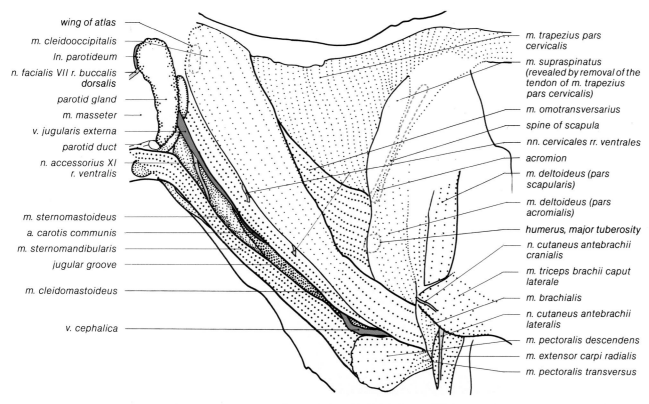

wing of atlas
m. cleidooccipitalis
ln. parotideum
n. facialis VII r. buccalis dorsalis
parotid gland
m. masseter
v. jugularis externa
parotid duct
n. accessorius XI r. ventralis

m. sternomastoideus
a. carotis communis
m. sternomandibularis
jugular groove
m. cleidomastoideus

v. cephalica

m. trapezius pars cervicalis
m. supraspinatus (revealed by removal of the tendon of m. trapezius pars cervicalis)
m. omotransversarius
spine of scapula
nn. cervicales rr. ventrales
acromion
m. deltoideus (pars scapularis)
m. deltoideus (pars acromialis)
humerus, major tuberosity
n. cutaneus antebrachii cranialis
m. triceps brachii caput laterale
m. brachialis
n. cutaneus antebrachii lateralis
m. pectoralis descendens
m. extensor carpi radialis
m. pectoralis transversus

Fig. 2.3 Superficial structures of the neck

This figure shows the details of the boundaries of the jugular groove. The external jugular vein has collapsed and no longer fills this groove.

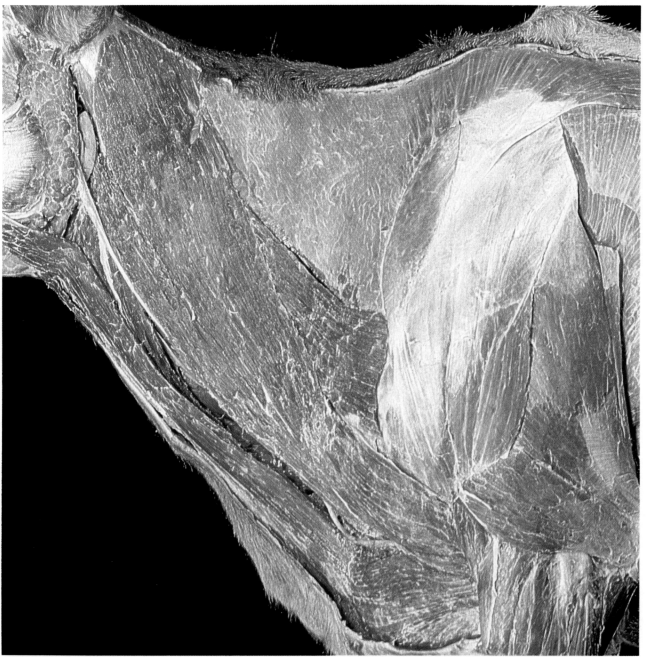

Fig. 2.4 The superficial cervical lymph node.

The omotransversarius muscle has been sectioned to show the position of the superficial cervical lymph node, deep to the omotransversarius muscle, on the cranial border of the supraspinatus muscle.

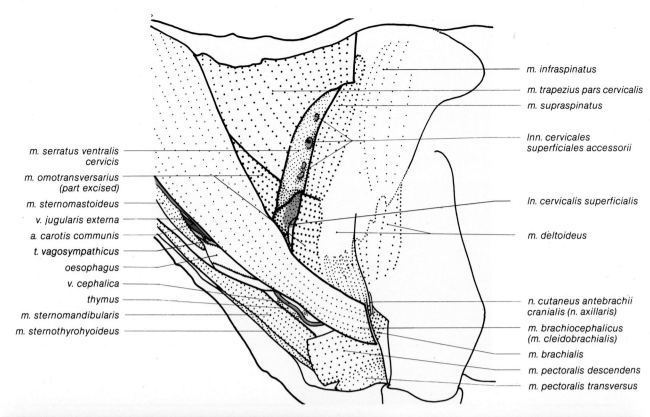

m. infraspinatus

m. trapezius pars cervicalis

m. supraspinatus

Inn. cervicales superficiales accessorii

m. serratus ventralis cervicis

m. omotransversarius (part excised)

m. sternomastoideus

v. jugularis externa

a. carotis communis

t. vagosympathicus

oesophagus

v. cephalica

thymus

m. sternomandibularis

m. sternothyrohyoideus

ln. cervicalis superficialis

m. deltoideus

n. cutaneus antebrachii cranialis (n. axillaris)

m. brachiocephalicus (m. cleidobrachialis)

m. brachialis

m. pectoralis descendens

m. pectoralis transversus

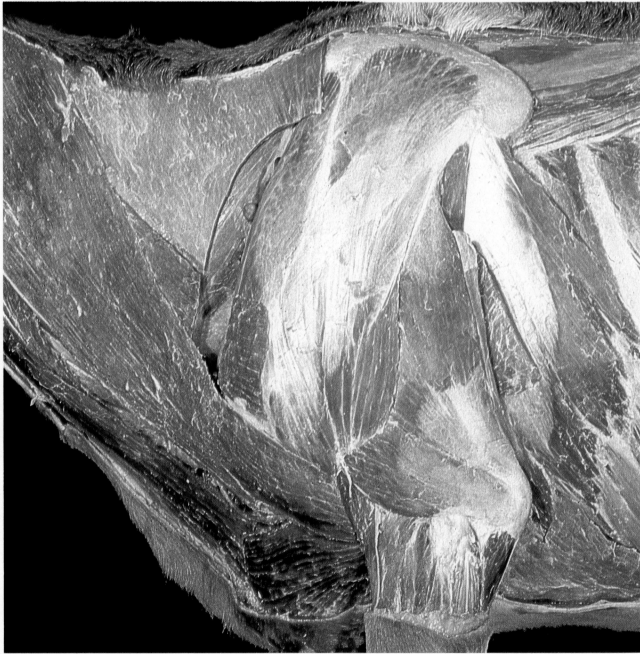

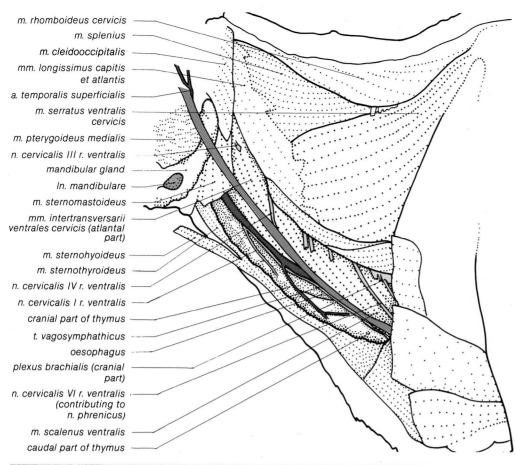

m. rhomboideus cervicis
m. splenius
m. cleidooccipitalis
mm. longissimus capitis et atlantis
a. temporalis superficialis
m. serratus ventralis cervicis
m. pterygoideus medialis
n. cervicalis III r. ventralis
mandibular gland
ln. mandibulare
m. sternomastoideus
mm. intertransversarii ventrales cervicis (atlantal part)
m. sternohyoideus
m. sternothyroideus
n. cervicalis IV r. ventralis
n. cervicalis I r. ventralis
cranial part of thymus
t. vagosymphathicus
oesophagus
plexus brachialis (cranial part)
n. cervicalis VI r. ventralis (contributing to n. phrenicus)
m. scalenus ventralis
caudal part of thymus

Fig. 2.5 The contents of the carotid sheath and the muscles of the neck.

The brachiocephalicus, sternocephalicus and cervical trapezius muscles have been removed. The carotid artery and the vagosympathetic trunk have been freed from the carotid sheath which normally encloses them.

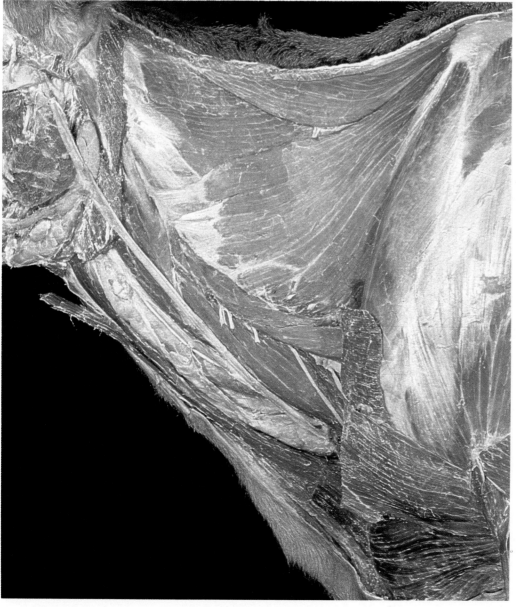

2.5

Fig. 2.6 The caudal part of the neck and the brachial plexus.

The forelimb has been removed, and the thorax dissected as shown in fig. 4.10.

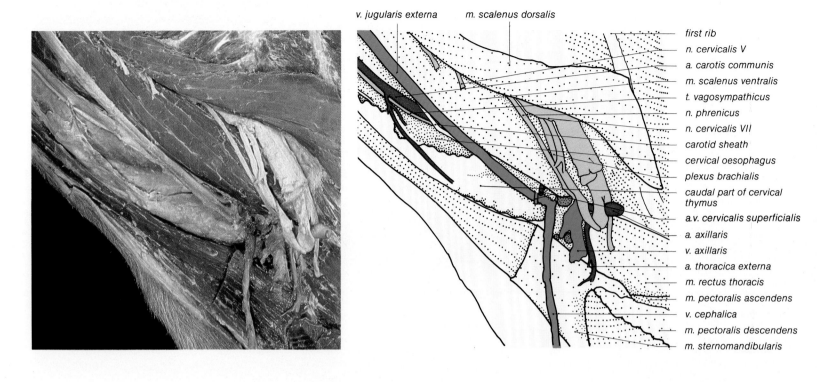

v. jugularis externa   m. scalenus dorsalis

first rib
n. cervicalis V
a. carotis communis
m. scalenus ventralis
t. vagosympathicus
n. phrenicus
n. cervicalis VII
carotid sheath
cervical oesophagus
plexus brachialis
caudal part of cervical thymus
a.v. cervicalis superficialis
a. axillaris
v. axillaris
a. thoracica externa
m. rectus thoracis
m. pectoralis ascendens
v. cephalica
m. pectoralis descendens
m. sternomandibularis

Fig. 2.7 The lateral relationships of the first rib.

The nerves of the brachial plexus have been reflected dorsally, and the axillary artery and vein have been tucked deep to the sternomandibularis muscle to show the lymph nodes and the relationships of the first rib to the muscles, nerves and artery.

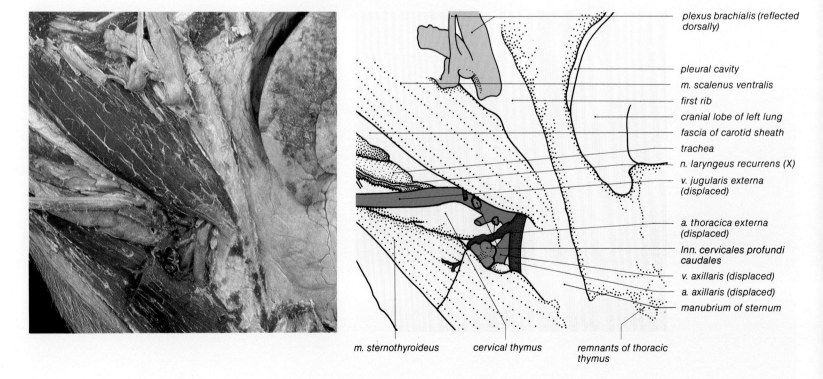

plexus brachialis (reflected dorsally)

pleural cavity
m. scalenus ventralis
first rib
cranial lobe of left lung
fascia of carotid sheath
trachea
n. laryngeus recurrens (X)
v. jugularis externa (displaced)

a. thoracica externa (displaced)
lnn. cervicales profundi caudales
v. axillaris (displaced)
a. axillaris (displaced)
manubrium of sternum

m. sternothyroideus   cervical thymus   remnants of thoracic thymus

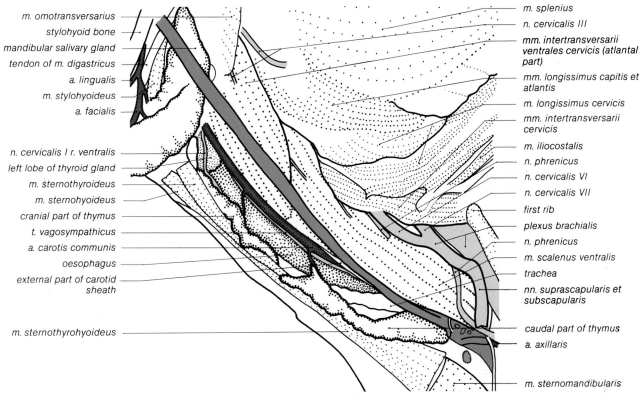

m. omotransversarius
stylohyoid bone
mandibular salivary gland
tendon of m. digastricus
a. lingualis
m. stylohyoideus
a. facialis

n. cervicalis I r. ventralis
left lobe of thyroid gland
m. sternothyroideus
m. sternohyoideus
cranial part of thymus
t. vagosympathicus
a. carotis communis
oesophagus
external part of carotid sheath

m. sternothyrohyoideus

m. splenius
n. cervicalis III
mm. intertransversarii ventrales cervicis (atlantal part)
mm. longissimus capitis et atlantis
m. longissimus cervicis
mm. intertransversarii cervicis
m. iliocostalis
n. phrenicus
n. cervicalis VI
n. cervicalis VII
first rib
plexus brachialis
n. phrenicus
m. scalenus ventralis
trachea
nn. suprascapularis et subscapularis
caudal part of thymus
a. axillaris

m. sternomandibularis

Fig. 2.8 The thymus gland in the neck.

The dorsal scalenus muscle has been removed and the fascia holding the thymus has been loosened to show the cranial and caudal parts of the cervical thymus. This cow was about six years of age.

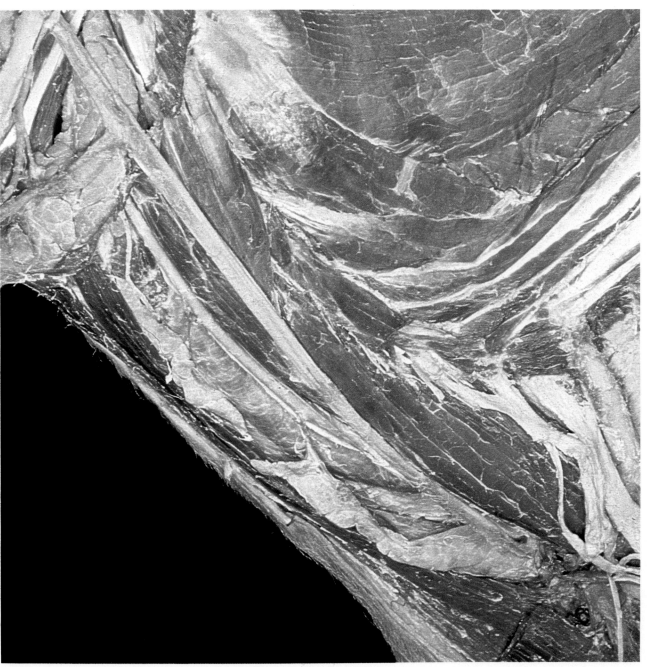

Fig. 2.9 Nerves, arteries, veins and visceral organs of the neck.

The external jugular vein and the 'strap muscles' of the neck have been removed.

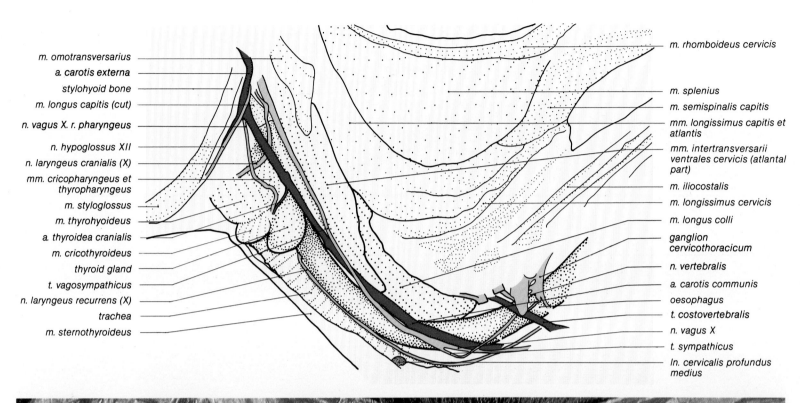

m. omotransversarius
a. carotis externa
stylohyoid bone
m. longus capitis (cut)
n. vagus X. r. pharyngeus
n. hypoglossus XII
n. laryngeus cranialis (X)
mm. cricopharyngeus et thyropharyngeus
m. styloglossus
m. thyrohyoideus
a. thyroidea cranialis
m. cricothyroideus
thyroid gland
t. vagosympathicus
n. laryngeus recurrens (X)
trachea
m. sternothyroideus

m. rhomboideus cervicis
m. splenius
m. semispinalis capitis
mm. longissimus capitis et atlantis
mm. intertransversarii ventrales cervicis (atlantal part)
m. iliocostalis
m. longissimus cervicis
m. longus colli
ganglion cervicothoracicum
n. vertebralis
a. carotis communis
oesophagus
t. costovertebralis
n. vagus X
t. sympathicus
ln. cervicalis profundus medius

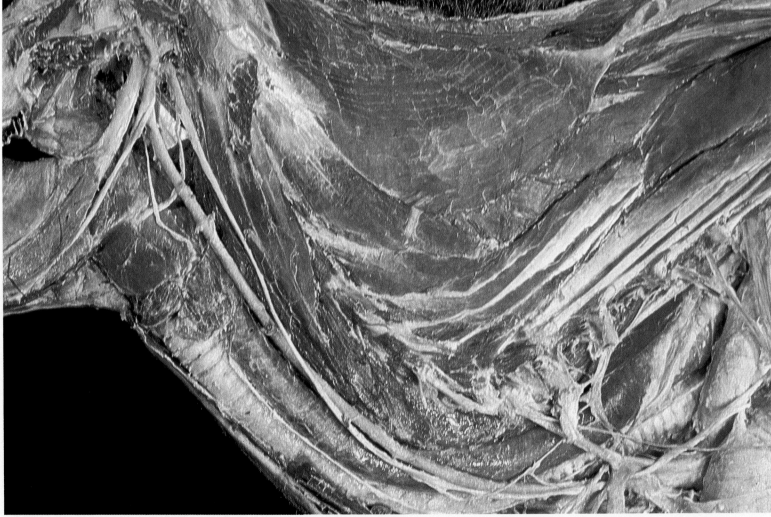

Fig. 2.10 The ligamentum nuchae and the epaxial muscles of the neck.

Removal of the splenius and rhomboideus muscles reveals the nuchal ligament, which is seen more fully in figs. 2.11 and 2.12.

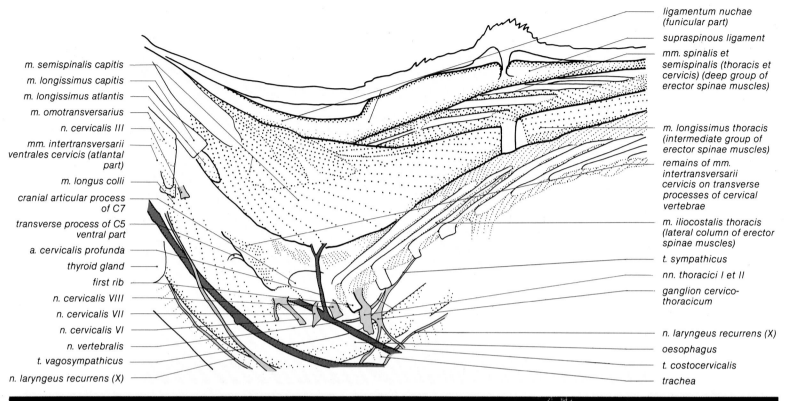

m. semispinalis capitis

m. longissimus capitis

m. longissimus atlantis

m. omotransversarius

n. cervicalis III

mm. intertransversarii ventrales cervicis (atlantal part)

m. longus colli

cranial articular process of C7

transverse process of C5 ventral part

a. cervicalis profunda

thyroid gland

first rib

n. cervicalis VIII

n. cervicalis VII

n. cervicalis VI

n. vertebralis

t. vagosympathicus

n. laryngeus recurrens (X)

ligamentum nuchae (funicular part)

supraspinous ligament

mm. spinalis et semispinalis (thoracis et cervicis) (deep group of erector spinae muscles)

m. longissimus thoracis (intermediate group of erector spinae muscles)

remains of mm. intertransversarii cervicis on transverse processes of cervical vertebrae

m. iliocostalis thoracis (lateral column of erector spinae muscles)

t. sympathicus

nn. thoracici I et II

ganglion cervico-thoracicum

n. laryngeus recurrens (X)

oesophagus

t. costocervicalis

trachea

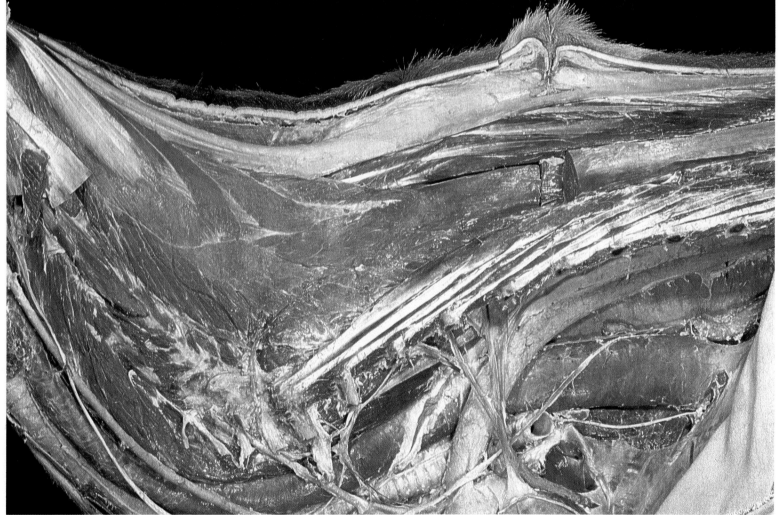

Fig. 2.11 The nuchal ligament and deep epaxial muscles of the neck.

Removal of the semispinalis capitis muscle reveals the nuchal ligament and the short segmental muscles of the neck, including those of the atlas and axis.

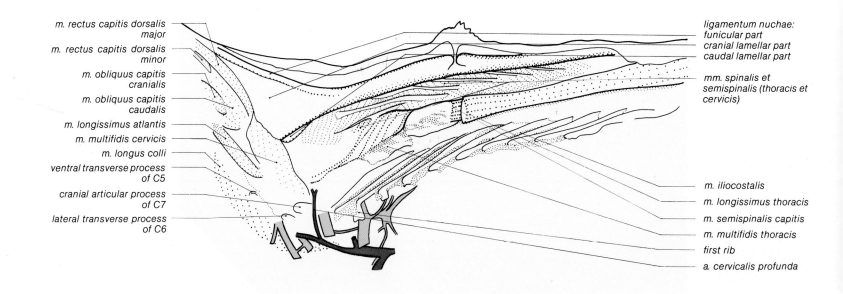

m. rectus capitis dorsalis major
m. rectus capitis dorsalis minor
m. obliquus capitis cranialis
m. obliquus capitis caudalis
m. longissimus atlantis
m. multifidis cervicis
m. longus colli
ventral transverse process of C5
cranial articular process of C7
lateral transverse process of C6

ligamentum nuchae:
funicular part
cranial lamellar part
caudal lamellar part

mm. spinalis et semispinalis (thoracis et cervicis)

m. iliocostalis
m. longissimus thoracis
m. semispinalis capitis
m. multifidis thoracis
first rib
a. cervicalis profunda

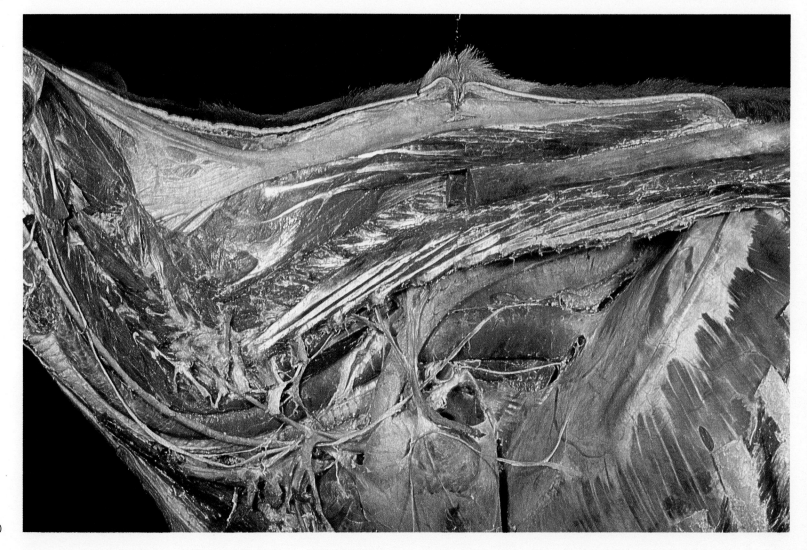

Fig. 2.12 The nuchal ligament, vertebral artery and cervical nerves.

The elastic nuchal ligament is fully revealed by removal of the epaxial muscle mass on the left side. The continuity with the supraspinous ligament is shown in fig. 2.10.

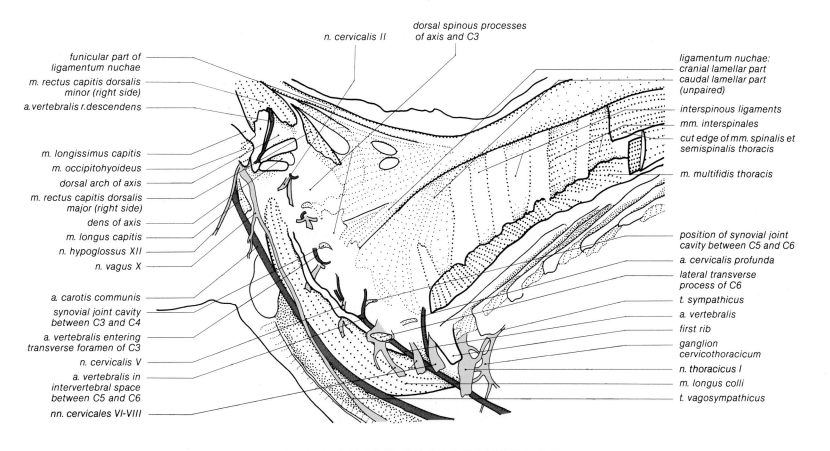

n. cervicalis II

dorsal spinous processes of axis and C3

funicular part of ligamentum nuchae

m. rectus capitis dorsalis minor (right side)

a. vertebralis r. descendens

m. longissimus capitis

m. occipitohyoideus

dorsal arch of axis

m. rectus capitis dorsalis major (right side)

dens of axis

m. longus capitis

n. hypoglossus XII

n. vagus X

a. carotis communis

synovial joint cavity between C3 and C4

a. vertebralis entering transverse foramen of C3

n. cervicalis V

a. vertebralis in intervertebral space between C5 and C6

nn. cervicales VI-VIII

ligamentum nuchae:
cranial lamellar part
caudal lamellar part (unpaired)

interspinous ligaments

mm. interspinales

cut edge of mm. spinalis et semispinalis thoracis

m. multifidis thoracis

position of synovial joint cavity between C5 and C6

a. cervicalis profunda

lateral transverse process of C6

t. sympathicus

a. vertebralis

first rib

ganglion cervicothoracicum

n. thoracicus I

m. longus colli

t. vagosympathicus

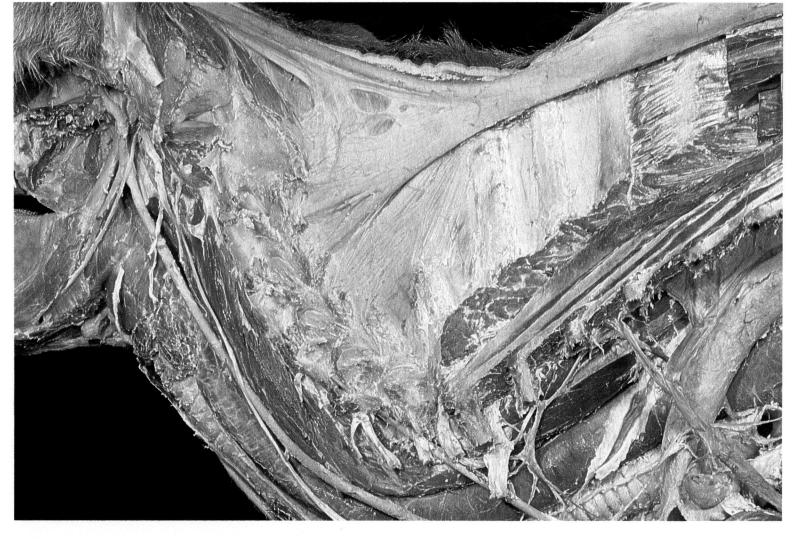

Fig. 2.13 Superficial structures of the neck in the calf.

The course of the dorsal branch of the spinal accessory nerve is unusual: the nerve usually lies deep to the cervical trapezius muscle.

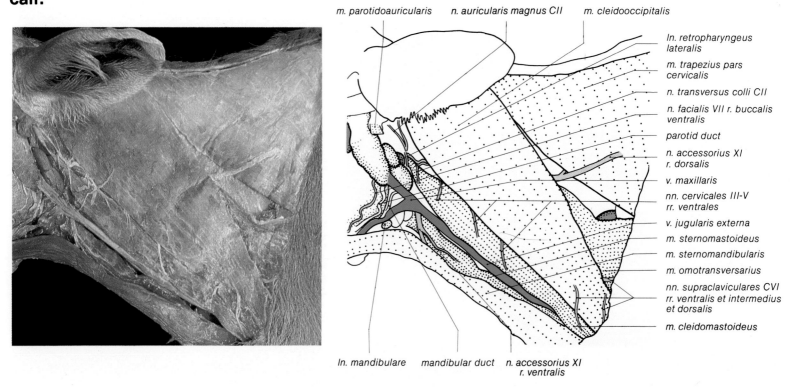

m. parotidoauricularis   n. auricularis magnus CII   m. cleidooccipitalis

ln. retropharyngeus lateralis
m. trapezius pars cervicalis
n. transversus colli CII
n. facialis VII r. buccalis ventralis
parotid duct
n. accessorius XI r. dorsalis
v. maxillaris
nn. cervicales III-V rr. ventrales
v. jugularis externa
m. sternomastoideus
m. sternomandibularis
m. omotransversarius
nn. supraclaviculares CVI rr. ventralis et intermedius et dorsalis
m. cleidomastoideus

ln. mandibulare   mandibular duct   n. accessorius XI r. ventralis

Fig. 2.14 The spinal accessory nerve and the thymus gland in the neck of the calf.

Removal of the brachiocephalicus and sternocephalicus muscles exposes the cervical thymus gland, which is large at one week of age. Compare with fig. 2.8.

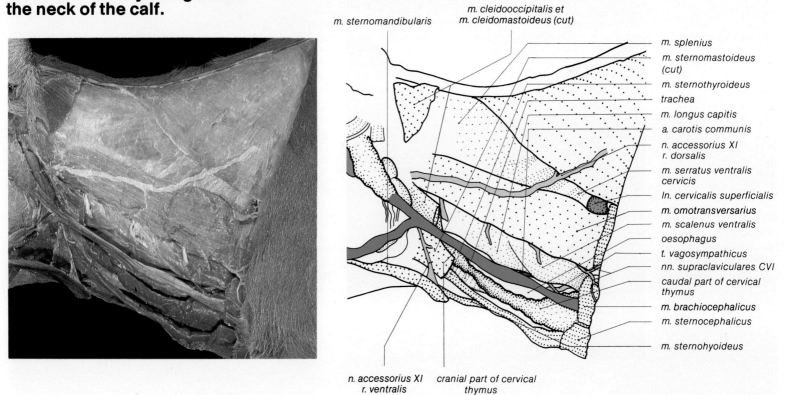

m. sternomandibularis   m. cleidooccipitalis et m. cleidomastoideus (cut)

m. splenius
m. sternomastoideus (cut)
m. sternothyroideus
trachea
m. longus capitis
a. carotis communis
n. accessorius XI r. dorsalis
m. serratus ventralis cervicis
ln. cervicalis superficialis
m. omotransversarius
m. scalenus ventralis
oesophagus
t. vagosympathicus
nn. supraclaviculares CVI
caudal part of cervical thymus
m. brachiocephalicus
m. sternocephalicus
m. sternohyoideus

n. accessorius XI r. ventralis   cranial part of cervical thymus

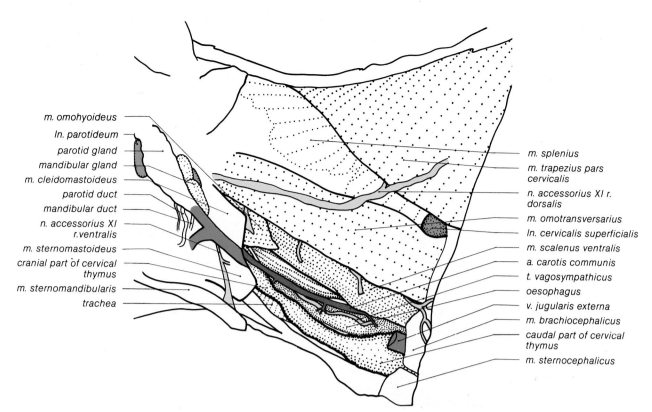

Fig. 2.15 The visceral and associated structures in the neck of the calf.

Removal of the external jugular vein displays the contents of the carotid sheath.

m. omohyoideus
ln. parotideum
parotid gland
mandibular gland
m. cleidomastoideus
parotid duct
mandibular duct
n. accessorius XI r.ventralis
m. sternomastoideus
cranial part of cervical thymus
m. sternomandibularis
trachea

m. splenius
m. trapezius pars cervicalis
n. accessorius XI r. dorsalis
m. omotransversarius
ln. cervicalis superficialis
m. scalenus ventralis
a. carotis communis
t. vagosympathicus
oesophagus
v. jugularis externa
m. brachiocephalicus
caudal part of cervical thymus
m. sternocephalicus

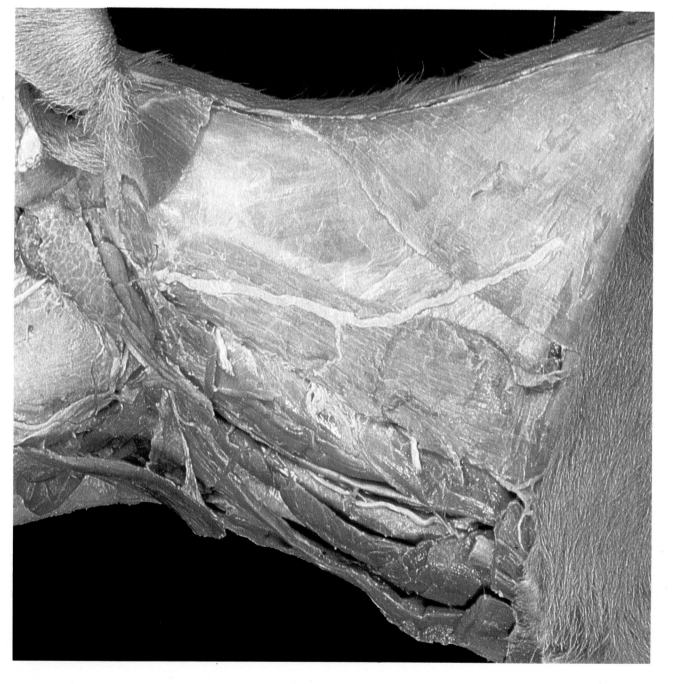

Fig. 2.16 The cervical vertebrae, vertebral artery and ligamentrum nuchae of the calf.

This dissection was performed on the right side, but the figure has been reversed to allow comparison with figs. 2.13, 2.14 and 2.15.

The entire epaxial musculature has been removed from this side to display the nuchal ligament.

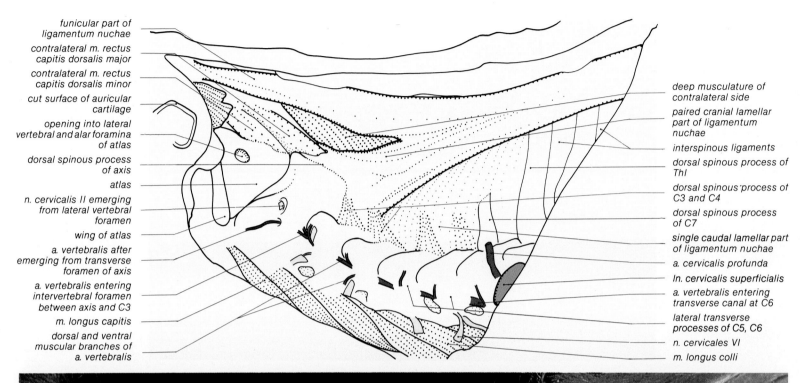

funicular part of ligamentum nuchae

contralateral m. rectus capitis dorsalis major

contralateral m. rectus capitis dorsalis minor

cut surface of auricular cartilage

opening into lateral vertebral and alar foramina of atlas

dorsal spinous process of axis

atlas

n. cervicalis II emerging from lateral vertebral foramen

wing of atlas

a. vertebralis after emerging from transverse foramen of axis

a. vertebralis entering intervertebral foramen between axis and C3

m. longus capitis

dorsal and ventral muscular branches of a. vertebralis

deep musculature of contralateral side

paired cranial lamellar part of ligamentum nuchae

interspinous ligaments

dorsal spinous process of ThI

dorsal spinous process of C3 and C4

dorsal spinous process of C7

single caudal lamellar part of ligamentum nuchae

a. cervicalis profunda

ln. cervicalis superficialis

a. vertebralis entering transverse canal at C6

lateral transverse processes of C5, C6

n. cervicales VI

m. longus colli

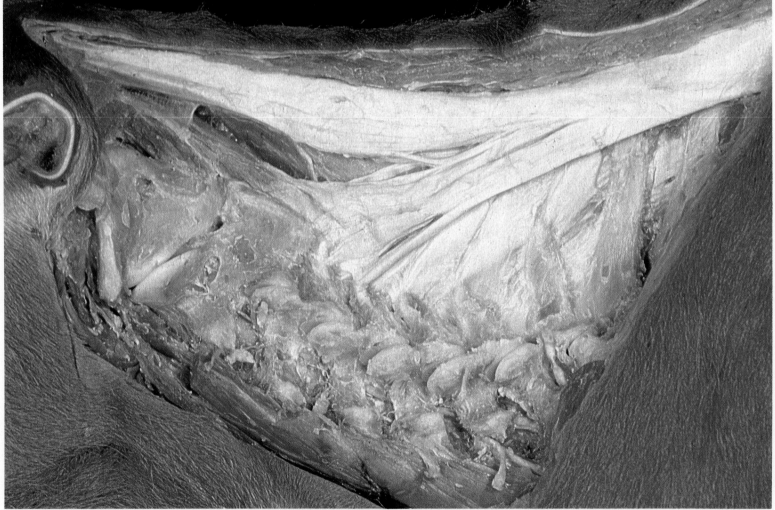

3 The Forelimb

Fig. 3.1 Surface features of the shoulder and forelimb, in left lateral view.

The palpable bony prominences have been shaved.

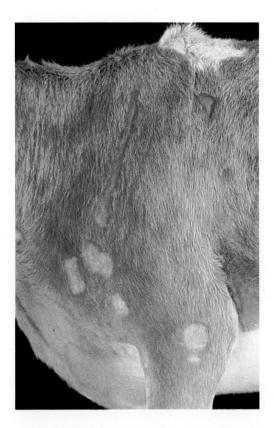

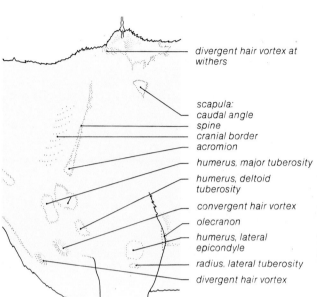

divergent hair vortex at withers

scapula:
caudal angle
spine
cranial border
acromion

humerus, major tuberosity

humerus, deltoid tuberosity

convergent hair vortex

olecranon

humerus, lateral epicondyle

radius. lateral tuberosity

divergent hair vortex

Fig. 3.2 Bones of the shoulder and forelimb.

The palpable features shown in fig. 3.1 are coloured red.

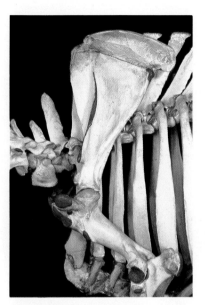

Fig. 3.3 Surface features of the forelimb, in left lateral view.

In normal level standing, the olecranon lies superficial to the costochondral junction of rib 5. There is a divergent hair whorl in the white hair immediately caudal to the olecranon, but it is not visible in this figure because of the hair colour.

Fig. 3.4 Bones of the forelimb.

The palpable features shown in fig. 3.3 are coloured red.

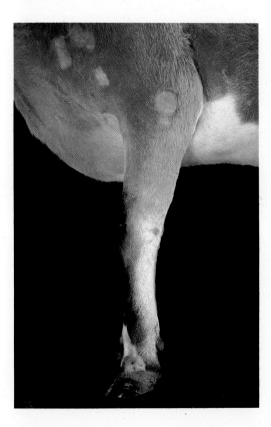

cranial and caudal divisions of major tuberosity of humerus

humerus, deltoid tuberosity

ulna, olecranon

humerus, lateral epicondyle

brachium

radius, lateral tuberosity

convergent hair vortex

divergent hair vortex

antebrachium

accessory carpal bone

position of radiocarpal joint

position of fetlock joint

digit V ('dew claw')

coronet

bulb of hoof

manus   digit IV (wall of hoof)

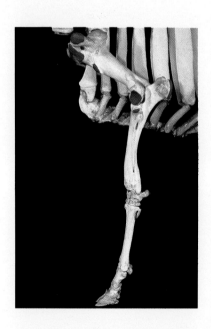

Fig. 3.5 Superficial muscles of the left scapular, brachial and antebrachial regions: (1).

The strong omobrachial and brachial fasciae which cover the muscles of these regions have been almost entirely removed.

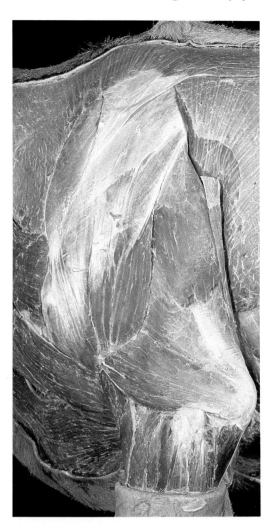

m. trapezius (pars cervicis) with tendon removed to show m. supraspinatus

scapula:
spine
acromion

m. omotransversarius

m. deltoideus:
pars acromialis
pars scapularis

humerus:
position of major tuberosity
position of deltoid tuberosity

m. brachiocephalicus

m. brachialis

n. cutaneus antebrachii lateralis (n. radialis r. superficialis)

m. pectoralis descendens

m. extensor carpi radialis

m. pectoralis transversus

m. trapezius (pars thoracica)

omobrachial fascia

scapula, caudal angle

m. latissimus dorsi

m. triceps brachii (caput longum)

m. tensor fasciae antebrachii

n. cutaneus brachii lateralis cranalis (n. axillaris)

m. triceps brachii (caput laterale)

n. cutaneus antebrachii cranialis (n. axillaris)

humerus, lateral epicondyle

m. extensor digitorum communis

m. flexor digitorum profundus (caput ulnare)

m. extensor digitorum lateralis

m. extensor carpi ulnaris

Fig. 3.6 Superficial muscles of the left scapular, brachial and antebrachial regions: (2).

The more cranial parts of this dissection are shown in fig. 2.5.

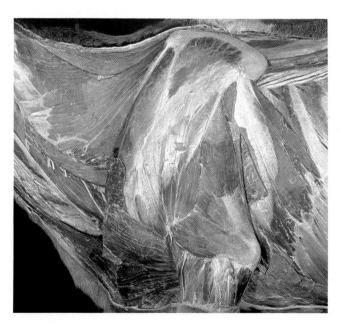

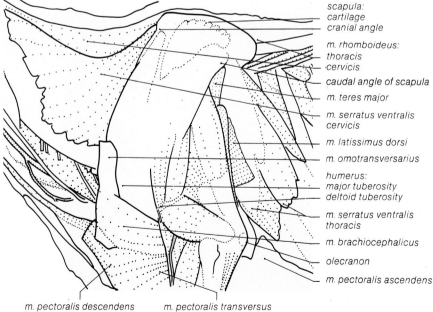

scapula:
cartilage
cranial angle

m. rhomboideus:
thoracis
cervicis

caudal angle of scapula

m. teres major

m. serratus ventralis cervicis

m. latissimus dorsi

m. omotransversarius

humerus:
major tuberosity
deltoid tuberosity

m. serratus ventralis thoracis

m. brachiocephalicus

olecranon

m. pectoralis ascendens

m. pectoralis descendens   m. pectoralis transversus

Fig. 3.7 Muscles of the scapular, brachial and antebrachial regions in the detached limb: lateral view.

The relationship of this limb to the thoracic structures is shown in fig. 4.12. The acromial part of the deltoid muscle has been removed and its scapular part cut, in order to show the tendon of insertion of the infraspinatus muscle.

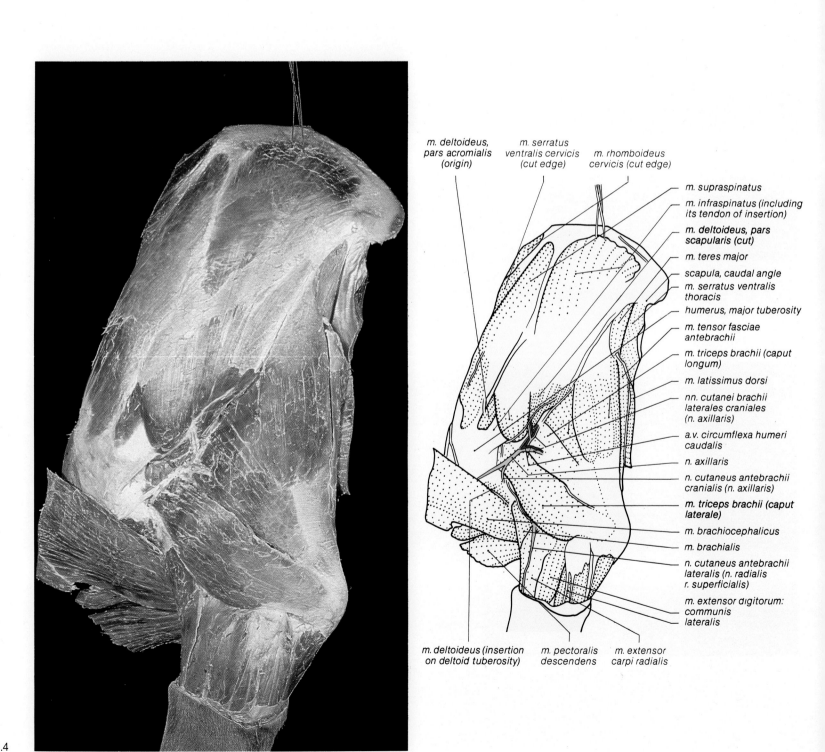

m. deltoideus, pars acromialis (origin)

m. serratus ventralis cervicis (cut edge)

m. rhomboideus cervicis (cut edge)

m. supraspinatus

m. infraspinatus (including its tendon of insertion)

m. deltoideus, pars scapularis (cut)

m. teres major

scapula, caudal angle

m. serratus ventralis thoracis

humerus, major tuberosity

m. tensor fasciae antebrachii

m. triceps brachii (caput longum)

m. latissimus dorsi

nn. cutanei brachii laterales craniales (n. axillaris)

a.v. circumflexa humeri caudalis

n. axillaris

n. cutaneus antebrachii cranialis (n. axillaris)

m. triceps brachii (caput laterale)

m. brachiocephalicus

m. brachialis

n. cutaneus antebrachii lateralis (n. radialis r. superficialis)

m. extensor digitorum: communis lateralis

m. deltoideus (insertion on deltoid tuberosity)

m. pectoralis descendens

m. extensor carpi radialis

3.4

Fig. 3.8 Superficial muscles and nerves of the antebrachium and carpus: lateral view.

The dense antebrachial fascia has been removed. The common digital extensor muscle has two tendons; that part of the muscle associated with the medial tendon is sometimes referred to as m. extensor digiti III proprius. The ulnar nerve runs superficially between the extensor carpi ulnaris and flexor carpi ulnaris muscles; it has been slightly displaced to reveal its position.

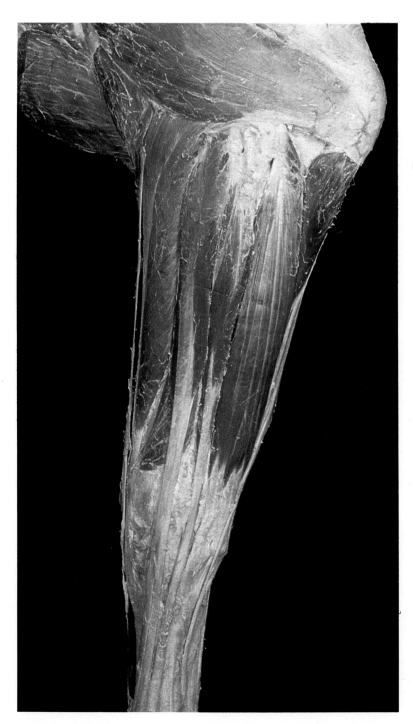

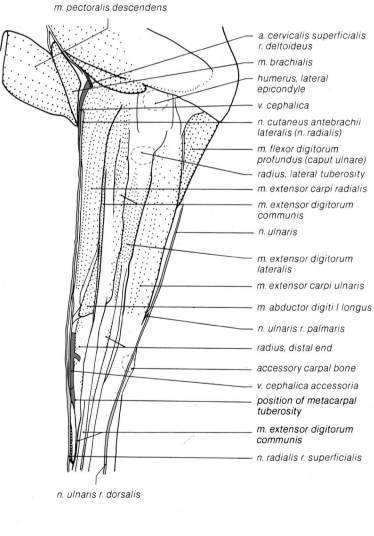

m. pectoralis descendens

a. cervicalis superficialis r. deltoideus

m. brachialis

humerus, lateral epicondyle

v. cephalica

n. cutaneus antebrachii lateralis (n. radialis)

m. flexor digitorum profundus (caput ulnare)

radius, lateral tuberosity

m. extensor carpi radialis

m. extensor digitorum communis

n. ulnaris

m. extensor digitorum lateralis

m. extensor carpi ulnaris

m. abductor digiti I longus

n. ulnaris r. palmaris

radius, distal end

accessory carpal bone

v. cephalica accessoria

position of metacarpal tuberosity

m. extensor digitorum communis

n. radialis r. superficialis

n. ulnaris r. dorsalis

Fig. 3.9 Muscles, vessels and nerves of the scapular and brachial regions: medial view.

The muscles that join the limb to the trunk have been cut, but their attachments to the scapula and humerus have been preserved. In this figure and fig. 3.10 no attempt has been made to display the axillary vessels and nerves in their topographical positions; these are shown in a separate series of dissections (figs. 3.25-3.28).

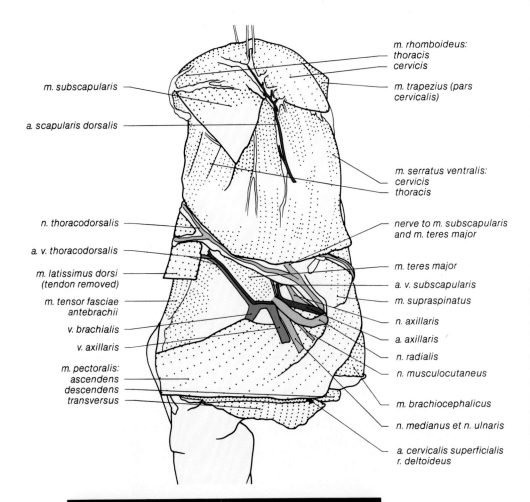

m. subscapularis

a. scapularis dorsalis

n. thoracodorsalis

a. v. thoracodorsalis

m. latissimus dorsi (tendon removed)

m. tensor fasciae antebrachii

v. brachialis

v. axillaris

m. pectoralis:
ascendens
descendens
transversus

m. rhomboideus:
thoracis
cervicis

m. trapezius (pars cervicalis)

m. serratus ventralis:
cervicis
thoracis

nerve to m. subscapularis and m. teres major

m. teres major

a. v. subscapularis

m. supraspinatus

n. axillaris

a. axillaris

n. radialis

n. musculocutaneus

m. brachiocephalicus

n. medianus et n. ulnaris

a. cervicalis superficialis
r. deltoideus

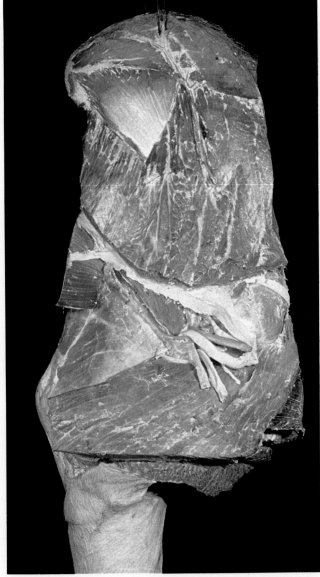

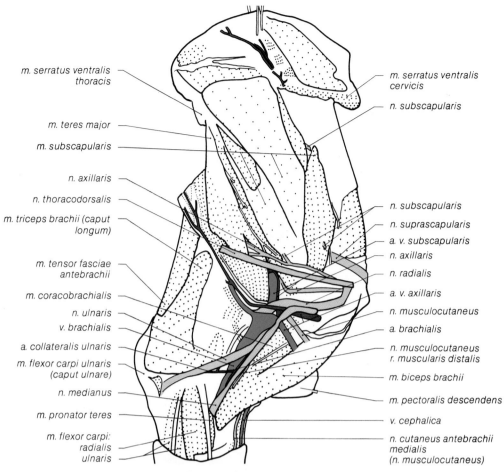

m. serratus ventralis thoracis

m. teres major

m. subscapularis

n. axillaris

n. thoracodorsalis

m. triceps brachii (caput longum)

m. tensor fasciae antebrachii

m. coracobrachialis

n. ulnaris

v. brachialis

a. collateralis ulnaris

m. flexor carpi ulnaris (caput ulnare)

n. medianus

m. pronator teres

m. flexor carpi:
radialis
ulnaris

m. serratus ventralis cervicis

n. subscapularis

n. subscapularis

n. suprascapularis

a. v. subscapularis

n. axillaris

n. radialis

a. v. axillaris

n. musculocutaneus

a. brachialis

n. musculocutaneus
r. muscularis distalis

m. biceps brachii

m. pectoralis descendens

v. cephalica

n. cutaneus antebrachii
medialis
(n. musculocutaneus)

Fig. 3.10 Muscles, vessels and nerves of the scapular, brachial and antebrachial regions: medial view.

Details of the nerves of the brachial plexus are exposed on cutting away the muscles joining the limb to the trunk. Removal of the limb makes it impossible to preserve the true topographical relationships of the nerves and blood vessels in the axilla, but these are shown in a separate series of dissections (figs. 3.25 – 3.28).

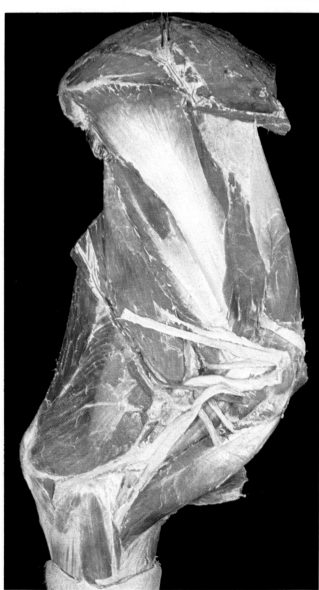

Fig. 3.11 Muscles of the antebrachium and carpus, in lateral view: (1).

The extensor carpi radialis and extensor carpi ulnaris muscles have been incised in preparation for removal as shown in the 2nd, 3rd and 4th dissections in this series (figs. 3.13 – 3.15). The extensor carpi ulnaris muscle is often called the m. ulnaris lateralis.

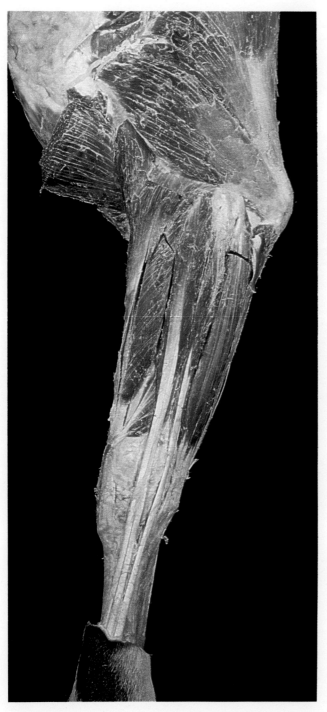

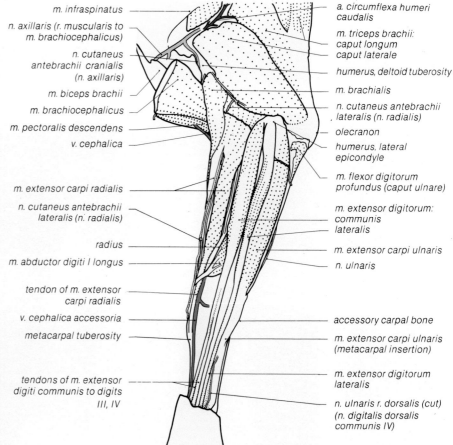

m. infraspinatus

n. axillaris (r. muscularis to m. brachiocephalicus)

n. cutaneus antebrachii cranialis (n. axillaris)

m. biceps brachii

m. brachiocephalicus

m. pectoralis descendens

v. cephalica

m. extensor carpi radialis

n. cutaneus antebrachii lateralis (n. radialis)

radius

m. abductor digiti I longus

tendon of m. extensor carpi radialis

v. cephalica accessoria

metacarpal tuberosity

tendons of m. extensor digiti communis to digits III, IV

a. circumflexa humeri caudalis

m. triceps brachii: caput longum caput laterale

humerus, deltoid tuberosity

m. brachialis

n. cutaneus antebrachii lateralis (n. radialis)

olecranon

humerus, lateral epicondyle

m. flexor digitorum profundus (caput ulnare)

m. extensor digitorum: communis lateralis

m. extensor carpi ulnaris

n. ulnaris

accessory carpal bone

m. extensor carpi ulnaris (metacarpal insertion)

m. extensor digitorum lateralis

n. ulnaris r. dorsalis (cut) (n. digitalis dorsalis communis IV)

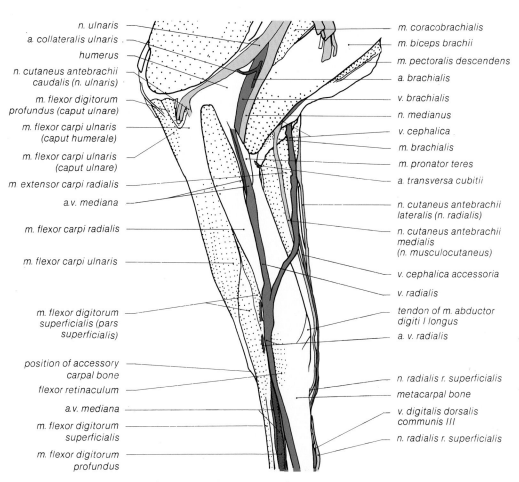

n. ulnaris
a. collateralis ulnaris
humerus
n. cutaneus antebrachii caudalis (n. ulnaris)
m. flexor digitorum profundus (caput ulnare)
m. flexor carpi ulnaris (caput humerale)
m. flexor carpi ulnaris (caput ulnare)
m. extensor carpi radialis
a.v. mediana
m. flexor carpi radialis
m. flexor carpi ulnaris
m. flexor digitorum superficialis (pars superficialis)
position of accessory carpal bone
flexor retinaculum
a.v. mediana
m. flexor digitorum superficialis
m. flexor digitorum profundus

m. coracobrachialis
m. biceps brachii
m. pectoralis descendens
a. brachialis
v. brachialis
n. medianus
v. cephalica
m. brachialis
m. pronator teres
a. transversa cubitii
n. cutaneus antebrachii lateralis (n. radialis)
n. cutaneus antebrachii medialis (n. musculocutaneus)
v. cephalica accessoria
v. radialis
tendon of m. abductor digiti I longus
a. v. radialis
n. radialis r. superficialis
metacarpal bone
v. digitalis dorsalis communis III
n. radialis r. superficialis

Fig. 3.12 Muscles, vessels and nerves of the antebrachium and carpus, in medial view.

The cut proximal ends of the ulnar median and radial nerves have fallen down into this figure and can be seen in the top right hand corner. Further dissections, shown in medial view, can be seen in figs. 3.16 and 3.17.

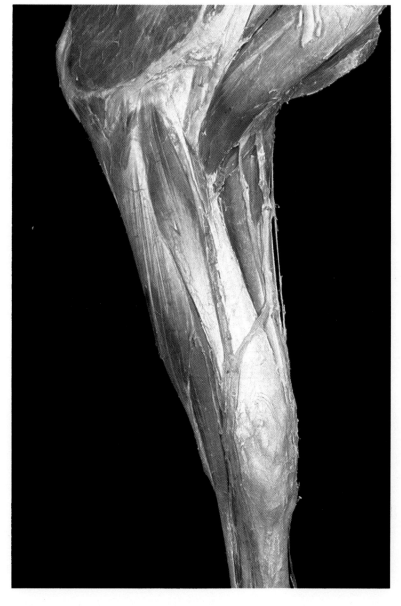

Fig. 3.13 Muscles of the antebrachium and carpus, in lateral view: (2).

The extensor carpi ulnaris muscle has been removed to expose the digital flexor muscles.

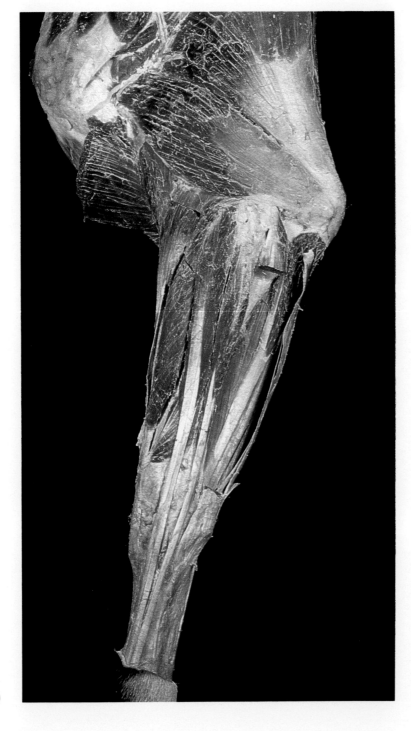

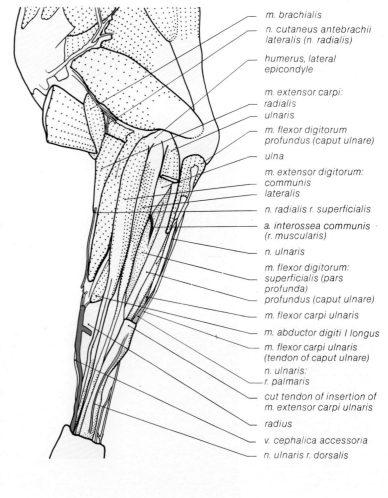

m. brachialis

n. cutaneus antebrachii lateralis (n. radialis)

humerus, lateral epicondyle

m. extensor carpi:
radialis
ulnaris

m. flexor digitorum profundus (caput ulnare)

ulna

m. extensor digitorum:
communis
lateralis

n. radialis r. superficialis

a. interossea communis (r. muscularis)

n. ulnaris

m. flexor digitorum:
superficialis (pars profunda)
profundus (caput ulnare)

m. flexor carpi ulnaris

m. abductor digiti I longus

m. flexor carpi ulnaris (tendon of caput ulnare)

n. ulnaris:
r. palmaris

cut tendon of insertion of m. extensor carpi ulnaris

radius

v. cephalica accessoria

n. ulnaris r. dorsalis

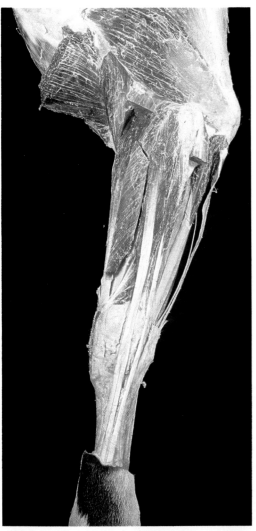
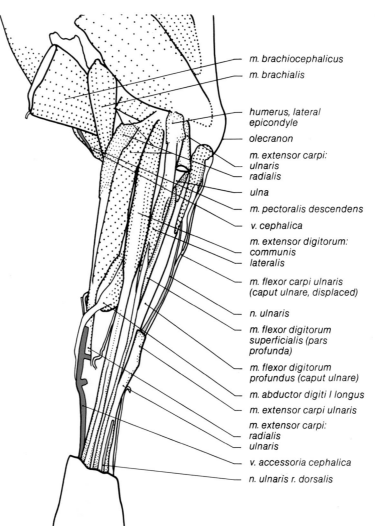

m. brachiocephalicus

m. brachialis

humerus, lateral epicondyle

olecranon

m. extensor carpi:
ulnaris
radialis

ulna

m. pectoralis descendens

v. cephalica

m. extensor digitorum:
communis
lateralis

m. flexor carpi ulnaris
(caput ulnare, displaced)

n. ulnaris

m. flexor digitorum
superficialis (pars
profunda)

m. flexor digitorum
profundus (caput ulnare)

m. abductor digiti I longus

m. extensor carpi ulnaris

m. extensor carpi:
radialis
ulnaris

v. accessoria cephalica

n. ulnaris r. dorsalis

Fig. 3.14 Muscles of the antebrachium and carpus, in lateral view: (3).

The part of the extensor carpi radialis muscle that originates from the lateral epicondylar crest of the humerus has been removed to show the brachialis muscle more clearly.

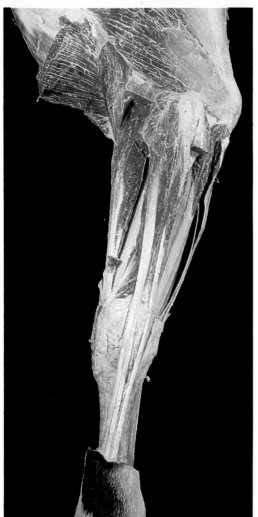
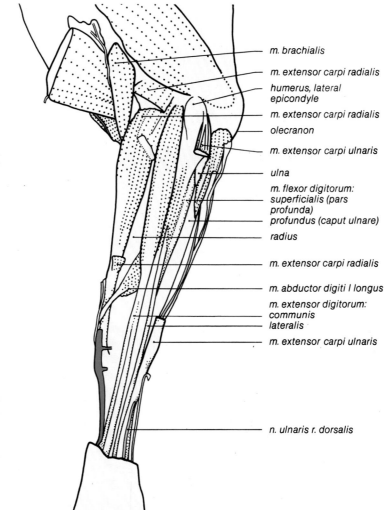

m. brachialis

m. extensor carpi radialis

humerus, lateral epicondyle

m. extensor carpi radialis

olecranon

m. extensor carpi ulnaris

ulna

m. flexor digitorum:
superficialis (pars
profunda)
profundus (caput ulnare)

radius

m. extensor carpi radialis

m. abductor digiti I longus

m. extensor digitorum:
communis
lateralis

m. extensor carpi ulnaris

n. ulnaris r. dorsalis

Fig. 3.15 Muscles of the ante-brachium and carpus, in lateral view: (4).

The part of the humeral head of the extensor carpi radialis muscle that originates from the intermuscular septum between the extensor carpi radialis and the common digital extensor muscle has now been removed to show more clearly the component originating from the radial fossa of the humerus.

Fig. 3.16 Muscles, vessels and nerves of the antebrachium and carpus, in medial view: (1).

The m. pronator teres has been removed to display the artery, vein and nerve at the cubital region more completely. The humeral origins of the carpal flexors have been incised in preparation for removal as shown in fig. 3.17. An earlier stage of this dissection is shown in fig. 3.12.

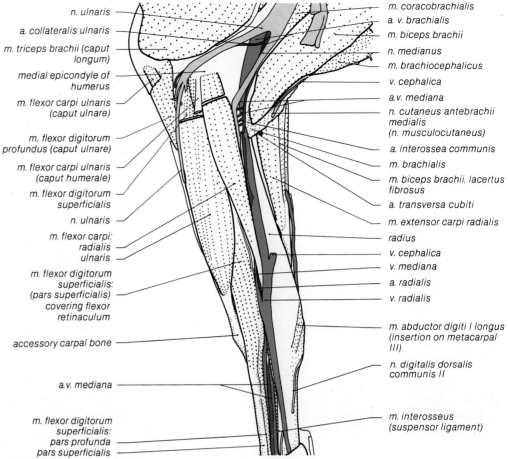

n. ulnaris
a. collateralis ulnaris
m. triceps brachii (caput longum)
medial epicondyle of humerus
m. flexor carpi ulnaris (caput ulnare)
m. flexor digitorum profundus (caput ulnare)
m. flexor carpi ulnaris (caput humerale)
m. flexor digitorum superficialis
n. ulnaris
m. flexor carpi: radialis ulnaris
m. flexor digitorum superficialis: (pars superficialis) covering flexor retinaculum
accessory carpal bone
a.v. mediana
m. flexor digitorum superficialis: pars profunda pars superficialis

m. coracobrachialis
a. v. brachialis
m. biceps brachii
n. medianus
m. brachiocephalicus
v. cephalica
a.v. mediana
n. cutaneus antebrachii medialis (n. musculocutaneus)
a. interossea communis
m. brachialis
m. biceps brachii, lacertus fibrosus
a. transversa cubiti
m. extensor carpi radialis
radius
v. cephalica
v. mediana
a. radialis
v. radialis
m. abductor digiti I longus (insertion on metacarpal III)
n. digitalis dorsalis communis II
m. interosseus (suspensor ligament)

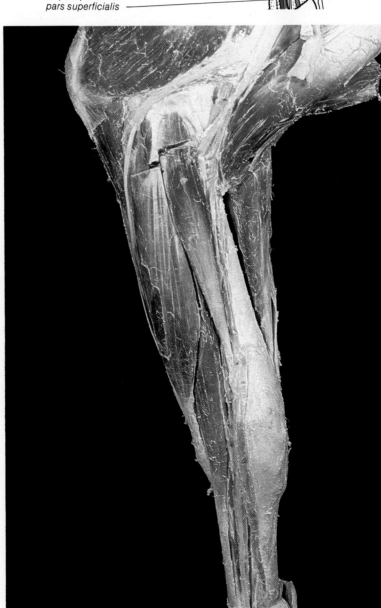

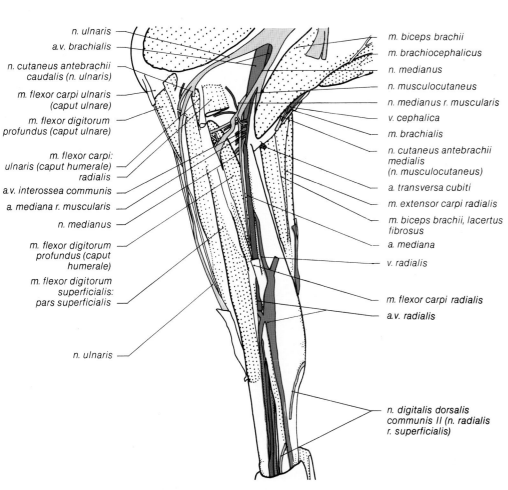

n. ulnaris
a.v. brachialis
n. cutaneus antebrachii caudalis (n. ulnaris)
m. flexor carpi ulnaris (caput ulnare)
m. flexor digitorum profundus (caput ulnare)
m. flexor carpi: ulnaris (caput humerale) radialis
a.v. interossea communis
a. mediana r. muscularis
n. medianus
m. flexor digitorum profundus (caput humerale)
m. flexor digitorum superficialis: pars superficialis
n. ulnaris

m. biceps brachii
m. brachiocephalicus
n. medianus
n. musculocutaneus
n. medianus r. muscularis
v. cephalica
m. brachialis
n. cutaneus antebrachii medialis (n. musculocutaneus)
a. transversa cubiti
m. extensor carpi radialis
m. biceps brachii, lacertus fibrosus
a. mediana
v. radialis
m. flexor carpi radialis
a.v. radialis
n. digitalis dorsalis communis II (n. radialis r. superficialis)

Fig. 3.17 Muscles, vessels and nerves of the antebrachium and carpus, in medial view: (2).

Removal of the humeral origins of the carpal flexors exposes further details of the cubital region and two heads of the deep digital flexor muscle. Further details of this muscle are shown in the third dissection in this series (fig. 3.22).

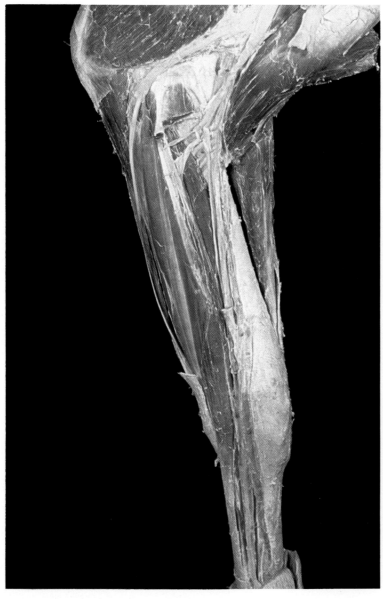

Fig. 3.18 Muscles, vessels and nerves of the carpal and metacarpal regions: (1), dorsal view.

The superficial ramus of the radial nerve was seen at antebrachial level in fig. 3.8. Its medial branch was seen in figs. 3.16, 3.17 and 3.21 and now its dorsal branch is seen as the third common dorsal digital nerve.

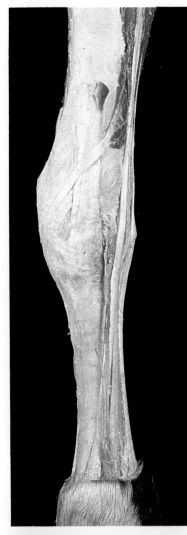

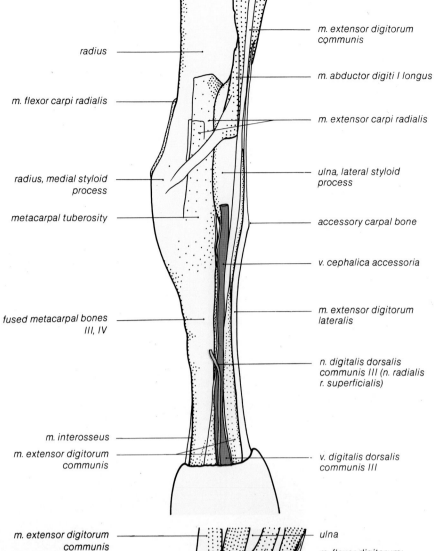

radius

m. flexor carpi radialis

radius, medial styloid process

metacarpal tuberosity

fused metacarpal bones III, IV

m. interosseus
m. extensor digitorum communis

m. extensor digitorum communis

m. abductor digiti I longus

m. extensor carpi radialis

ulna, lateral styloid process

accessory carpal bone

v. cephalica accessoria

m. extensor digitorum lateralis

n. digitalis dorsalis communis III (n. radialis r. superficialis)

v. digitalis dorsalis communis III

Fig. 3.19 Muscles, vessels and nerves of the carpal and metacarpal regions: (2), lateral view.

The origin of the fourth common dorsal digital nerve from the dorsal branch of the ulnar nerve is shown by dotted lines. This origin is clearly revealed in fig. 3.8 but in all subsequent dissections has been removed.

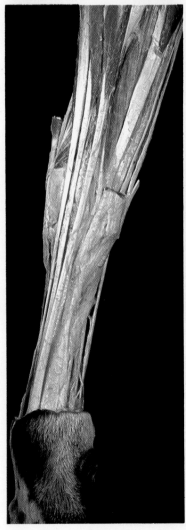

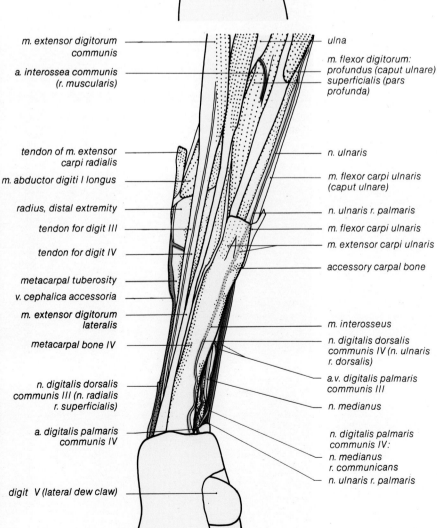

m. extensor digitorum communis

a. interossea communis (r. muscularis)

tendon of m. extensor carpi radialis

m. abductor digiti I longus

radius, distal extremity

tendon for digit III

tendon for digit IV

metacarpal tuberosity

v. cephalica accessoria

m. extensor digitorum lateralis

metacarpal bone IV

n. digitalis dorsalis communis III (n. radialis r. superficialis)

a. digitalis palmaris communis IV

digit V (lateral dew claw)

ulna

m. flexor digitorum: profundus (caput ulnare) superficialis (pars profunda)

n. ulnaris

m. flexor carpi ulnaris (caput ulnare)

n. ulnaris r. palmaris

m. flexor carpi ulnaris

m. extensor carpi ulnaris

accessory carpal bone

m. interosseus

n. digitalis dorsalis communis IV (n. ulnaris r. dorsalis)

a.v. digitalis palmaris communis III

n. medianus

n. digitalis palmaris communis IV: n. medianus r. communicans n. ulnaris r. palmaris

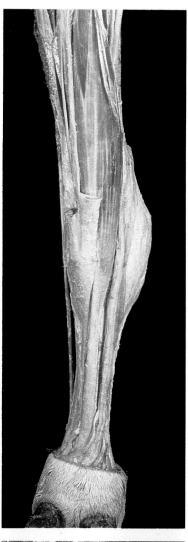

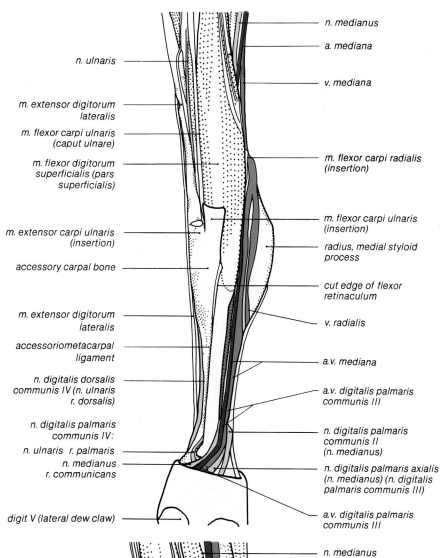

n. ulnaris

m. extensor digitorum
lateralis

m. flexor carpi ulnaris
(caput ulnare)

m. flexor digitorum
superficialis (pars
superficialis)

m. extensor carpi ulnaris
(insertion)

accessory carpal bone

m. extensor digitorum
lateralis

accessoriometacarpal
ligament

n. digitalis dorsalis
communis IV (n. ulnaris
r. dorsalis)

n. digitalis palmaris
communis IV:
n. ulnaris r. palmaris
n. medianus
r. communicans

digit V (lateral dew claw)

n. medianus

a. mediana

v. mediana

m. flexor carpi radialis
(insertion)

m. flexor carpi ulnaris
(insertion)

radius, medial styloid
process

cut edge of flexor
retinaculum

v. radialis

a.v. mediana

a.v. digitalis palmaris
communis III

n. digitalis palmaris
communis II
(n. medianus)

n. digitalis palmaris axialis
(n. medianus) (n. digitalis
palmaris communis III)

a.v. digitalis palmaris
communis III

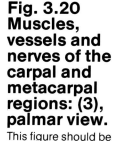

Fig. 3.20 Muscles, vessels and nerves of the carpal and metacarpal regions: (3), palmar view.
This figure should be compared with other views of the dissection, shown in figs. 3.18, 3.19 and 3.21.

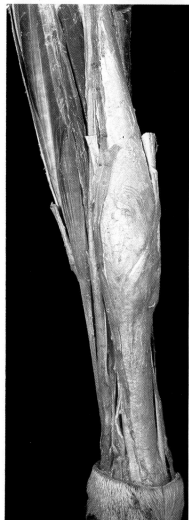

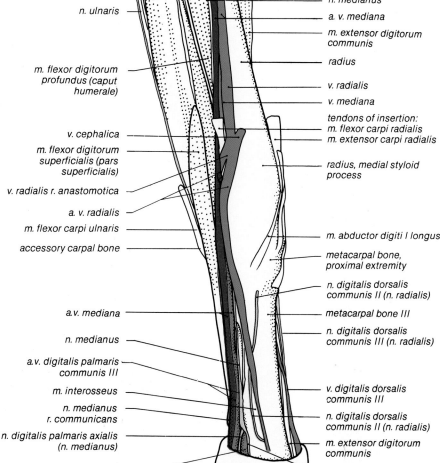

n. ulnaris

m. flexor digitorum
profundus (caput
humerale)

v. cephalica

m. flexor digitorum
superficialis (pars
superficialis)

v. radialis r. anastomotica

a. v. radialis

m. flexor carpi ulnaris

accessory carpal bone

a.v. mediana

n. medianus

a.v. digitalis palmaris
communis III

m. interosseus

n. medianus
r. communicans

n. digitalis palmaris axialis
(n. medianus)

v. digitalis palmaris
communis II

n. medianus

a. v. mediana

m. extensor digitorum
communis

radius

v. radialis

v. mediana

tendons of insertion:
m. flexor carpi radialis
m. extensor carpi radialis

radius, medial styloid
process

m. abductor digiti I longus

metacarpal bone,
proximal extremity

n. digitalis dorsalis
communis II (n. radialis)

metacarpal bone III

n. digitalis dorsalis
communis III (n. radialis)

v. digitalis dorsalis
communis III

n. digitalis dorsalis
communis II (n. radialis)

m. extensor digitorum
communis

n. digitalis palmaris
communis II
(n. medianus)

Fig. 3.21 Muscles, vessels and nerves of the carpal and metacarpal regions: (4), medial view.
The medial branch of the superficial ramus of the radial nerve, (n. cutaneus antebrachii lateralis) seen below carpal level in this dissection, also includes fibres derived from the musculocutaneous nerve (n. cutaneus antebrachii medialis) (see fig. 3.12). Radial and musculocutaneous nerves combine to supply the dorsal aspect of the skin at carpal, metacarpal and digital levels.

Fig. 3.22 Muscles of the antebrachium and carpus, in medial view.

Removal of the superficial part of the superficial digital flexor has exposed the deep part of this muscle and all three heads are now visible. The union between the tendons of superficial and deep parts of the superficial flexor muscle has been cut; it is located just proximal to the fetlock region.

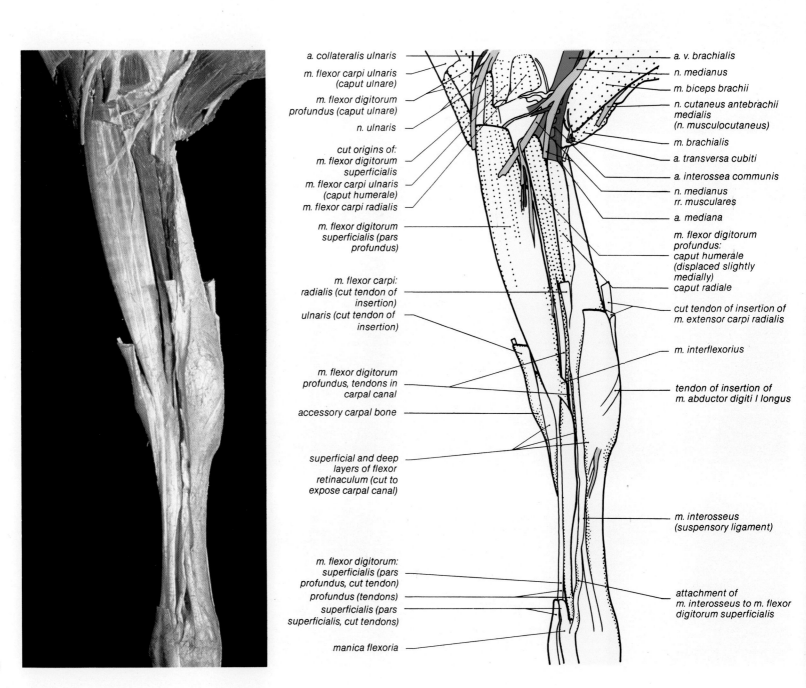

a. collateralis ulnaris

m. flexor carpi ulnaris (caput ulnare)

m. flexor digitorum profundus (caput ulnare)

n. ulnaris

cut origins of:
m. flexor digitorum superficialis
m. flexor carpi ulnaris (caput humerale)
m. flexor carpi radialis

m. flexor digitorum superficialis (pars profundus)

m. flexor carpi:
radialis (cut tendon of insertion)
ulnaris (cut tendon of insertion)

m. flexor digitorum profundus, tendons in carpal canal

accessory carpal bone

superficial and deep layers of flexor retinaculum (cut to expose carpal canal)

m. flexor digitorum:
superficialis (pars profundus, cut tendon)
profundus (tendons)
superficialis (pars superficialis, cut tendons)

manica flexoria

a. v. brachialis

n. medianus

m. biceps brachii

n. cutaneus antebrachii medialis (n. musculocutaneus)

m. brachialis

a. transversa cubiti

a. interossea communis

n. medianus rr. musculares

a. mediana

m. flexor digitorum profundus:
caput humerale (displaced slightly medially)
caput radiale

cut tendon of insertion of m. extensor carpi radialis

m. interflexorius

tendon of insertion of m. abductor digiti I longus

m. interosseus (suspensory ligament)

attachment of m. interosseus to m. flexor digitorum superficialis

Fig. 3.23 Superficial features of the right manus, in dorsal view.

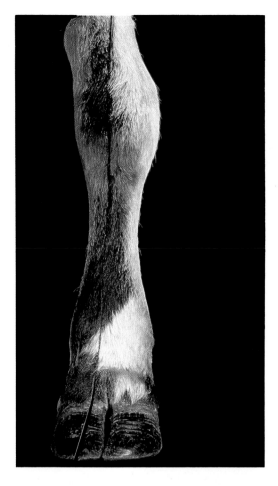

The saw cut used for the sagittal section in fig. 3.24 passes through the axis of the fourth digit and then through the axis of the limb in metacarpal, carpal and antebrachial regions.

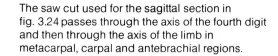

antebrachium

carpus

line of saw cut

metacarpus

fetlock

digit IV

digit III

interdigital cleft

coronet

wall of hoof

Fig. 3.24 Bones and muscles of the right manus seen in sagittal section

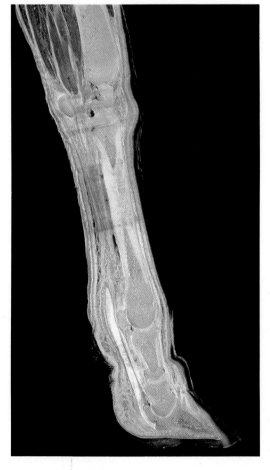

The detailed anatomy of the manus and pes is dealt with in a separate chapter, but this figure is included here to show the insertions of some of the muscles dealt with in the forelimb, and the

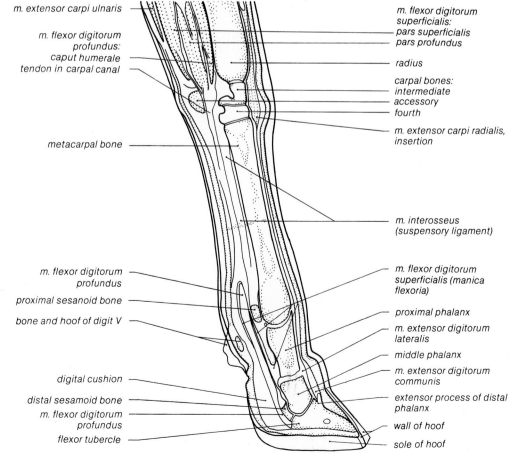

m. extensor carpi ulnaris

m. flexor digitorum profundus:
caput humerale
tendon in carpal canal

metacarpal bone

m. flexor digitorum profundus

proximal sesanoid bone

bone and hoof of digit V

digital cushion

distal sesanoid bone

m. flexor digitorum profundus

flexor tubercle

m. flexor digitorum superficialis:
pars superficialis
pars profundus

radius

carpal bones:
intermediate
accessory
fourth

m. extensor carpi radialis, insertion

m. interosseus (suspensory ligament)

m. flexor digitorum superficialis (manica flexoria)

proximal phalanx

m. extensor digitorum lateralis

middle phalanx

m. extensor digitorum communis

extensor process of distal phalanx

wall of hoof

sole of hoof

3.17

Fig. 3.25 The left axilla and brachial plexus in the 4-month bull calf: medial view.

Earlier stages of this dissection are shown in figs. 4.29-4.34. The left rib cage and the ventral serrate muscle have been removed to display the normal topographical relationships of the axillary structures on the left side in the standing animal.

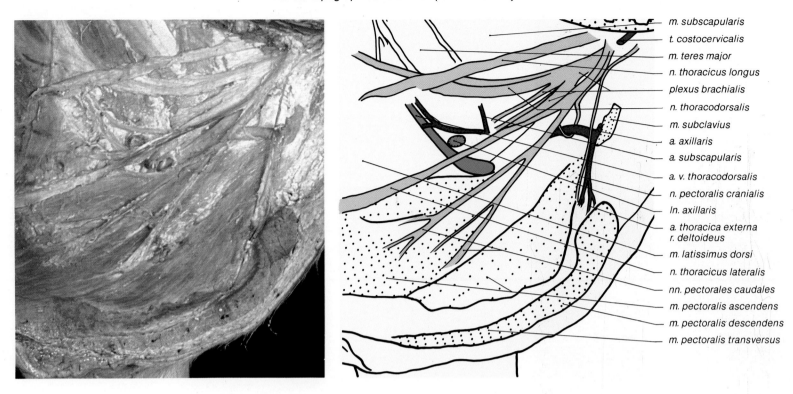

— m. subscapularis
— t. costocervicalis
— m. teres major
— n. thoracicus longus
— plexus brachialis
— n. thoracodorsalis
— m. subclavius
— a. axillaris
— a. subscapularis
— a. v. thoracodorsalis
— n. pectoralis cranialis
— ln. axillaris
— a. thoracica externa
  r. deltoideus
— m. latissimus dorsi
— n. thoracicus lateralis
— nn. pectorales caudales
— m. pectoralis ascendens
— m. pectoralis descendens
— m. pectoralis transversus

Fig. 3.26 The left axilla to show nerves of the forelimb in the calf: medial view.

The nerves supplying the muscles of the synsarcotic union (long thoracic, thoracodorsal and pectoral nerves) have been removed together with the lateral thoracic nerve. Note that the main trunk of the thoracodorsal nerve supplies branches to the teres major (axillary nerve) and subscapular (subscapular nerve) muscles.

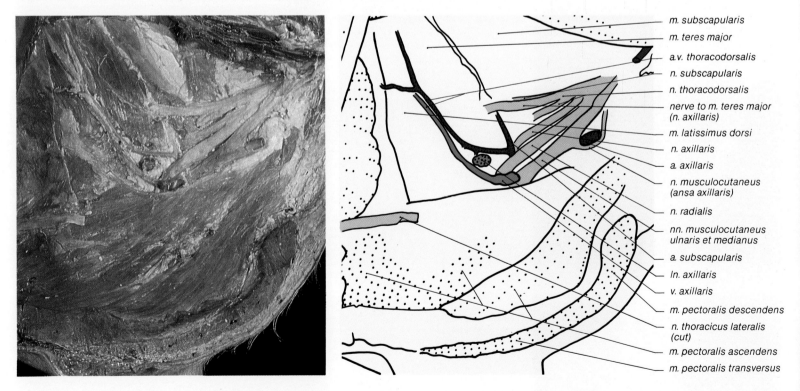

— m. subscapularis
— m. teres major
— a.v. thoracodorsalis
— n. subscapularis
— n. thoracodorsalis
— nerve to m. teres major
  (n. axillaris)
— m. latissimus dorsi
— n. axillaris
— a. axillaris
— n. musculocutaneus
  (ansa axillaris)
— n. radialis
— nn. musculocutaneus
  ulnaris et medianus
— a. subscapularis
— ln. axillaris
— v. axillaris
— m. pectoralis descendens
— n. thoracicus lateralis
  (cut)
— m. pectoralis ascendens
— m. pectoralis transversus

Fig. 3.27 Vascular structures of the axillary and brachial regions in the calf: medial view.

Removal of most of the pectoral muscle mass exposes the medial brachial structures. The muscles and nerves of the region are shown in fig. 3.28. Compare the relationships of the structures in these dissections with those seen in the excised limb (fig. 3.10) where the correct topographical relationships cannot be preserved.

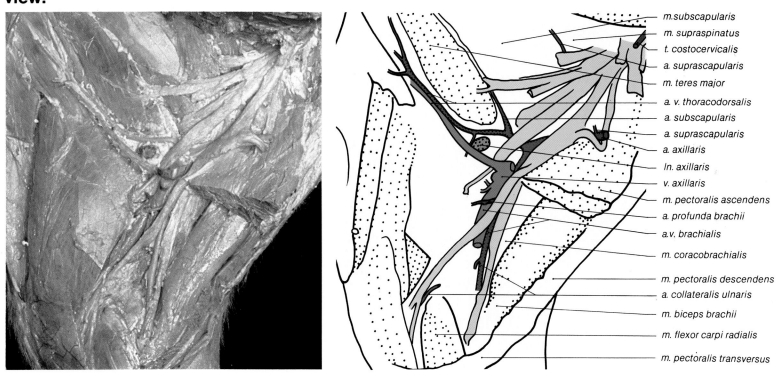

m.subscapularis
m. supraspinatus
t. costocervicalis
a. suprascapularis
m. teres major
a. v. thoracodorsalis
a. subscapularis
a. suprascapularis
a. axillaris
ln. axillaris
v. axillaris
m. pectoralis ascendens
a. profunda brachii
a.v. brachialis
m. coracobrachialis
m. pectoralis descendens
a. collateralis ulnaris
m. biceps brachii
m. flexor carpi radialis
m. pectoralis transversus

Fig. 3.28 Muscles and nerves of the axillary and brachial regions in the calf: medial view.

Removal of the remainder of the ascending pectoral muscle completes the dissection of this region with the limb still attached to the trunk.

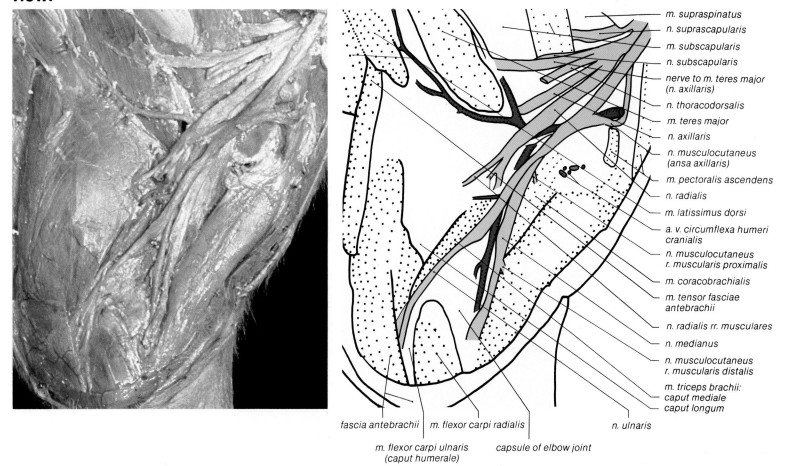

m. supraspinatus
n. suprascapularis
m. subscapularis
n. subscapularis
nerve to m. teres major (n. axillaris)
n. thoracodorsalis
m. teres major
n. axillaris
n. musculocutaneus (ansa axillaris)
m. pectoralis ascendens
n. radialis
m. latissimus dorsi
a. v. circumflexa humeri cranialis
n. musculocutaneus r. muscularis proximalis
m. coracobrachialis
m. tensor fasciae antebrachii
n. radialis rr. musculares
n. medianus
n. musculocutaneus r. muscularis distalis
m. triceps brachii:
caput mediale
caput longum

fascia antebrachii | m. flexor carpi radialis | n. ulnaris

m. flexor carpi ulnaris (caput humerale)   capsule of elbow joint

3.19

4 The Thorax

Fig. 4.1 Surface features of the neck, shoulder and thorax, in left lateral view.

The hair over the palpable surface features was shaved before embalming commenced. The surface projections of the thoracic and cervical vertebrae, cupola of the diaphragm and diaphragmatic line of pleural reflection are based on the dissection shown in fig. 4.15.

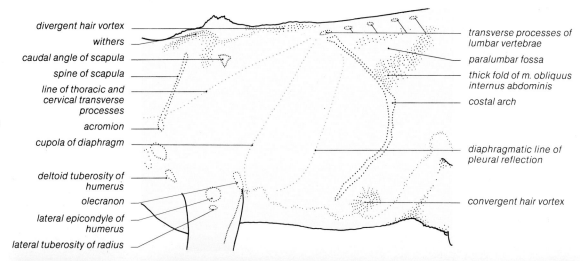

divergent hair vortex
withers
caudal angle of scapula
spine of scapula
line of thoracic and cervical transverse processes
acromion
cupola of diaphragm

deltoid tuberosity of humerus
olecranon
lateral epicondyle of humerus
lateral tuberosity of radius

transverse processes of lumbar vertebrae
paralumbar fossa
thick fold of m. obliquus internus abdominis
costal arch

diaphragmatic line of pleural reflection

convergent hair vortex

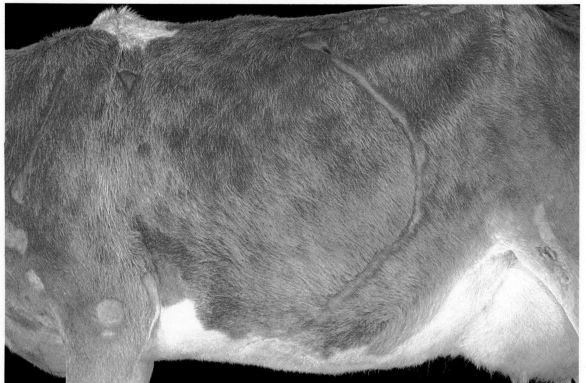

Fig. 4.2 Scapula, humerus, thoracic vertebrae and costal arch.

The palpable features shown in fig. 4.1 are coloured red.

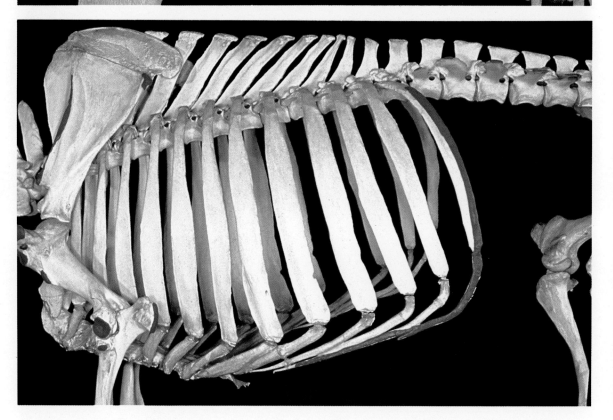

Fig. 4.3 Surface features of the caudal neck and shoulder regions, in left lateral view.

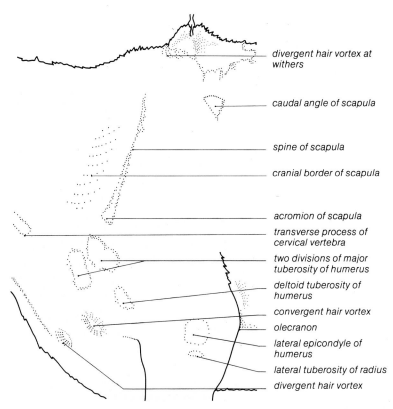

- divergent hair vortex at withers
- caudal angle of scapula
- spine of scapula
- cranial border of scapula
- acromion of scapula
- transverse process of cervical vertebra
- two divisions of major tuberosity of humerus
- deltoid tuberosity of humerus
- convergent hair vortex
- olecranon
- lateral epicondyle of humerus
- lateral tuberosity of radius
- divergent hair vortex

Fig. 4.4 Scapula, humerus and caudal cervical vertebrae.

The palpable features shown in fig. 4.3 are coloured red.

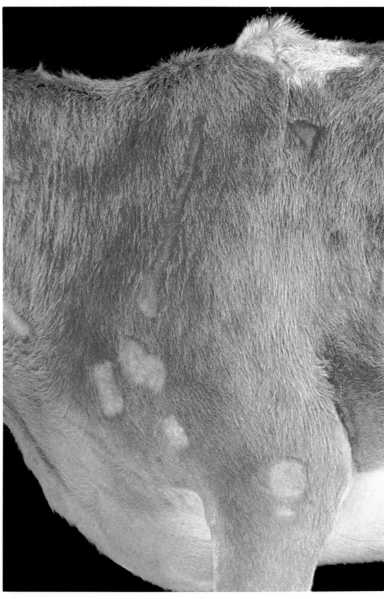

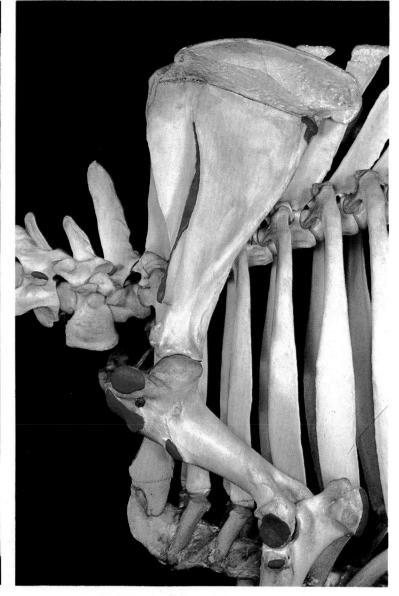

4.3

**Fig. 4.5
Superficial features of the neck, shoulder and thorax, in left lateral view.**

Muscles of the antebrachium are labelled in fig. 4.7.

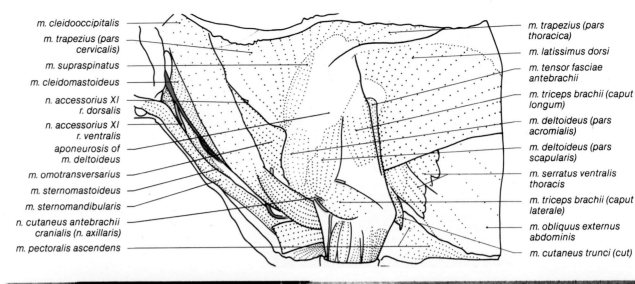

m. cleidooccipitalis

m. trapezius (pars cervicalis)

m. supraspinatus

m. cleidomastoideus

n. accessorius XI r. dorsalis

n. accessorius XI r. ventralis

aponeurosis of m. deltoideus

m. omotransversarius

m. sternomastoideus

m. sternomandibularis

n. cutaneus antebrachii cranialis (n. axillaris)

m. pectoralis ascendens

m. trapezius (pars thoracica)

m. latissimus dorsi

m. tensor fasciae antebrachii

m. triceps brachii (caput longum)

m. deltoideus (pars acromialis)

m. deltoideus (pars scapularis)

m. serratus ventralis thoracis

m. triceps brachii (caput laterale)

m. obliquus externus abdominis

m. cutaneus trunci (cut)

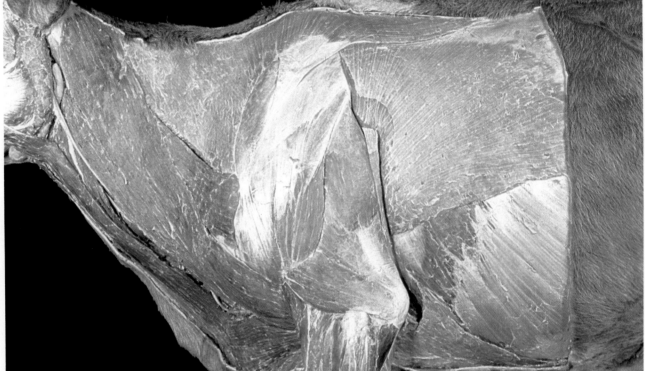

**Fig. 4.6
Muscles of the shoulder and elbow, in left lateral view.**

For further details of the anatomy of the forelimb, Chapter 3 should be consulted.

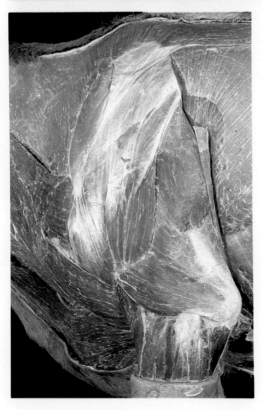

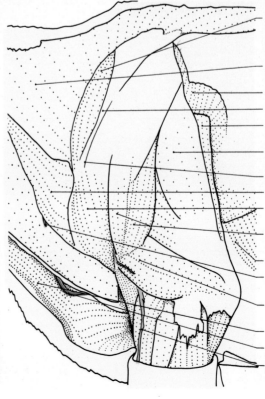

m. supraspinatus (exposed by removal of part of m. trapezius tendon)

m. trapezius (pars cervicalis)

m. latissimus dorsi

spine of scapula

m. tensor fasciae antebrachii

m. triceps brachii (caput longum)

position of acromion

m. omotransversarius

m. deltoideus (pars acromialis)

m. deltoideus (pars scapularis)

m. serratus ventralis

n. supraclavicularis dorsalis (CVI)

m. triceps brachii (caput laterale)

m. sternocephalicus

v. cephalica

n. cutaneus antebrachii lateralis (n. radialis)

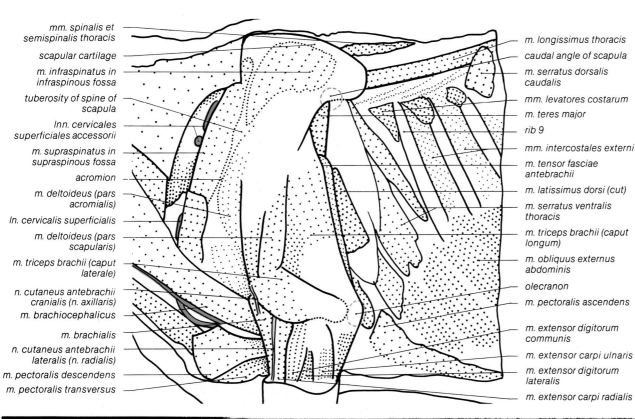

mm. spinalis et semispinalis thoracis
scapular cartilage
m. infraspinatus in infraspinous fossa
tuberosity of spine of scapula
lnn. cervicales superficiales accessorii
m. supraspinatus in supraspinous fossa
acromion
m. deltoideus (pars acromialis)
ln. cervicalis superficialis
m. deltoideus (pars scapularis)
m. triceps brachii (caput laterale)
n. cutaneus antebrachii cranialis (n. axillaris)
m. brachiocephalicus
m. brachialis
n. cutaneus antebrachii lateralis (n. radialis)
m. pectoralis descendens
m. pectoralis transversus

m. longissimus thoracis
caudal angle of scapula
m. serratus dorsalis caudalis
mm. levatores costarum
m. teres major
rib 9
mm. intercostales externi
m. tensor fasciae antebrachii
m. latissimus dorsi (cut)
m. serratus ventralis thoracis
m. triceps brachii (caput longum)
m. obliquus externus abdominis
olecranon
m. pectoralis ascendens
m. extensor digitorum communis
m. extensor carpi ulnaris
m. extensor digitorum lateralis
m. extensor carpi radialis

Fig. 4.7 The left thoracic wall after removal of the latissimus dorsi muscle.

The caudal border of the triceps muscle is the cranial limit of the area of auscultation and percussion.

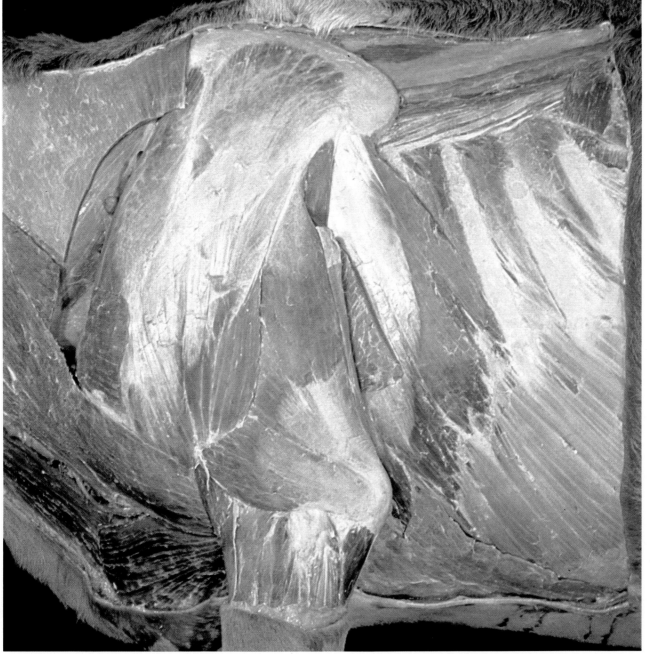

4.5

Fig. 4.8 The caudal neck and shoulder region in craniolateral view.

The axillary vessels have been displaced to reveal the lymph node more clearly. The rostral dissection of the neck is shown in fig. 2.5.

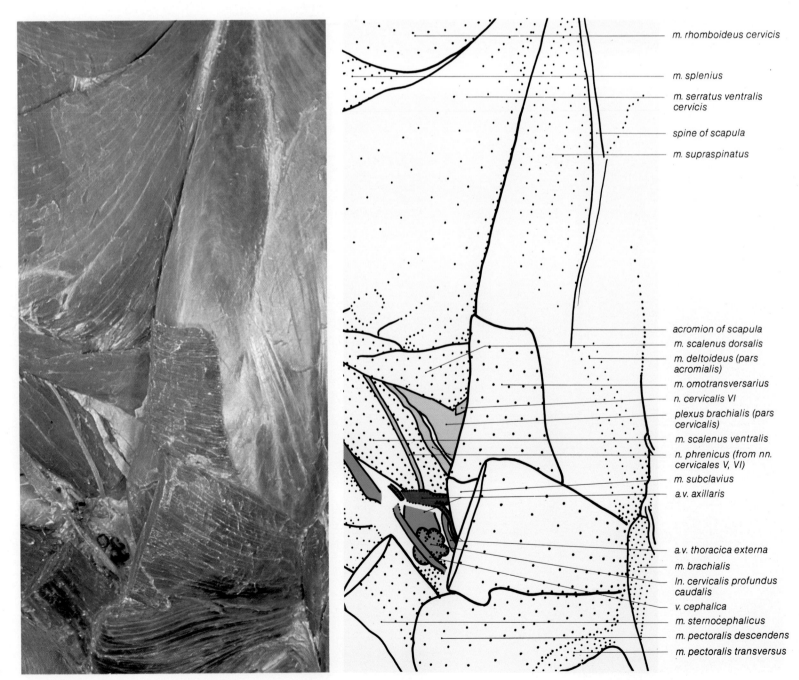

m. rhomboideus cervicis

m. splenius

m. serratus ventralis cervicis

spine of scapula

m. supraspinatus

acromion of scapula

m. scalenus dorsalis

m. deltoideus (pars acromialis)

m. omotransversarius

n. cervicalis VI

plexus brachialis (pars cervicalis)

m. scalenus ventralis

n. phrenicus (from nn. cervicales V, VI)

m. subclavius

a.v. axillaris

a.v. thoracica externa

m. brachialis

ln. cervicalis profundus caudalis

v. cephalica

m. sternocephalicus

m. pectoralis descendens

m. pectoralis transversus

Fig. 4.9 The long thoracic and lateral thoracic nerves.

The right forelimb has been removed with a part of the ventral serrate muscle. This figure has been laterally reversed to facilitate comparison with fig. 4.8.

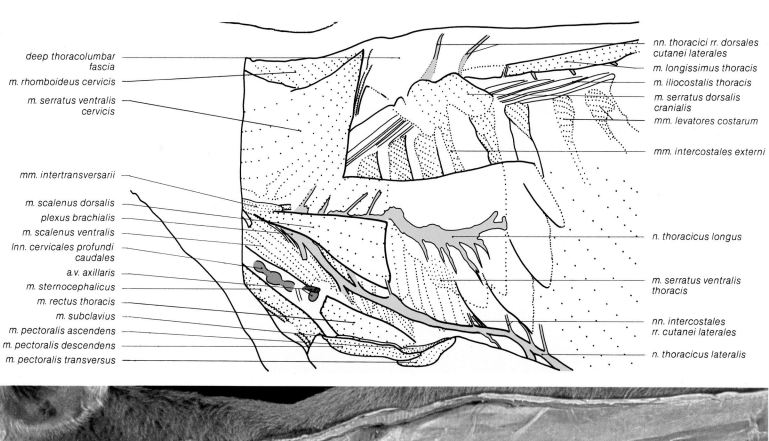

deep thoracolumbar fascia

m. rhomboideus cervicis

m. serratus ventralis cervicis

mm. intertransversarii

m. scalenus dorsalis

plexus brachialis

m. scalenus ventralis

lnn. cervicales profundi caudales

a.v. axillaris

m. sternocephalicus

m. rectus thoracis

m. subclavius

m. pectoralis ascendens

m. pectoralis descendens

m. pectoralis transversus

nn. thoracici rr. dorsales cutanei laterales

m. longissimus thoracis

m. iliocostalis thoracis

m. serratus dorsalis cranialis

mm. levatores costarum

mm. intercostales externi

n. thoracicus longus

m. serratus ventralis thoracis

nn. intercostales rr. cutanei laterales

n. thoracicus lateralis

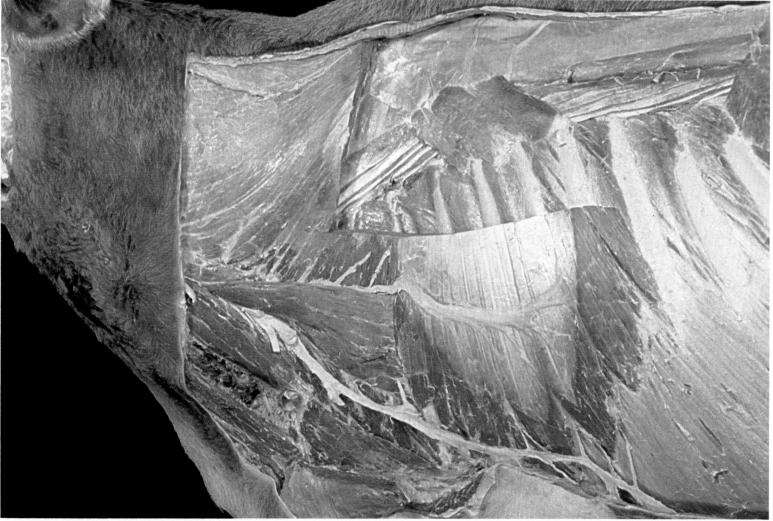

Fig. 4.10 The rib cage and muscles of the left thoracic wall.

The left forelimb has been removed.

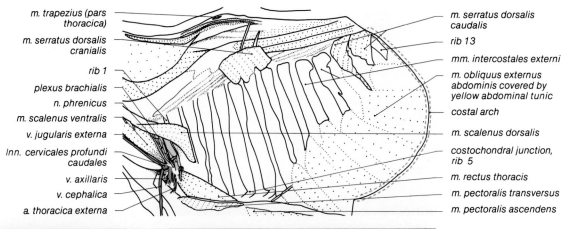

m. trapezius (pars thoracica)
m. serratus dorsalis cranialis
rib 1
plexus brachialis
n. phrenicus
m. scalenus ventralis
v. jugularis externa
lnn. cervicales profundi caudales
v. axillaris
v. cephalica
a. thoracica externa

m. serratus dorsalis caudalis
rib 13
mm. intercostales externi
m. obliquus externus abdominis covered by yellow abdominal tunic
costal arch
m. scalenus dorsalis
costochondral junction, rib 5
m. rectus thoracis
m. pectoralis transversus
m. pectoralis ascendens

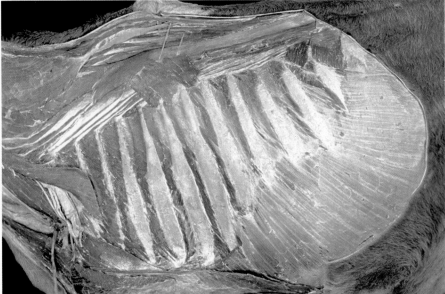

Fig. 4.11 The left lung *in situ.*

The intercostal muscles, pleura and endothoracic fascia of the intercostal spaces have been removed.

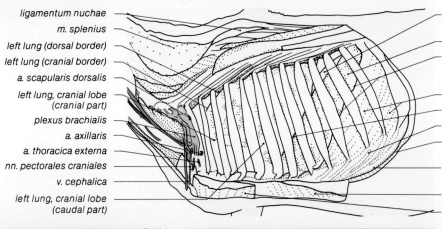

ligamentum nuchae
m. splenius
left lung (dorsal border)
left lung (cranial border)
a. scapularis dorsalis
left lung, cranial lobe (cranial part)
plexus brachialis
a. axillaris
a. thoracica externa
nn. pectorales craniales
v. cephalica
left lung, cranial lobe (caudal part)

diaphragm (central tendon)
diaphragm (costal part)
mm. intercostales cut away along diaphragmatic line of pleural reflection
mm. intercostales interni
left lung (caudal border)
costal cartilage, rib 11
m. obliquus externus abdominis
m. transversus abdominis
m. pectoralis ascendens
m. pectoralis transversus

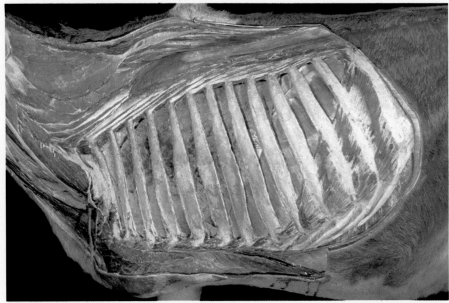

Fig. 4.12 Topography of the left lung and forelimb.

The dissected left forelimb, which was removed in fig. 4.10 has been replaced to show the relationships between thoracic and appendicular structures (see also fig. 4.11). This figure shows the restricted region available in the standing animal for pulmonary auscultation and percussion.

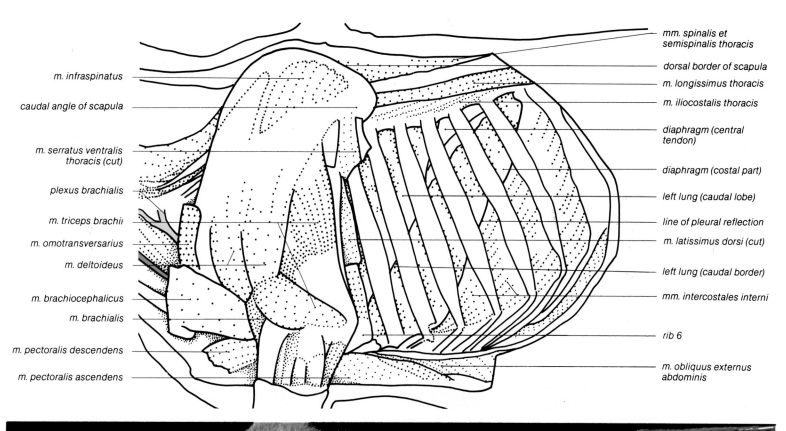

m. infraspinatus

caudal angle of scapula

m. serratus ventralis thoracis (cut)

plexus brachialis

m. triceps brachii

m. omotransversarius

m. deltoideus

m. brachiocephalicus

m. brachialis

m. pectoralis descendens

m. pectoralis ascendens

mm. spinalis et semispinalis thoracis

dorsal border of scapula

m. longissimus thoracis

m. iliocostalis thoracis

diaphragm (central tendon)

diaphragm (costal part)

left lung (caudal lobe)

line of pleural reflection

m. latissimus dorsi (cut)

left lung (caudal border)

mm. intercostales interni

rib 6

m. obliquus externus abdominis

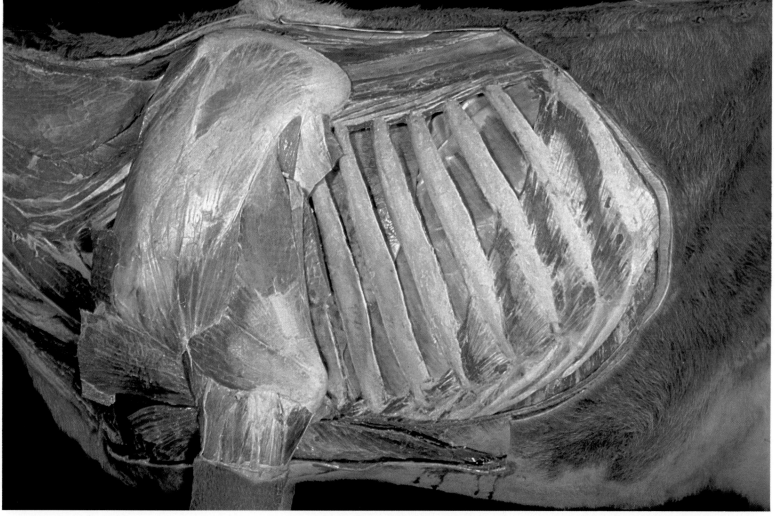

Fig. 4.13 Thoracic viscera *in situ*, **in left lateral view.**

The ribs have been removed close to their costochondral junctions except for three important "marker" ribs (1, 3 and 6) and those parts that do not enclose the left pleural cavity.

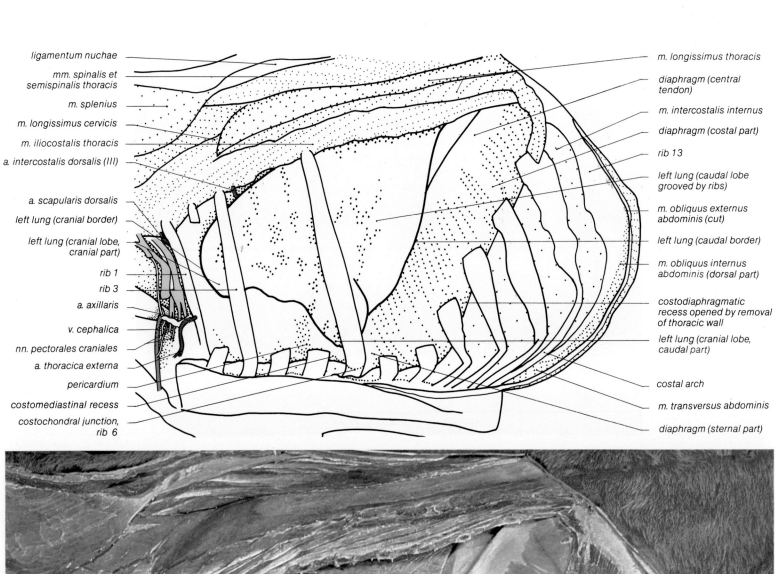

ligamentum nuchae

mm. spinalis et semispinalis thoracis

m. splenius

m. longissimus cervicis

m. iliocostalis thoracis

a. intercostalis dorsalis (III)

a. scapularis dorsalis

left lung (cranial border)

left lung (cranial lobe, cranial part)

rib 1

rib 3

a. axillaris

v. cephalica

nn. pectorales craniales

a. thoracica externa

pericardium

costomediastinal recess

costochondral junction, rib 6

m. longissimus thoracis

diaphragm (central tendon)

m. intercostalis internus

diaphragm (costal part)

rib 13

left lung (caudal lobe grooved by ribs)

m. obliquus externus abdominis (cut)

left lung (caudal border)

m. obliquus internus abdominis (dorsal part)

costodiaphragmatic recess opened by removal of thoracic wall

left lung (cranial lobe, caudal part)

costal arch

m. transversus abdominis

diaphragm (sternal part)

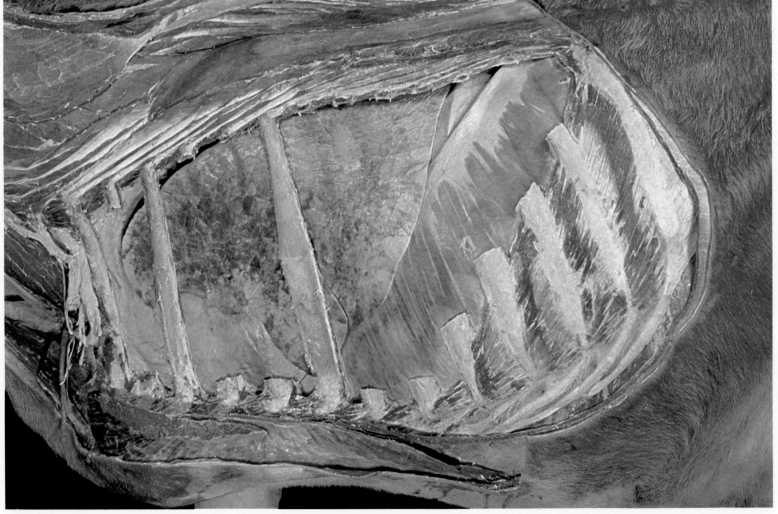

Fig. 4.14 The left lung; lobation, lobulation and topography.

Removal of ribs 1, 3 and 6 shows the lung and the cranial mediastinum more clearly.

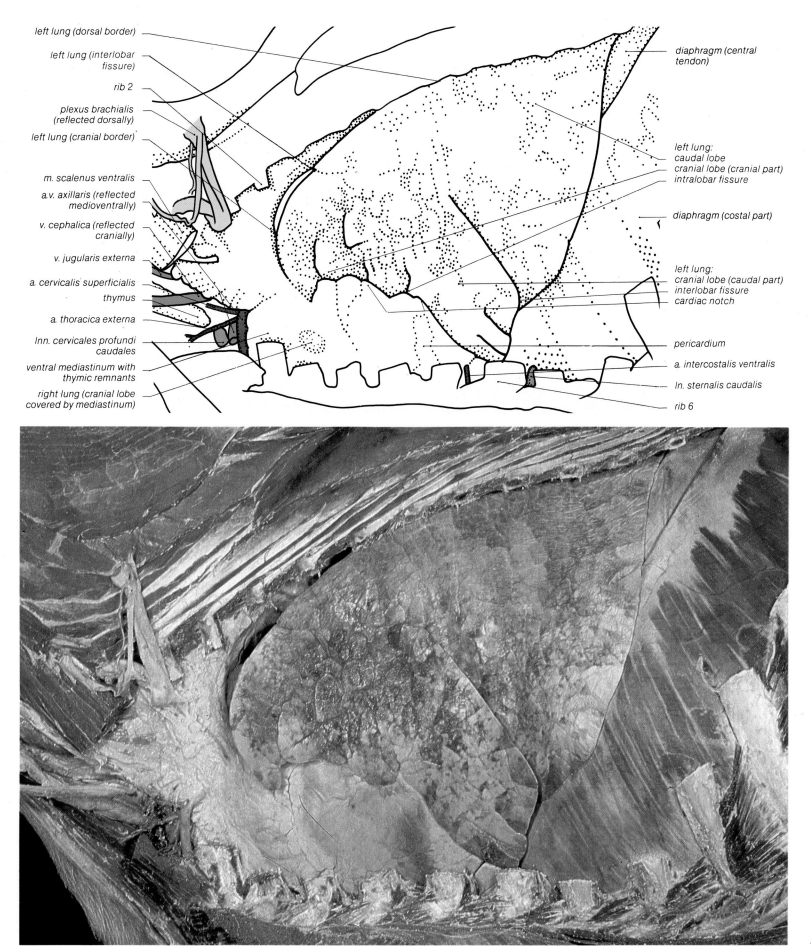

left lung (dorsal border)

left lung (interlobar fissure)

rib 2

plexus brachialis (reflected dorsally)

left lung (cranial border)

m. scalenus ventralis

a.v. axillaris (reflected medioventrally)

v. cephalica (reflected cranially)

v. jugularis externa

a. cervicalis superficialis

thymus

a. thoracica externa

lnn. cervicales profundi caudales

ventral mediastinum with thymic remnants

right lung (cranial lobe covered by mediastinum)

diaphragm (central tendon)

left lung:
caudal lobe
cranial lobe (cranial part)
intralobar fissure

diaphragm (costal part)

left lung:
cranial lobe (caudal part)
interlobar fissure
cardiac notch

pericardium

a. intercostalis ventralis

ln. sternalis caudalis

rib 6

Fig. 4.15 Thoracic structures after removal of the left lung.

For further details of the structures found in the left side of the mediastinum figs. 4.16, 4.19 and 4.20 should be consulted. The phrenic nerve has been displaced in figs. 4.15 – 4.17 and 4.19; its true course is shown by the dotted lines in these figures, and by the dissections shown in figs. 4.29 and 4.30.

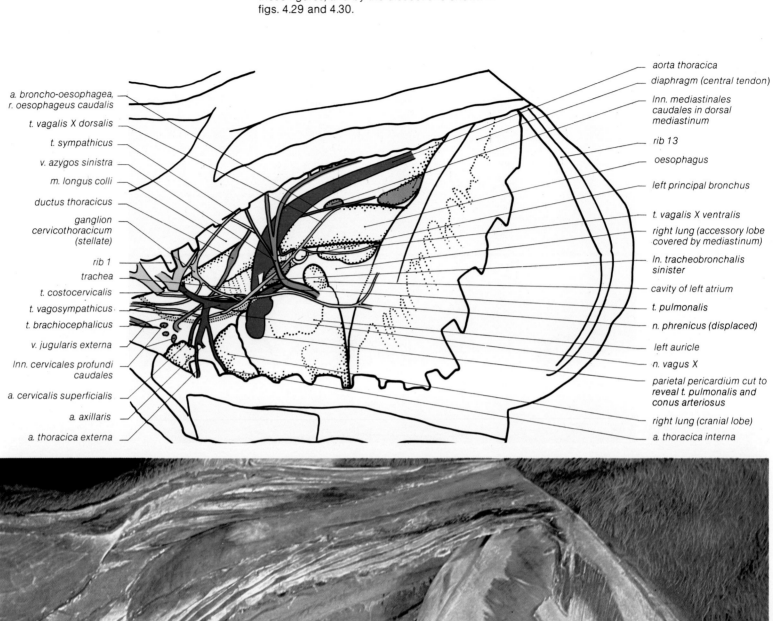

a. broncho-oesophagea, r. oesophageus caudalis

t. vagalis X dorsalis

t. sympathicus

v. azygos sinistra

m. longus colli

ductus thoracicus

ganglion cervicothoracicum (stellate)

rib 1

trachea

t. costocervicalis

t. vagosympathicus

t. brachiocephalicus

v. jugularis externa

lnn. cervicales profundi caudales

a. cervicalis superficialis

a. axillaris

a. thoracica externa

aorta thoracica

diaphragm (central tendon)

lnn. mediastinales caudales in dorsal mediastinum

rib 13

oesophagus

left principal bronchus

t. vagalis X ventralis

right lung (accessory lobe covered by mediastinum)

ln. tracheobronchalis sinister

cavity of left atrium

t. pulmonalis

n. phrenicus (displaced)

left auricle

n. vagus X

parietal pericardium cut to reveal t. pulmonalis and conus arteriosus

right lung (cranial lobe)

a. thoracica interna

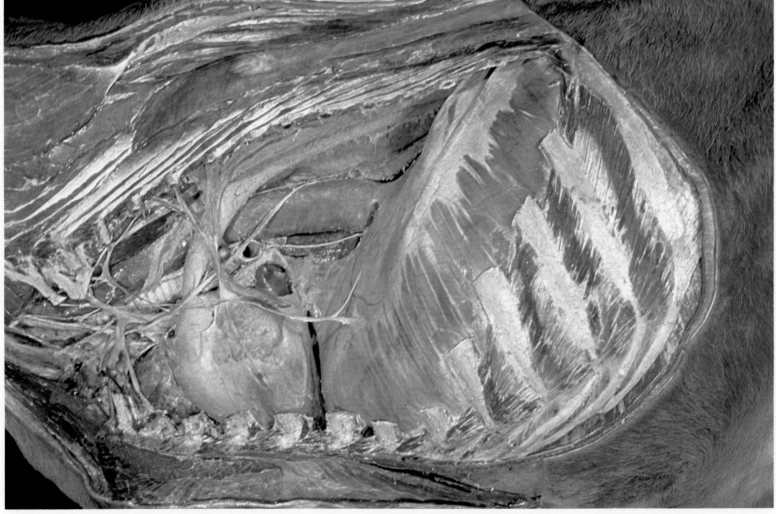

Fig. 4.16 Thoracic vessels, nerves and lymph nodes, in left lateral view.

The phrenic nerve is displaced but its true course is shown by the dotted lines.

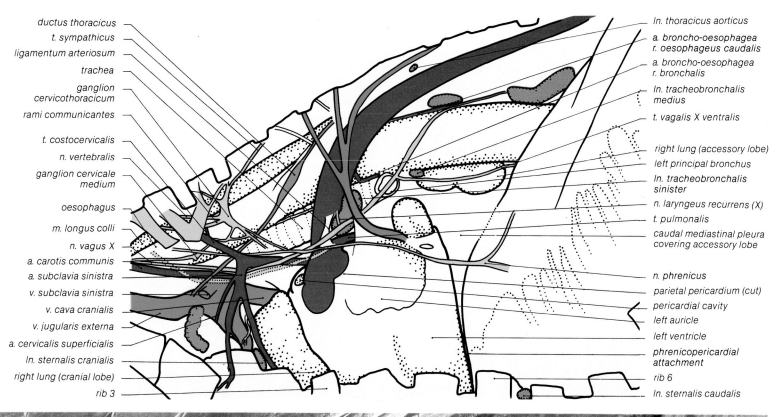

ductus thoracicus
t. sympathicus
ligamentum arteriosum
trachea
ganglion cervicothoracicum
rami communicantes
t. costocervicalis
n. vertebralis
ganglion cervicale medium
oesophagus
m. longus colli
n. vagus X
a. carotis communis
a. subclavia sinistra
v. subclavia sinistra
v. cava cranialis
v. jugularis externa
a. cervicalis superficialis
ln. sternalis cranialis
right lung (cranial lobe)
rib 3

ln. thoracicus aorticus
a. broncho-oesophagea r. oesophageus caudalis
a. broncho-oesophagea r. bronchalis
ln. tracheobronchalis medius
t. vagalis X ventralis
right lung (accessory lobe)
left principal bronchus
ln. tracheobronchalis sinister
n. laryngeus recurrens (X)
t. pulmonalis
caudal mediastinal pleura covering accessory lobe
n. phrenicus
parietal pericardium (cut)
pericardial cavity
left auricle
left ventricle
phrenicopericardial attachment
rib 6
ln. sternalis caudalis

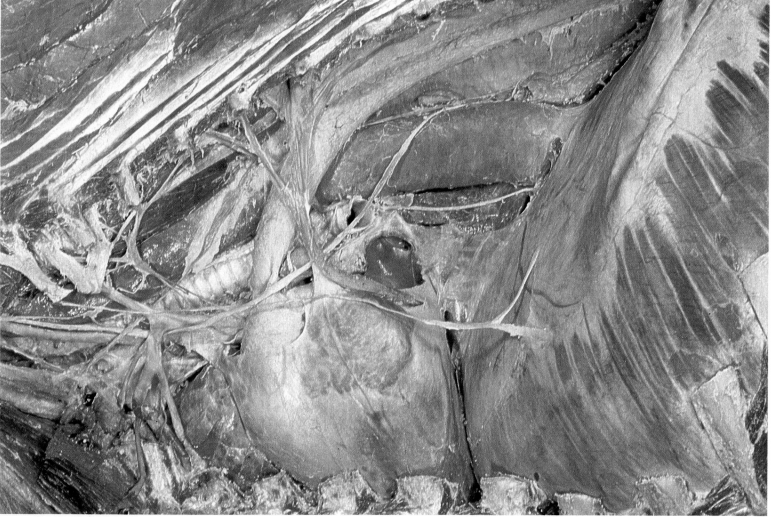

Fig. 4.17 The heart: topography in left lateral view.

Ribs 1, 3 and 6, which were removed in fig. 4.14, have been replaced to show their relationships to the dissected structures of the thorax. The true course of the phrenic nerve is shown by the dotted lines.

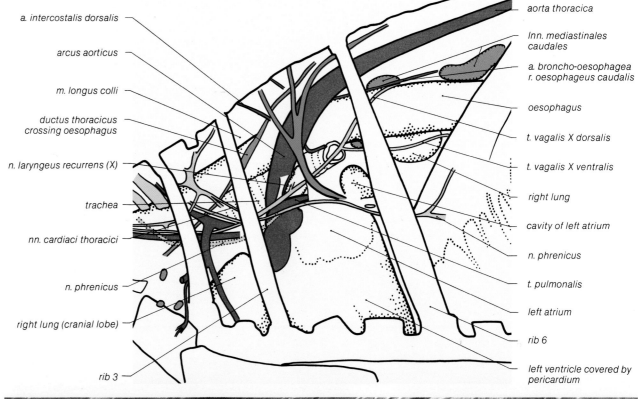

a. intercostalis dorsalis

arcus aorticus

m. longus colli

ductus thoracicus crossing oesophagus

n. laryngeus recurrens (X)

trachea

nn. cardiaci thoracici

n. phrenicus

right lung (cranial lobe)

rib 3

aorta thoracica

lnn. mediastinales caudales

a. broncho-oesophagea r. oesophageus caudalis

oesophagus

t. vagalis X dorsalis

t. vagalis X ventralis

right lung

cavity of left atrium

n. phrenicus

t. pulmonalis

left atrium

rib 6

left ventricle covered by pericardium

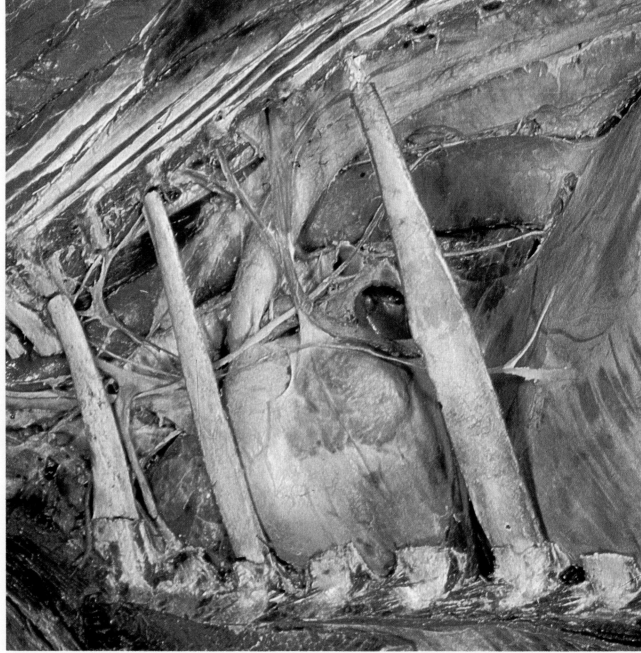

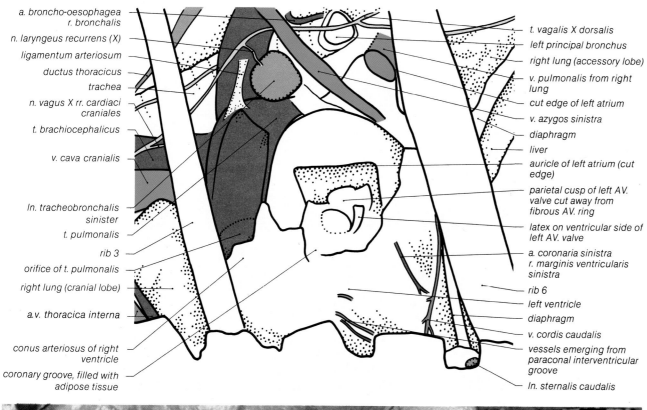

a. broncho-oesophagea r. bronchialis
n. laryngeus recurrens (X)
ligamentum arteriosum
ductus thoracicus
trachea
n. vagus X rr. cardiaci craniales
t. brachiocephalicus
v. cava cranialis
ln. tracheobronchalis sinister
t. pulmonalis
rib 3
orifice of t. pulmonalis
right lung (cranial lobe)
a.v. thoracica interna
conus arteriosus of right ventricle
coronary groove, filled with adipose tissue

t. vagalis X dorsalis
left principal bronchus
right lung (accessory lobe)
v. pulmonalis from right lung
cut edge of left atrium
v. azygos sinistra
diaphragm
liver
auricle of left atrium (cut edge)
parietal cusp of left AV. valve cut away from fibrous AV. ring
latex on ventricular side of left AV. valve
a. coronaria sinistra r. marginis ventricularis sinistra
rib 6
left ventricle
diaphragm
v. cordis caudalis
vessels emerging from paraconal interventricular groove
ln. sternalis caudalis

Fig. 4.18 The positions of the left atrioventricular and pulmonary heart valves.

Red latex, injected into the common carotid artery, has filled the left ventricle but not the left atrium. The pulmonary valve is just visible at the orifice of the pulmonary trunk.

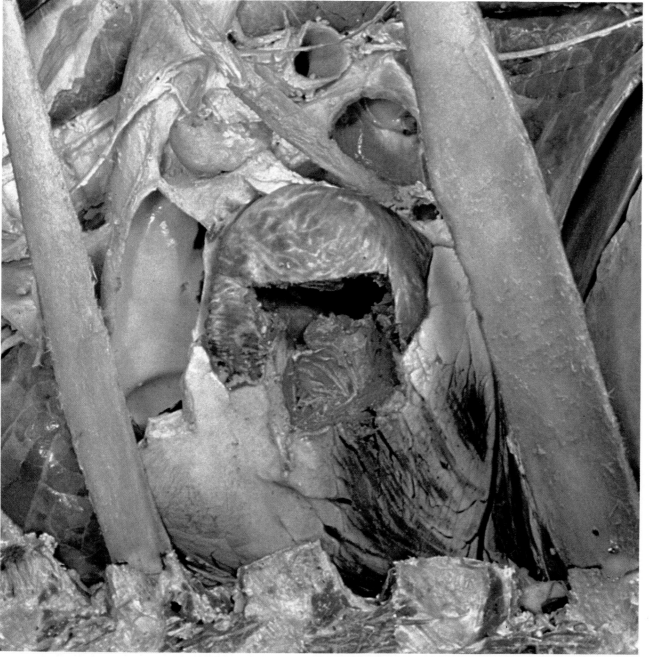

Fig. 4.19 The vessels and nerves of the cranial mediastinum.

This is a closer view of the dissection shown in fig. 4.16. The true course of the phrenic nerve is shown by the dotted lines.

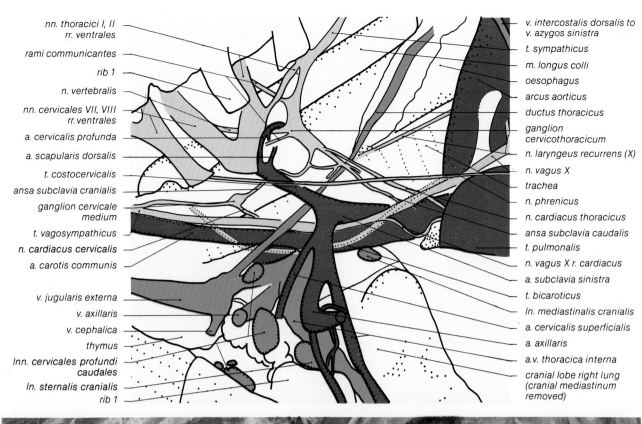

nn. thoracici I, II rr. ventrales
rami communicantes
rib 1
n. vertebralis
nn. cervicales VII, VIII rr. ventrales
a. cervicalis profunda
a. scapularis dorsalis
t. costocervicalis
ansa subclavia cranialis
ganglion cervicale medium
t. vagosympathicus
n. cardiacus cervicalis
a. carotis communis
v. jugularis externa
v. axillaris
v. cephalica
thymus
lnn. cervicales profundi caudales
ln. sternalis cranialis
rib 1

v. intercostalis dorsalis to v. azygos sinistra
t. sympathicus
m. longus colli
oesophagus
arcus aorticus
ductus thoracicus
ganglion cervicothoracicum
n. laryngeus recurrens (X)
n. vagus X
trachea
n. phrenicus
n. cardiacus thoracicus
ansa subclavia caudalis
t. pulmonalis
n. vagus X r. cardiacus
a. subclavia sinistra
t. bicaroticus
ln. mediastinalis cranialis
a. cervicalis superficialis
a. axillaris
a.v. thoracica interna
cranial lobe right lung (cranial mediastinum removed)

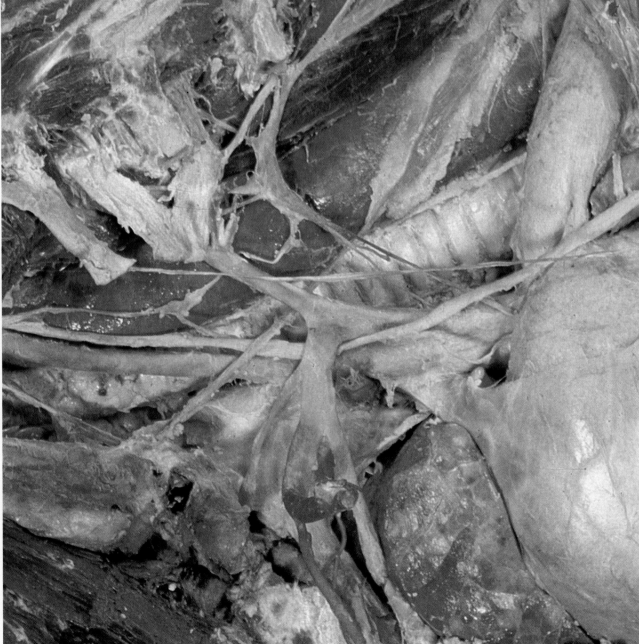

Fig. 4.20 The dorsal part of the caudal mediastinum.

This is a closer view of the dissection shown in fig. 4.16.

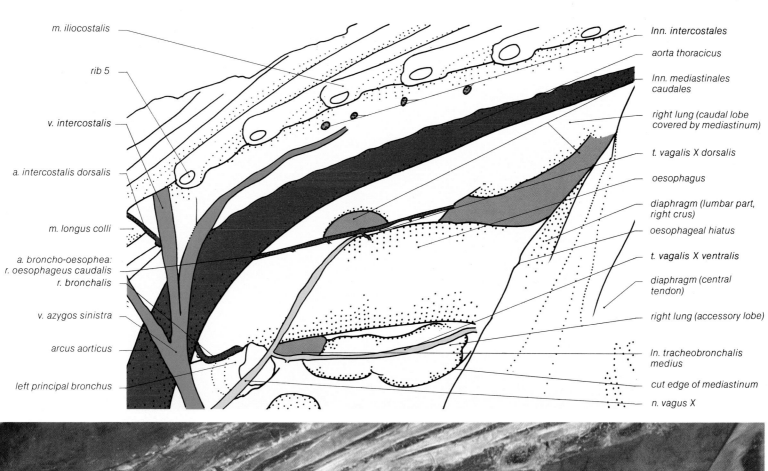

m. iliocostalis

rib 5

v. intercostalis

a. intercostalis dorsalis

m. longus colli

a. broncho-oesophea:
r. oesophageus caudalis
r. bronchalis

v. azygos sinistra

arcus aorticus

left principal bronchus

lnn. intercostales

aorta thoracicus

lnn. mediastinales caudales

right lung (caudal lobe covered by mediastinum)

t. vagalis X dorsalis

oesophagus

diaphragm (lumbar part, right crus)

oesophageal hiatus

t. vagalis X ventralis

diaphragm (central tendon)

right lung (accessory lobe)

ln. tracheobronchalis medius

cut edge of mediastinum

n. vagus X

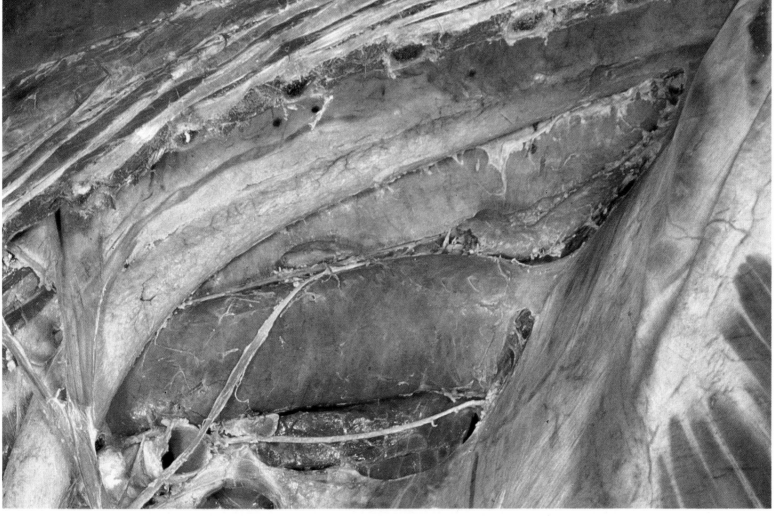

Fig. 4.21 The rib cage with the right lung in situ: right lateral view.

This dissection of the right side corresponds with that of the left shown in fig. 4.11.

mm. spinalis et semispinalis thoracis
m. longissimus thoracis et lumborum
m. iliocostalis thoracis
nn. thoracici rr. cutanei laterales dorsales
diaphragm
diaphragmatic line of pleural reflection
right lung (caudal lobe)
mm. intercostales interni
right lung (caudal part of cranial lobe)
right lung (middle lobe)

m. rhomboideus
m. splenius
a. cervicalis profunda
dorsal border of right lung
a. scapularis dorsalis
m. scalenus dorsalis
plexus brachialis
m. scalenus ventralis
right lung (cranial part of cranial lobe)
rib 1
right lung (cardiac notch)
a. axillaris
m. rectus thoracis

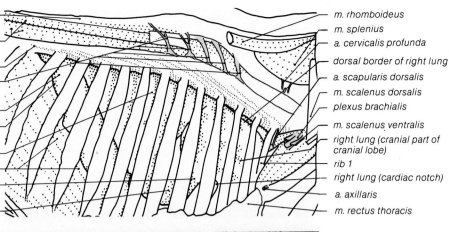

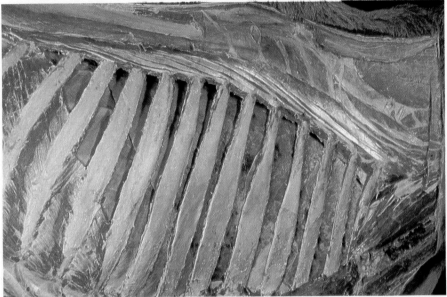

Fig. 4.22 Right lung: lobation, lobulation and topography.

This dissection of the right side corresponds with that of the left shown in fig. 4.13.

right lung (cranial lobe, caudal part)
interlobar fissures
right lung (caudal lobe)
diaphragm (central tendon)
diaphragm (costal part)
diaphragmatic line of pleural reflection
intralobar fissure
cardiac notch of right lung
right lung (middle lobe)
pericardium
rib 6

m. rhomboideus
m. splenius
m. iliocostalis thoracis
right lung (dorsal border)
right lung, cranial lobe (cranial part)
a. scapularis dorsalis
m. scalenus ventralis
rib 1
a. axillaris
rib 3

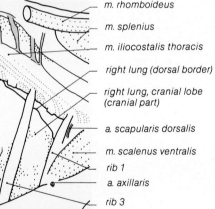

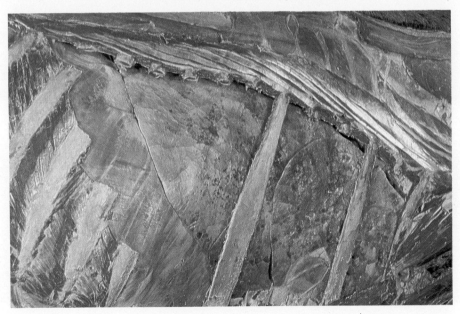

Fig. 4.23 The right side of the mediastinum after removal of the right lung

The right azygos vein is not always present in the ruminants. The mediastinum has not yet been dissected, but it has suffered some damage to the dorsocaudal part, which is very thin, during dissection to the left side.

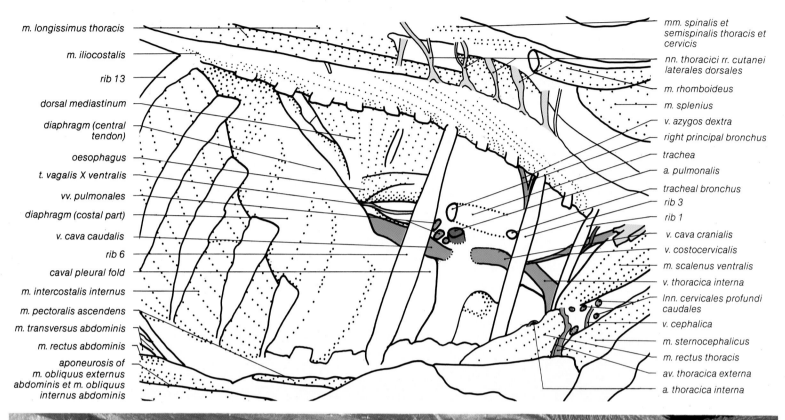

m. longissimus thoracis

m. iliocostalis

rib 13

dorsal mediastinum

diaphragm (central tendon)

oesophagus

t. vagalis X ventralis

vv. pulmonales

diaphragm (costal part)

v. cava caudalis

rib 6

caval pleural fold

m. intercostalis internus

m. pectoralis ascendens

m. transversus abdominis

m. rectus abdominis

aponeurosis of m. obliquus externus abdominis et m. obliquus internus abdominis

mm. spinalis et semispinalis thoracis et cervicis

nn. thoracici rr. cutanei laterales dorsales

m. rhomboideus

m. splenius

v. azygos dextra

right principal bronchus

trachea

a. pulmonalis

tracheal bronchus

rib 3

rib 1

v. cava cranialis

v. costocervicalis

m. scalenus ventralis

v. thoracica interna

lnn. cervicales profundi caudales

v. cephalica

m. sternocephalicus

m. rectus thoracis

av. thoracica externa

a. thoracica interna

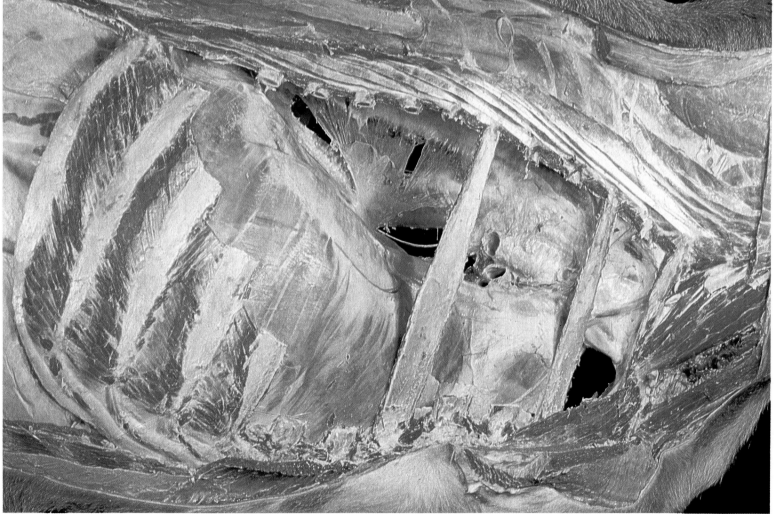

**Fig. 4.24
Thoracic
structures
after removal
of the right
lung: right
lateral view.**

This dissection of the
right side corresponds
with that of the left side
shown in fig. 4.17.

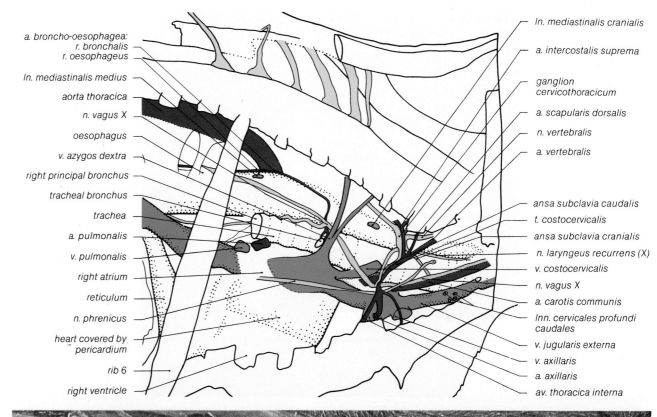

a. broncho-oesophagea:
r. bronchialis
r. oesophageus

ln. mediastinalis medius

aorta thoracica

n. vagus X

oesophagus

v. azygos dextra

right principal bronchus

tracheal bronchus

trachea

a. pulmonalis

v. pulmonalis

right atrium

reticulum

n. phrenicus

heart covered by
pericardium

rib 6

right ventricle

ln. mediastinalis cranialis

a. intercostalis suprema

ganglion
cervicothoracicum

a. scapularis dorsalis

n. vertebralis

a. vertebralis

ansa subclavia caudalis

t. costocervicalis

ansa subclavia cranialis

n. laryngeus recurrens (X)

v. costocervicalis

n. vagus X

a. carotis communis

lnn. cervicales profundi
caudales

v. jugularis externa

v. axillaris

a. axillaris

av. thoracica interna

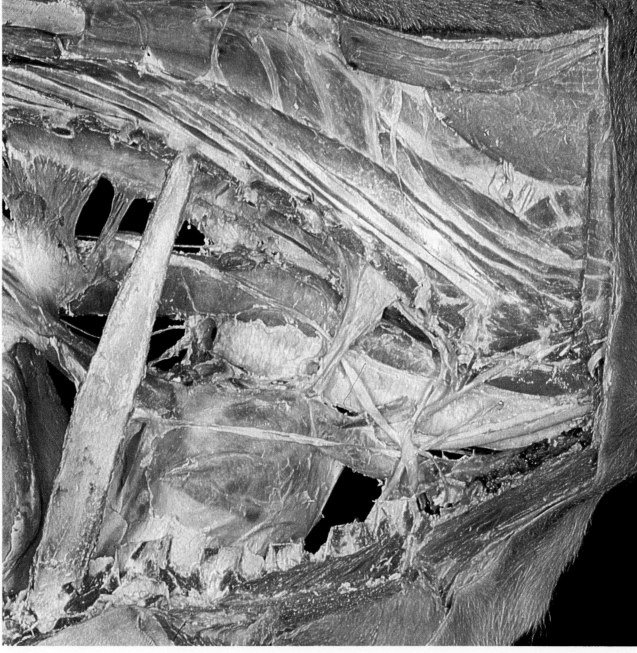

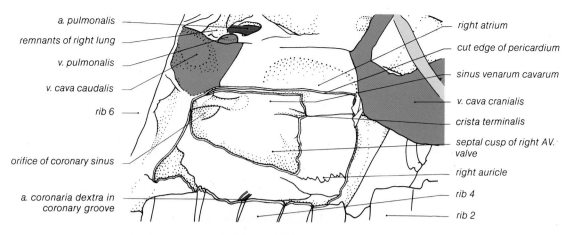

a. pulmonalis
remnants of right lung
v. pulmonalis
v. cava caudalis
rib 6
orifice of coronary sinus
a. coronaria dextra in coronary groove

right atrium
cut edge of pericardium
sinus venarum cavarum
v. cava cranialis
crista terminalis
septal cusp of right AV. valve
right auricle
rib 4
rib 2

Fig. 4.25 The cavity of the right atrium.

The lateral wall of the atrium has been removed, but the general topography of this part of the thorax can be seen in fig. 4.24.

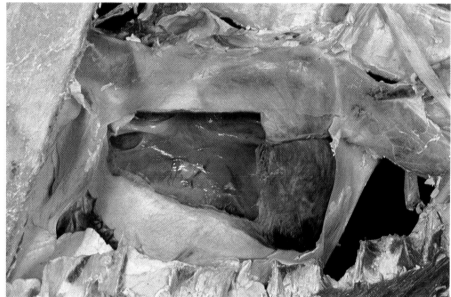

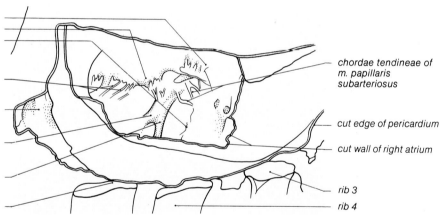

cusps of right AV valve:
angular
septal
parietal

chordae tendineae of mm. papillares parvi
pericardial cavity
m. papillaris subarteriosus
trabecula septomarginalis
rib 5

chordae tendineae of m. papillaris subarteriosus
cut edge of pericardium
cut wall of right atrium
rib 3
rib 4

Fig. 4.26 The right atrioventricular valve.

This is a dorsolateral view of the dissection shown in fig. 4.25. The parietal cusp and its associated great papillary muscle arise from the outer wall of the ventricle and are therefore not visible in either figure.

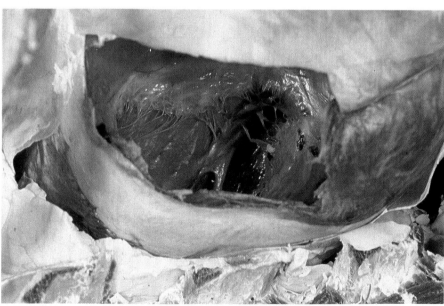

Fig. 4.27 The diaphragmatic line of pleural reflection in the calf: left lateral view.

Compare this figure with fig. 4.28.

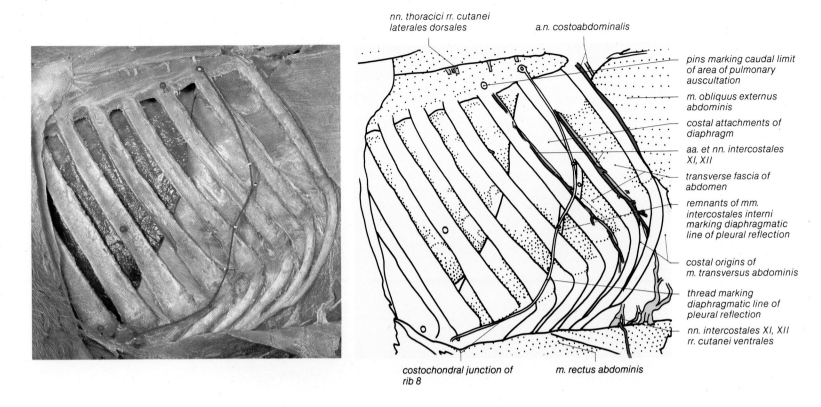

nn. thoracici rr. cutanei laterales dorsales

a.n. costoabdominalis

pins marking caudal limit of area of pulmonary auscultation

m. obliquus externus abdominis

costal attachments of diaphragm

aa. et nn. intercostales XI, XII

transverse fascia of abdomen

remnants of mm. intercostales interni marking diaphragmatic line of pleural reflection

costal origins of m. transversus abdominis

thread marking diaphragmatic line of pleural reflection

nn. intercostales XI, XII rr. cutanei ventrales

costochondral junction of rib 8

m. rectus abdominis

Fig. 4.28 The diaphragmatic line of pleural reflection in the calf: right lateral view.

In this and the preceding figure the diaphragmatic lines of pleural reflection were carefully defined; note the differences between left and right sides in this individual.

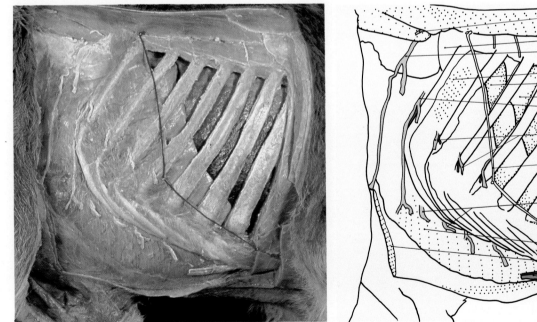
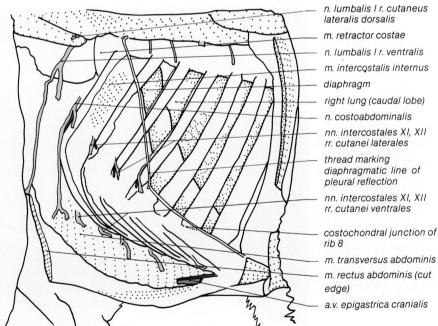

n. lumbalis I r. cutaneus lateralis dorsalis

m. retractor costae

n. lumbalis I r. ventralis

m. intercostalis internus

diaphragm

right lung (caudal lobe)

n. costoabdominalis

nn. intercostales XI, XII rr. cutanei laterales

thread marking diaphragmatic line of pleural reflection

nn. intercostales XI, XII rr. cutanei ventrales

costochondral junction of rib 8

m. transversus abdominis

m. rectus abdominis (cut edge)

a.v. epigastrica cranialis

Fig.4.29 The thoracic surface of the diaphragm of the calf; oblique craniolateral view.

Figs. 4.29 – 4.34 show a series of dissections in which the left thoracic wall was removed to provide a medial view of the axilla. The dissections of the forelimb in this series are shown in figs. 3.26–3.29.

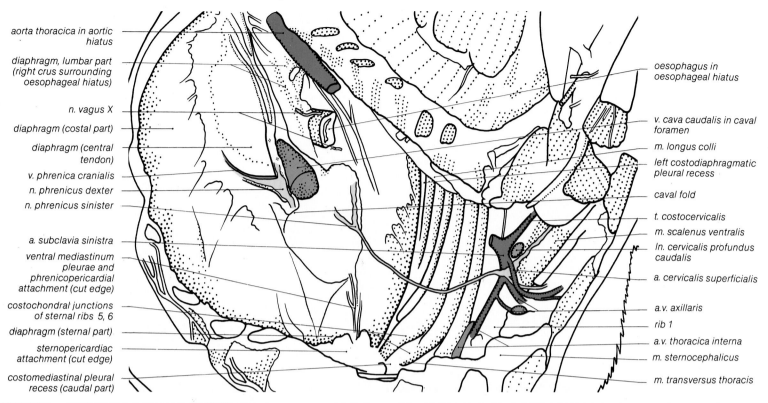

aorta thoracica in aortic hiatus

diaphragm, lumbar part (right crus surrounding oesophageal hiatus)

n. vagus X

diaphragm (costal part)

diaphragm (central tendon)

v. phrenica cranialis

n. phrenicus dexter

n. phrenicus sinister

a. subclavia sinistra

ventral mediastinum pleurae and phrenicopericardial attachment (cut edge)

costochondral junctions of sternal ribs 5, 6

diaphragm (sternal part)

sternopericardiac attachment (cut edge)

costomediastinal pleural recess (caudal part)

oesophagus in oesophageal hiatus

v. cava caudalis in caval foramen

m. longus colli

left costodiaphragmatic pleural recess

caval fold

t. costocervicalis

m. scalenus ventralis

ln. cervicalis profundus caudalis

a. cervicalis superficialis

a.v. axillaris

rib 1

a.v. thoracica interna

m. sternocephalicus

m. transversus thoracis

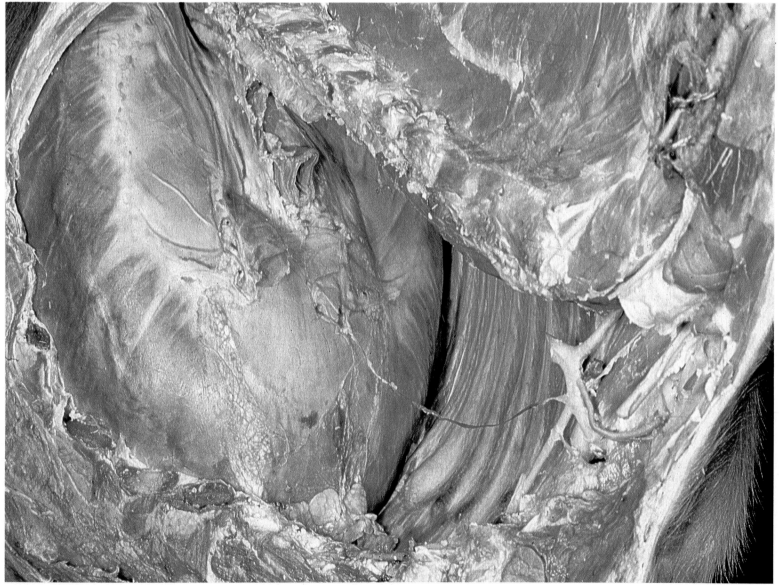

Fig. 4.30 The thoracic wall of the calf, in medial view (1).

In this figure, the pleura and endothoracic fascia are shown lining the thoracic wall. The course of the phrenic nerve is topographically correct (compare with fig. 4.15 et seq.)

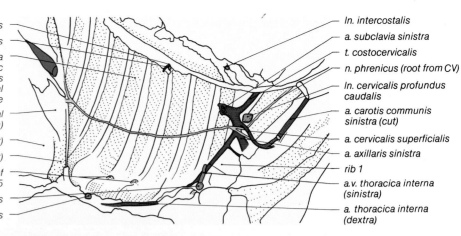

a. intercostalis dorsalis
ln. thoracicus aorticus
parietal (costal) pleura covering endothoracic fascia and m. intercostalis internus of 5th intercostal space
diaphragm (central tendon)
diaphragm (costal part)
diaphragm (sternal part)
costochondral junctions of ribs 4 and 5
ln. sternalis cranialis
ln. sternalis caudalis

ln. intercostalis
a. subclavia sinistra
t. costocervicalis
n. phrenicus (root from CV)
ln. cervicalis profundus caudalis
a. carotis communis sinistra (cut)
a. cervicalis superficialis
a. axillaris sinistra
rib 1
a.v. thoracica interna (sinistra)
a. thoracica interna (dextra)

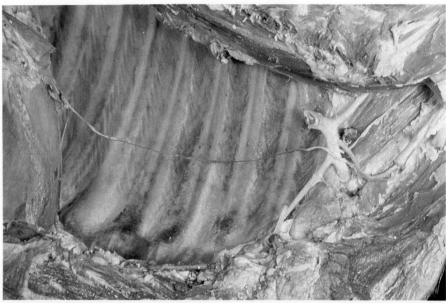

Fig. 4.31 The thoracic wall of the calf, in medial view (2).

Removal of fascial and muscular layers from some intercostal spaces reveals the structures of the thoracic wall. The external intercostal muscle is shown in the first intercostal space. The internal intercostal muscle is shown in the second space, and both muscles have been removed from the fourth space.

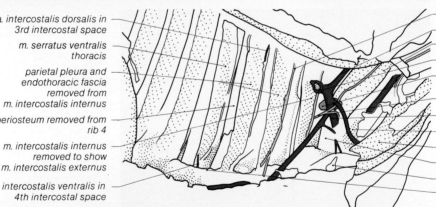

a. intercostalis dorsalis in 3rd intercostal space
m. serratus ventralis thoracis
parietal pleura and endothoracic fascia removed from m. intercostalis internus
periosteum removed from rib 4
m. intercostalis internus removed to show m. intercostalis externus
a. intercostalis ventralis in 4th intercostal space

n. intercostalis (Th.II)
t. costocervicalis
m. scalenus ventralis
a. subclavia sinistra
ln. cervicalis profundus caudalis
n. phrenicus (cut)
a. axillaris
m. subclavius
m. sternothyrohyoideus
rib 1
manubrium of sternum
cut edge of endothoracic fascia, parietal pleura and m. transversus thoracis

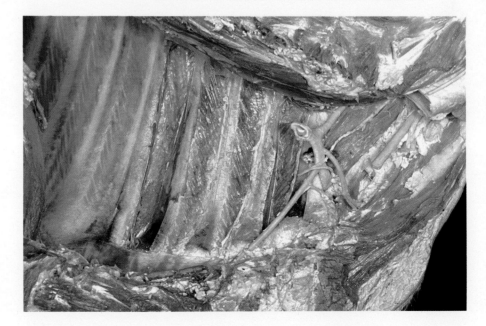

Fig. 4.32 Structures of the axilla of the calf, in medial view.

The left thoracic wall and the ventral serrate muscle have been removed to show the contents of the axilla.

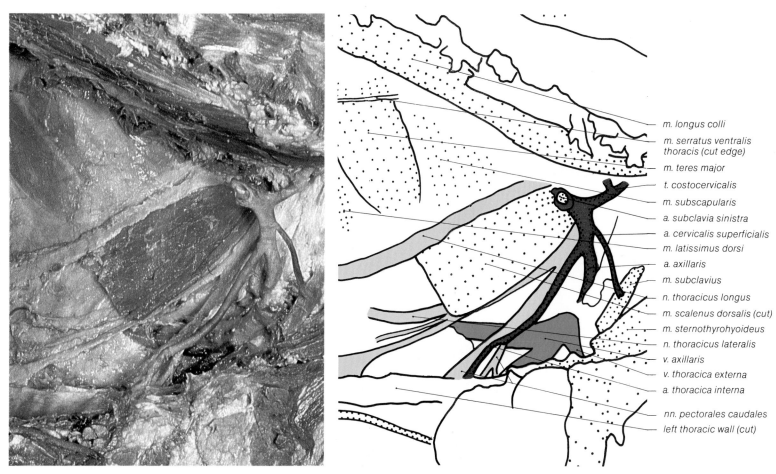

m. longus colli
m. serratus ventralis thoracis (cut edge)
m. teres major
t. costocervicalis
m. subscapularis
a. subclavia sinistra
a. cervicalis superficialis
m. latissimus dorsi
a. axillaris
m. subclavius
n. thoracicus longus
m. scalenus dorsalis (cut)
m. sternothyrohyoideus
n. thoracicus lateralis
v. axillaris
v. thoracica externa
a. thoracica interna
nn. pectorales caudales
left thoracic wall (cut)

Fig. 4.33 Nerves of the thoracic wall and brachial plexus in the calf: medial view.

The removal of the dorsal scalenus muscle exposes the nerves of the brachial plexus. Further dissections of the forelimb are shown in Chapter 3 (figs. 3.26 – 3.29).

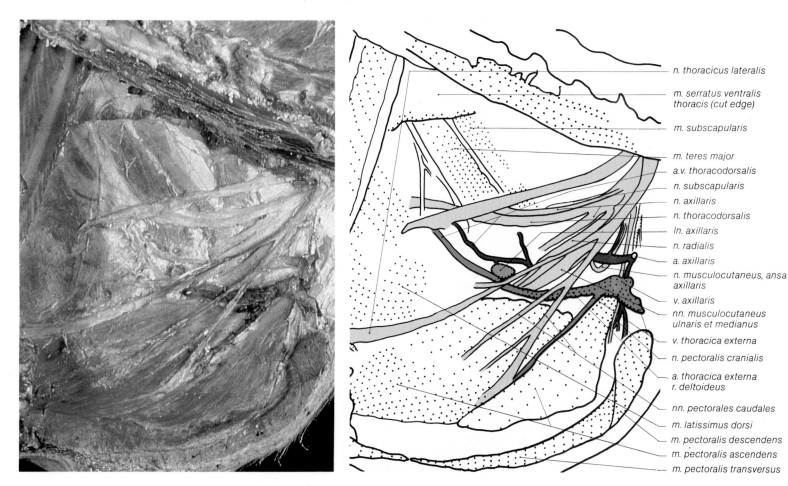

n. thoracicus lateralis
m. serratus ventralis thoracis (cut edge)
m. subscapularis
m. teres major
a.v. thoracodorsalis
n. subscapularis
n. axillaris
n. thoracodorsalis
ln. axillaris
n. radialis
a. axillaris
n. musculocutaneus, ansa axillaris
v. axillaris
nn. musculocutaneus ulnaris et medianus
v. thoracica externa
n. pectoralis cranialis
a. thoracica externa
r. deltoideus
nn. pectorales caudales
m. latissimus dorsi
m. pectoralis descendens
m. pectoralis ascendens
m. pectoralis transversus

4.25

Fig.4.34 The thoracic surface of the diaphragm of the calf: cranial view.

Removal of both left and right sides of the thorax shows the costal and sternal attachments of the diaphragm, and permits a full cranial view of the diaphragm.

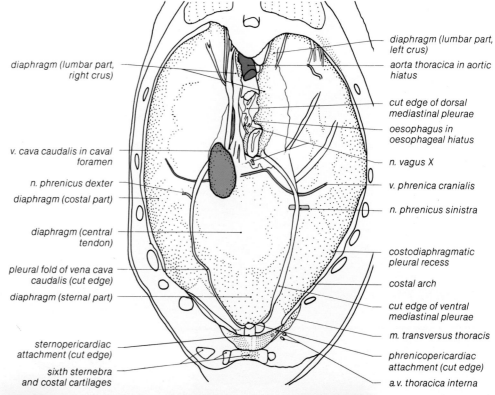

diaphragm (lumbar part, right crus)

v. cava caudalis in caval foramen

n. phrenicus dexter

diaphragm (costal part)

diaphragm (central tendon)

pleural fold of vena cava caudalis (cut edge)

diaphragm (sternal part)

sternopericardiac attachment (cut edge)

sixth sternebra and costal cartilages

diaphragm (lumbar part, left crus)

aorta thoracica in aortic hiatus

cut edge of dorsal mediastinal pleurae

oesophagus in oesophageal hiatus

n. vagus X

v. phrenica cranialis

n. phrenicus sinistra

costodiaphragmatic pleural recess

costal arch

cut edge of ventral mediastinal pleurae

m. transversus thoracis

phrenicopericardiac attachment (cut edge)

a.v. thoracica interna

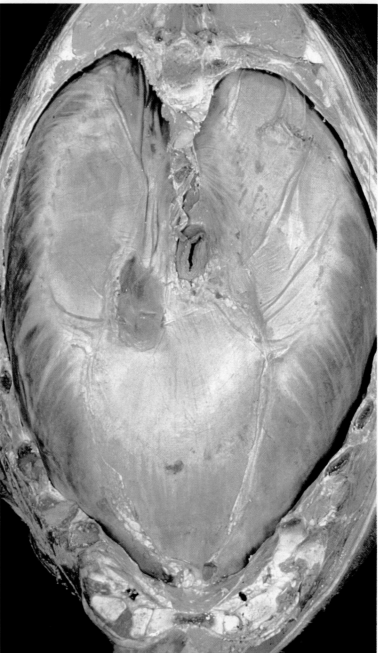

5 The Abdomen

**Fig.5.1
Surface
features of
the
abdomen, in
left lateral
view.**
The palpable bony
prominences have
been shaved.

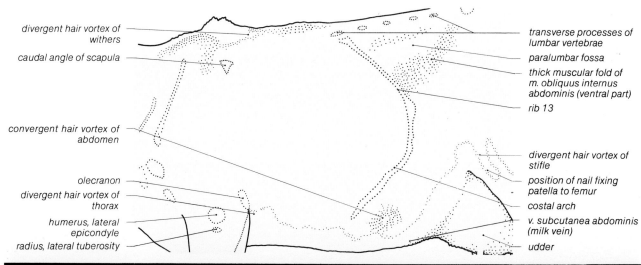

divergent hair vortex of
withers

caudal angle of scapula

convergent hair vortex of
abdomen

olecranon

divergent hair vortex of
thorax

humerus, lateral
epicondyle

radius, lateral tuberosity

transverse processes of
lumbar vertebrae

paralumbar fossa

thick muscular fold of
m. obliquus internus
abdominis (ventral part)

rib 13

divergent hair vortex of
stifle

position of nail fixing
patella to femur

costal arch

v. subcutanea abdominis
(milk vein)

udder

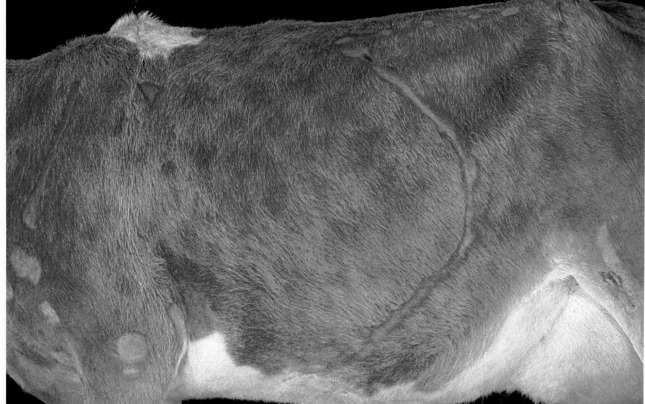

**Fig.5.2
Bones
related to the
abdomen, in
left lateral
view.**
The palpable bony
prominences shown in
fig. 5.1 are coloured
red.

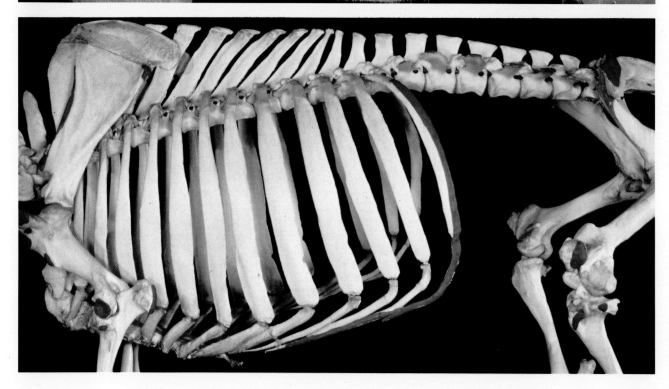

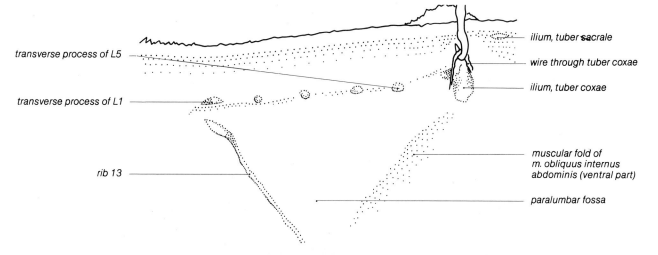

transverse process of L5

ilium, tuber sacrale

wire through tuber coxae

ilium, tuber coxae

transverse process of L1

muscular fold of
m. obliquus internus
abdominis (ventral part)

rib 13

paralumbar fossa

Fig. 5.3 The boundaries of the left paralumbar fossa.
The palpable prominences have been shaved. The transverse process of the first lumbar vertebra is palpable only in thin animals; that of the sixth is hidden by the tuber coxae.

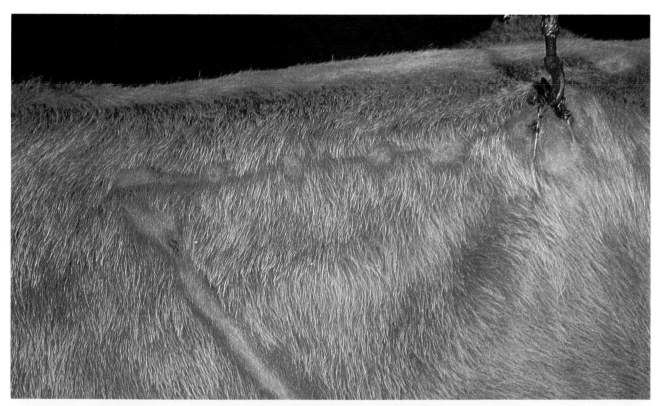

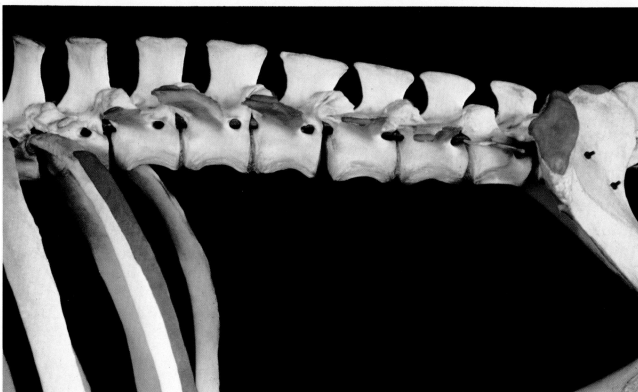

Fig. 5.4 Bones related to the left paralumbar fossa.
The palpable bony prominences shown in fig. 5.3 are coloured red.

Fig.5.5 The cutaneous nerves of the lateral abdominal wall.

A flap of skin and cutaneous muscle has been reflected ventrally and the cutaneous nerves in the superficial fascia have been traced. This dissection, and those shown in figs. 5.6-5.8 were made on the right side, but the photographs have been laterally reversed

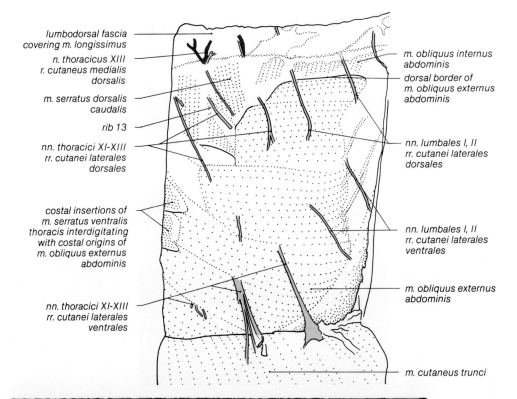

lumbodorsal fascia covering m. longissimus

n. thoracicus XIII r. cutaneus medialis dorsalis

m. serratus dorsalis caudalis

rib 13

nn. thoracici XI-XIII rr. cutanei laterales dorsales

costal insertions of m. serratus ventralis thoracis interdigitating with costal origins of m. obliquus externus abdominis

nn. thoracici XI-XIII rr. cutanei laterales ventrales

m. obliquus internus abdominis

dorsal border of m. obliquus externus abdominis

nn. lumbales I, II rr. cutanei laterales dorsales

nn. lumbales I, II rr. cutanei laterales ventrales

m. obliquus externus abdominis

m. cutaneus trunci

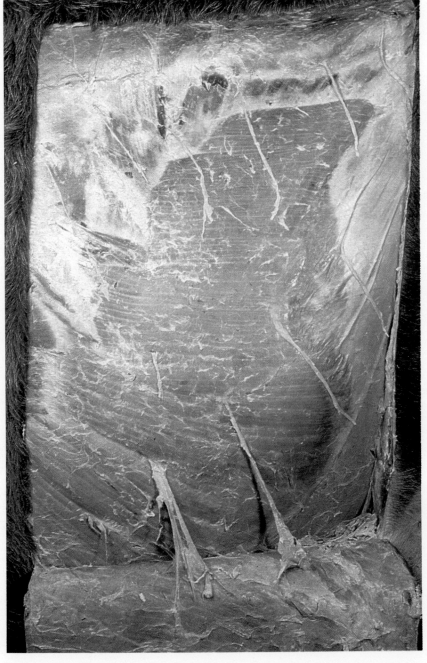

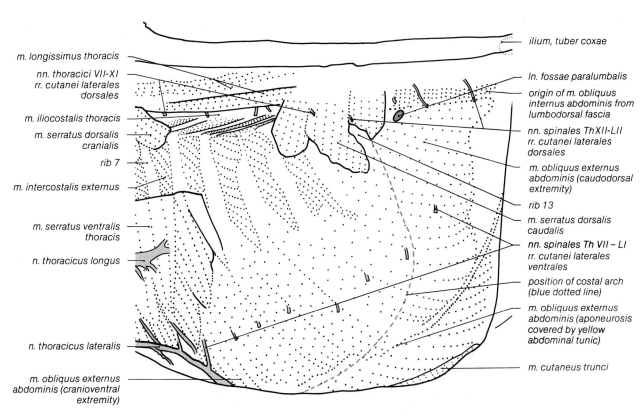

m. longissimus thoracis

nn. thoracici VII-XI
rr. cutanei laterales
dorsales

m. iliocostalis thoracis

m. serratus dorsalis
cranialis

rib 7

m. intercostalis externus

m. serratus ventralis
thoracis

n. thoracicus longus

n. thoracicus lateralis

m. obliquus externus
abdominis (cranioventral
extremity)

ilium, tuber coxae

ln. fossae paralumbalis

origin of m. obliquus
internus abdominis from
lumbodorsal fascia

nn. spinales ThXII-LII
rr. cutanei laterales
dorsales

m. obliquus externus
abdominis (caudodorsal
extremity)

rib 13

m. serratus dorsalis
caudalis

nn. spinales Th VII – LI
rr. cutanei laterales
ventrales

position of costal arch
(blue dotted line)

m. obliquus externus
abdominis (aponeurosis
covered by yellow
abdominal tunic)

m. cutaneus trunci

Fig.5.6 The external oblique abdominal muscle.
The cutaneous muscle of the trunk has been removed (see fig. 5.9) and the cutaneous nerves are shown emerging from the deep fascia.

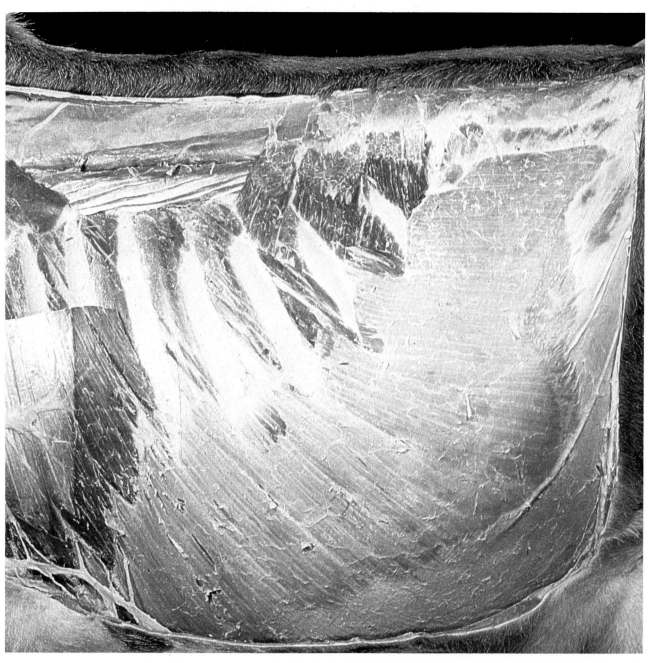

Fig.5.7 The left internal oblique abdominal muscle.

In this and the following figure, the full ventral extent of the straight abdominal muscle is not displayed (see figs. 5.11 and 5.12).

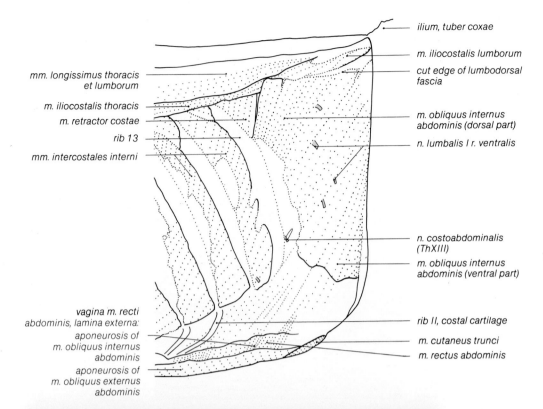

- ilium, tuber coxae
- m. iliocostalis lumborum
- cut edge of lumbodorsal fascia
- mm. longissimus thoracis et lumborum
- m. iliocostalis thoracis
- m. retractor costae
- rib 13
- mm. intercostales interni
- m. obliquus internus abdominis (dorsal part)
- n. lumbalis I r. ventralis
- n. costoabdominalis (ThXIII)
- m. obliquus internus abdominis (ventral part)
- vagina m. recti abdominis, lamina externa: aponeurosis of m. obliquus internus abdominis
- rib II, costal cartilage
- m. cutaneus trunci
- m. rectus abdominis
- aponeurosis of m. obliquus externus abdominis

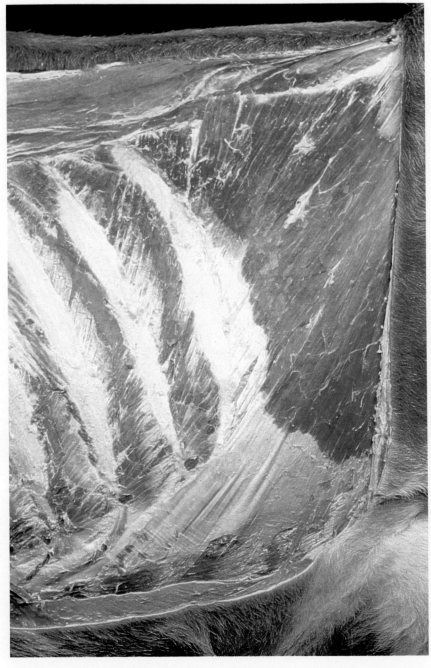

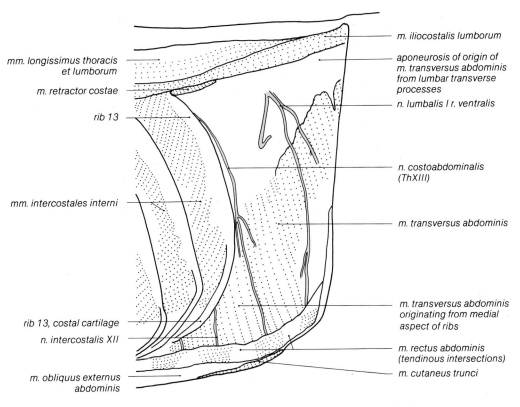

mm. longissimus thoracis
et lumborum

m. retractor costae

rib 13

mm. intercostales interni

rib 13, costal cartilage

n. intercostalis XII

m. obliquus externus
abdominis

m. iliocostalis lumborum

aponeurosis of origin of
m. transversus abdominis
from lumbar transverse
processes

n. lumbalis I r. ventralis

n. costoabdominalis
(ThXIII)

m. transversus abdominis

m. transversus abdominis
originating from medial
aspect of ribs

m. rectus abdominis
(tendinous intersections)

m. cutaneus trunci

Fig.5.8 The left transverse abdominal muscle.

The abdominal viscera lying deep to this muscle, caudal to the last rib, are shown in fig. 5.16.

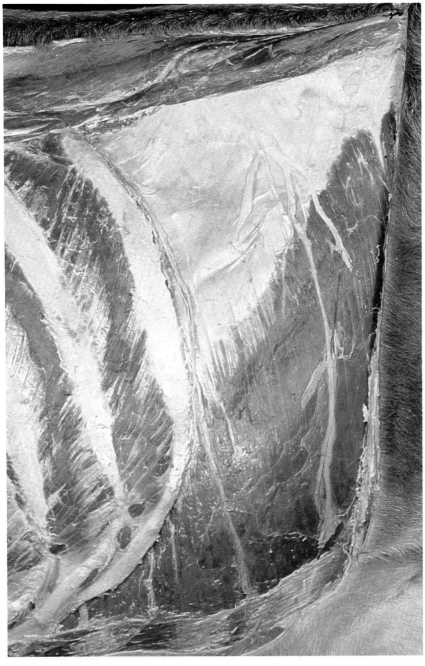

5.7

Fig. 5.9 The cutaneous muscle of the trunk in the 1-week old bull calf, in right lateral view.

The cranial muscle of the prepuce is more clearly seen in fig. 5.10. The surface of the cutaneous muscle is obscured by remnants of the dermis.

Figs. 5.10 – 5.15 show further dissections of the abdominal wall of this calf.

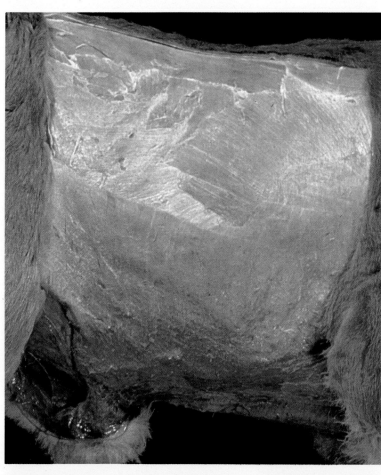

m. longissimus lumborum
m. iliocostalis lumborum
m. obliquus internus abdominis
m. trapezius (pars thoracica)
m. serratus dorsalis caudalis
nn. spinales rr. cutanei laterales dorsales
rib 13
m. cutaneus omobrachialis
m. latissimus dorsi
m. obliquus externus abdominis
nn. spinales rr. cutanei laterales ventrales
m. cutaneus trunci
m. pectoralis ascendens
m. preputialis cranialis

Fig. 5.10 The right external oblique abdominal muscle in the bull calf.

The origins from ribs 10 and 11 are covered by the latissimus dorsi muscle but the interdigitations with the serratus ventralis muscle at ribs 7, 8 and 9 are visible.

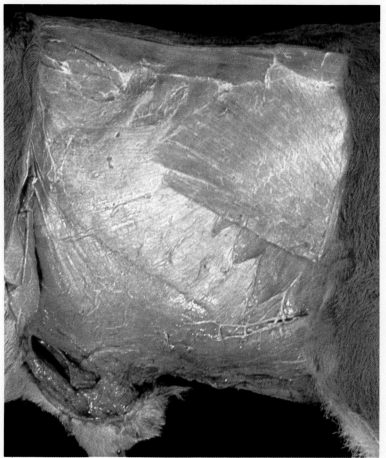

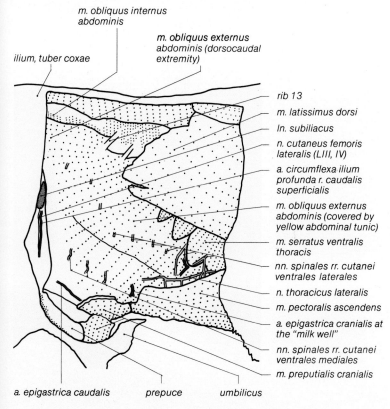

m. obliquus internus abdominis
m. obliquus externus abdominis (dorsocaudal extremity)
ilium, tuber coxae
rib 13
m. latissimus dorsi
ln. subiliacus
n. cutaneus femoris lateralis (LIII, IV)
a. circumflexa ilium profunda r. caudalis superficialis
m. obliquus externus abdominis (covered by yellow abdominal tunic)
m. serratus ventralis thoracis
nn. spinales rr. cutanei ventrales laterales
n. thoracicus lateralis
m. pectoralis ascendens
a. epigastrica cranialis at the "milk well"
nn. spinales rr. cutanei ventrales mediales
m. preputialis cranialis

a. epigastrica caudalis   prepuce   umbilicus

5.8

Fig. 5.11 The right internal oblique and straight abdominal muscles in the bull calf.

The full extent of the straight muscle is shown in this figure and should be compared with fig. 5.7, in which only the lateral part of the muscle is displayed.

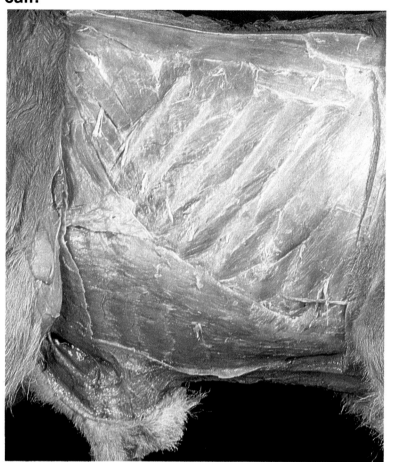

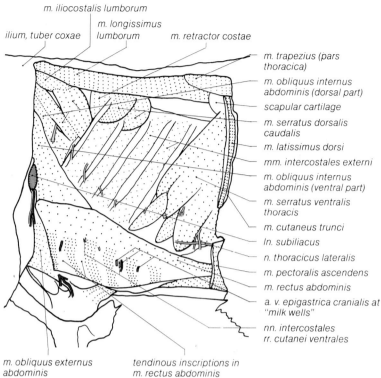

m. iliocostalis lumborum

m. longissimus lumborum

ilium, tuber coxae

m. retractor costae

m. trapezius (pars thoracica)

m. obliquus internus abdominis (dorsal part)

scapular cartilage

m. serratus dorsalis caudalis

m. latissimus dorsi

mm. intercostales externi

m. obliquus internus abdominis (ventral part)

m. serratus ventralis thoracis

m. cutaneus trunci

ln. subiliacus

n. thoracicus lateralis

m. pectoralis ascendens

m. rectus abdominis

a. v. epigastrica cranialis at "milk wells"

nn. intercostales rr. cutanei ventrales

m. obliquus externus abdominis

tendinous inscriptions in m. rectus abdominis

Fig. 5.12 The right transverse abdominal muscle, the rectus sheath and the nerves of the abdominal wall in the bull calf.

The middle portion of the straight muscle has been removed, showing the thin aponeurosis of the transverse abdominal muscle which forms the medial lamina of the rectus sheath. The abdominal viscera lying deep to the right transverse abdominal muscle are shown in fig. 5.54.

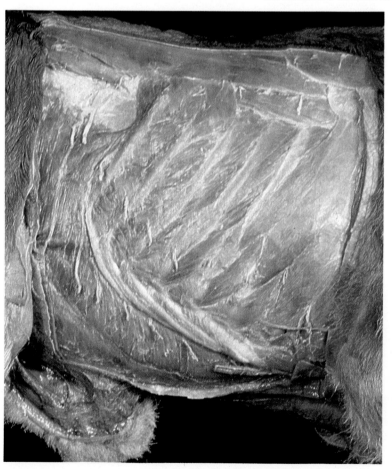

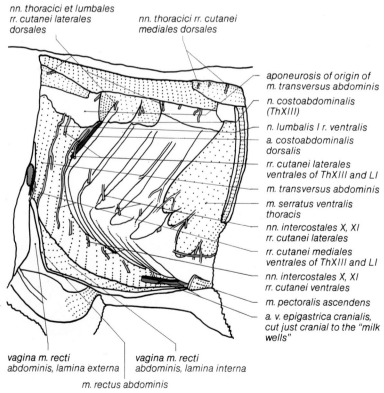

nn. thoracici et lumbales rr. cutanei laterales dorsales

nn. thoracici rr. cutanei mediales dorsales

aponeurosis of origin of m. transversus abdominis

n. costoabdominalis (ThXIII)

n. lumbalis I r. ventralis

a. costoabdominalis dorsalis

rr. cutanei laterales ventrales of ThXIII and LI

m. transversus abdominis

m. serratus ventralis thoracis

nn. intercostales X, XI rr. cutanei laterales

rr. cutanei mediales ventrales of ThXIII and LI

nn. intercostales X, XI rr. cutanei ventrales

m. pectoralis ascendens

a. v. epigastrica cranialis, cut just cranial to the "milk wells"

vagina m. recti abdominis, lamina externa

vagina m. recti abdominis, lamina interna

m. rectus abdominis

Fig. 5.13 Cutaneous nerves of the left abdominal and thoracic wall in the bull calf.

The cutaneous branches of the thoracic and lumbar nerves emerge from the deep fascia in three oblique rows; only the last thoracic components have been labelled in each of the rows.

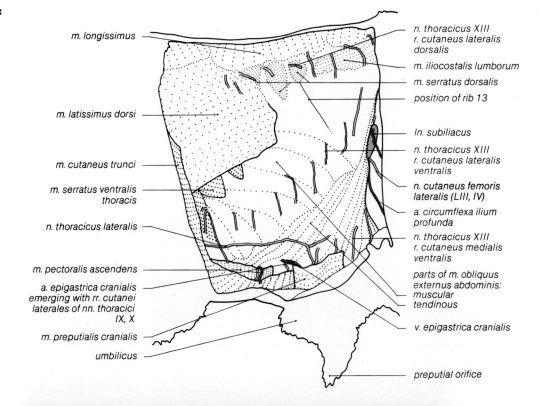

m. longissimus

n. thoracicus XIII
r. cutaneus lateralis
dorsalis

m. iliocostalis lumborum

m. serratus dorsalis

position of rib 13

m. latissimus dorsi

ln. subiliacus

n. thoracicus XIII
r. cutaneus lateralis
ventralis

m. cutaneus trunci

n. cutaneus femoris
lateralis (LIII, IV)

m. serratus ventralis
thoracis

a. circumflexa ilium
profunda

n. thoracicus lateralis

n. thoracicus XIII
r. cutaneus medialis
ventralis

m. pectoralis ascendens

parts of m. obliquus
externus abdominis:
muscular
tendinous

a. epigastrica cranialis
emerging with rr. cutanei
laterales of nn. thoracici
IX, X

v. epigastrica cranialis

m. preputialis cranialis

umbilicus

preputial orifice

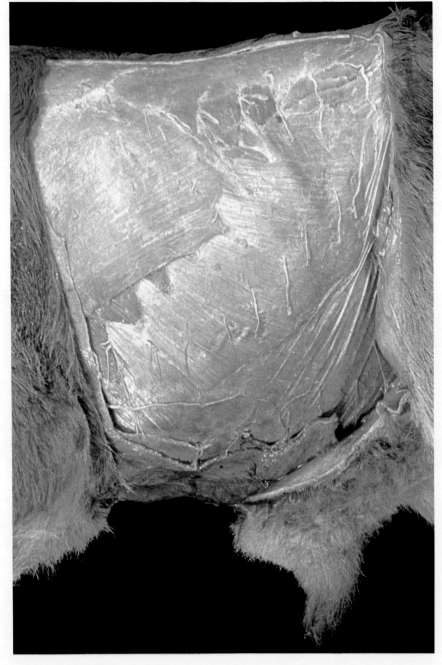

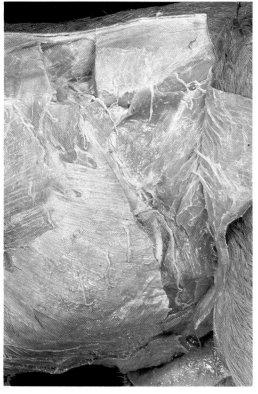

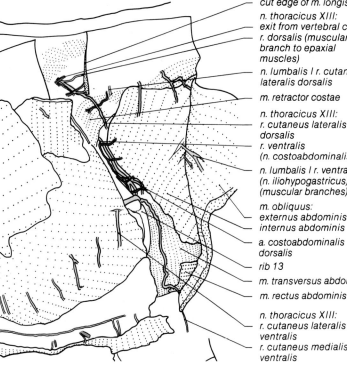

cut edge of m. longissimus
n. thoracicus XIII:
exit from vertebral canal
r. dorsalis (muscular branch to epaxial muscles)
n. lumbalis I r. cutaneus lateralis dorsalis
m. retractor costae
n. thoracicus XIII:
r. cutaneus lateralis dorsalis
r. ventralis (n. costoabdominalis)
n. lumbalis I r. ventralis (n. iliohypogastricus) (muscular branches)
m. obliquus:
externus abdominis
internus abdominis
a. costoabdominalis dorsalis
rib 13
m. transversus abdominis
m. rectus abdominis
n. thoracicus XIII:
r. cutaneus lateralis ventralis
r. cutaneus medialis ventralis

Fig. 5.14 The course of the last thoracic nerve and its cutaneous branches in the bull calf: left lateral view.
The muscles of the abdominal wall have been cut just caudal to the costal arch and displaced in order to demonstrate the course of a typical segmental nerve supplying the trunk. The details of the full series of nerves in the right abdominal wall can be seen by referring to figs. 5.10 and 5.12.

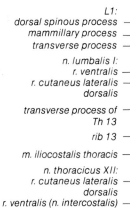

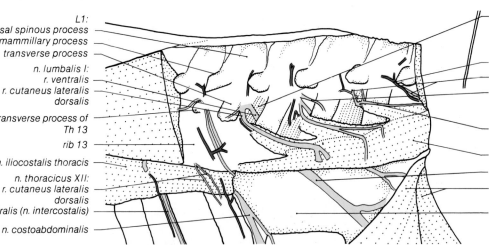

L1:
dorsal spinous process
mammillary process
transverse process
n. lumbalis I:
r. ventralis
r. cutaneus lateralis dorsalis
transverse process of Th 13
rib 13
m. iliocostalis thoracis
n. thoracicus XII:
r. cutaneus lateralis dorsalis
r. ventralis (n. intercostalis)
n. costoabdominalis

m. psoas revealed at intertransverse space by removal of mm. intertransversarii
a. lumbalis IV r. dorsalis
nn. lumbales III, IV
n. lumbalis II r. dorsalis (muscular branch to epaxial muscles)
n. lumbalis III r. cutaneus lateralis dorsalis
m. iliocostalis lumbalis
n. lumbalis I r. ventralis
m. obliquus internus abdominis
tendon of origin of m. transversus abdominis

Fig. 5.15 The thoracic and lumbar nerves of the left paravertebral region in the bull calf.
The ventral rami of the third and fourth lumbar nerves are not visible because they run longitudinally across the deepest parts of the intertransverse spaces. The abdominal viscera lying deep to the left transverse abdominal muscle are shown in fig. 5.46.

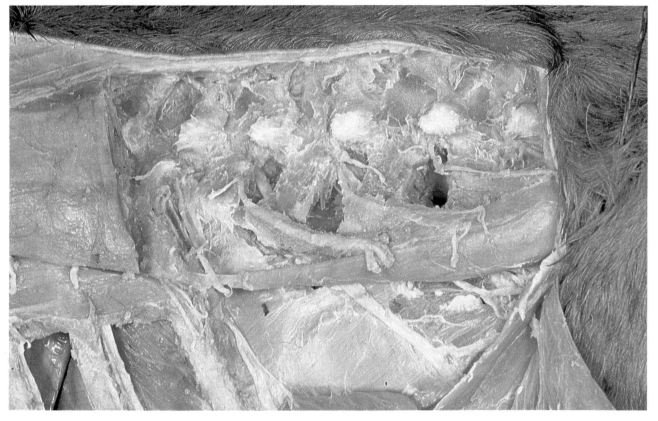

Fig. 5.16 The abdominal viscera caudal to the costal arch, in left lateral view.

The dorsal part of the external oblique abdominal muscle has been removed to reveal the muscle belly of the internal oblique muscle. The subiliac lymph node, which lies in the superficial fascia, is now in contact with the internal oblique muscle. This lymph node is displaced cranially from the cover of the tensor muscle of the fascia lata.

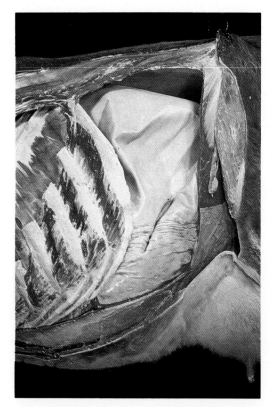

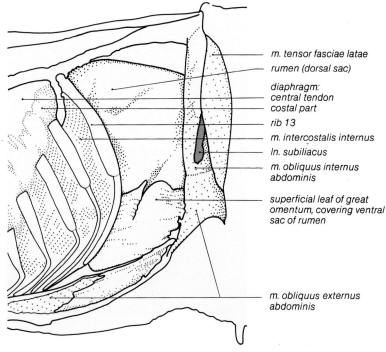

m. tensor fasciae latae
rumen (dorsal sac)
diaphragm:
central tendon
costal part
rib 13
m. intercostalis internus
ln. subiliacus
m. obliquus internus abdominis
superficial leaf of great omentum, covering ventral sac of rumen
m. obliquus externus abdominis

Fig. 5.17 The abdominal viscera after removal of the rib cage and diaphragm, in left lateral view.

The stomach has been moderately inflated to imitate its shape and position in life.

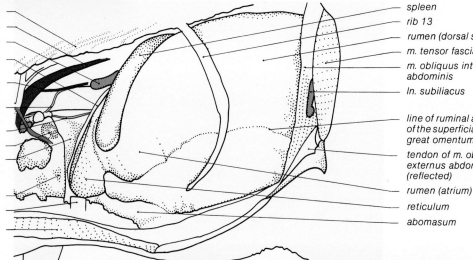

m. iliocostalis thoracis
aorta thoracica
ln. mediastinalis caudalis
diaphragm
a. broncho-oesophagea
r. oesophageus
t. vagalis X dorsalis
t. vagalis X ventralis
left atrium
accessory lobe of right lung, covered by mediastinum
left ventricle
rib 6
m. pectoralis ascendens

spleen
rib 13
rumen (dorsal sac)
m. tensor fasciae latae
m. obliquus internus abdominis
ln. subiliacus
line of ruminal attachment of the superficial leaf of the great omentum
tendon of m. obliquus externus abdominis (reflected)
rumen (atrium)
reticulum
abomasum

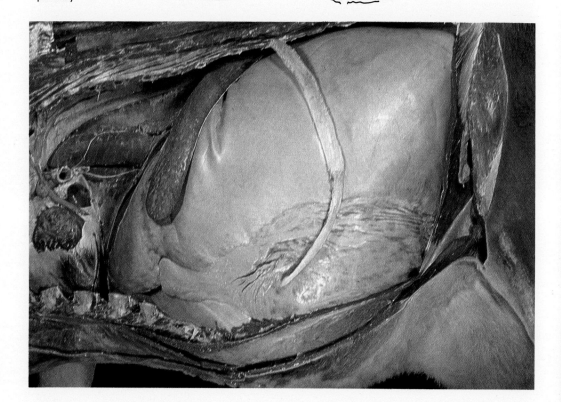

Fig. 5.18 The relationships of the reticulum, in left lateral view.

This figure has been taken from a slightly more cranial position than fig. 5.17 in order to show the liver more clearly.

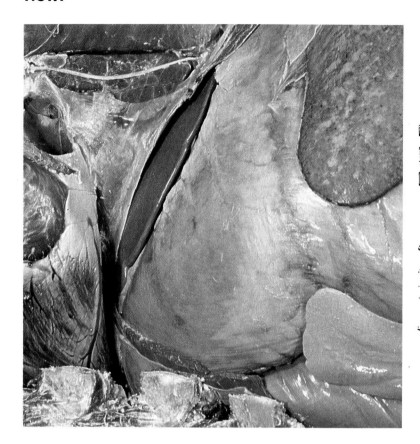

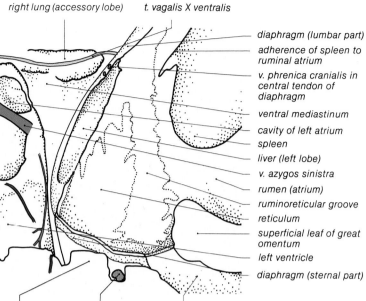

right lung (accessory lobe) t. vagalis X ventralis

diaphragm (lumbar part)

adherence of spleen to ruminal atrium

v. phrenica cranialis in central tendon of diaphragm

ventral mediastinum

cavity of left atrium

spleen

liver (left lobe)

v. azygos sinistra

rumen (atrium)

ruminoreticular groove

reticulum

superficial leaf of great omentum

left ventricle

diaphragm (sternal part)

rib 6 ln. sternalis caudalis abomasum

Fig. 5.19 The abdominal viscera after removal of the spleen, in left lateral view.

The view is from a slightly cranial angle, to show the small part of the liver that extends into the left half of the abdomen. The right lung has been removed.

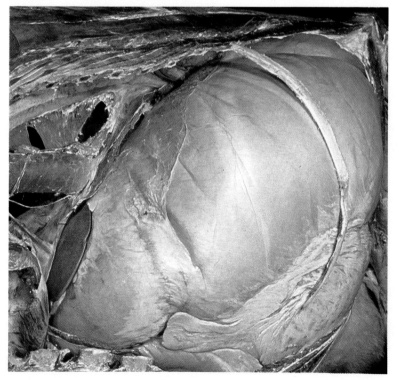

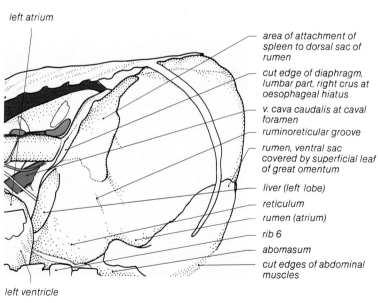

left atrium

area of attachment of spleen to dorsal sac of rumen

cut edge of diaphragm, lumbar part, right crus at oesophageal hiatus

v. cava caudalis at caval foramen

ruminoreticular groove

rumen, ventral sac covered by superficial leaf of great omentum

liver (left lobe)

reticulum

rumen (atrium)

rib 6

abomasum

cut edges of abdominal muscles

left ventricle

Fig. 5.20 The interior of the rumen, in left lateral view.

The dorsal part of the rumen has been stitched to the abdominal roof to preserve the topographical relationships. A small part of the cavity of the reticulum is also displayed. The solid contents have been entirely removed but a puddle of fluid remains in the ventral sac of the rumen.

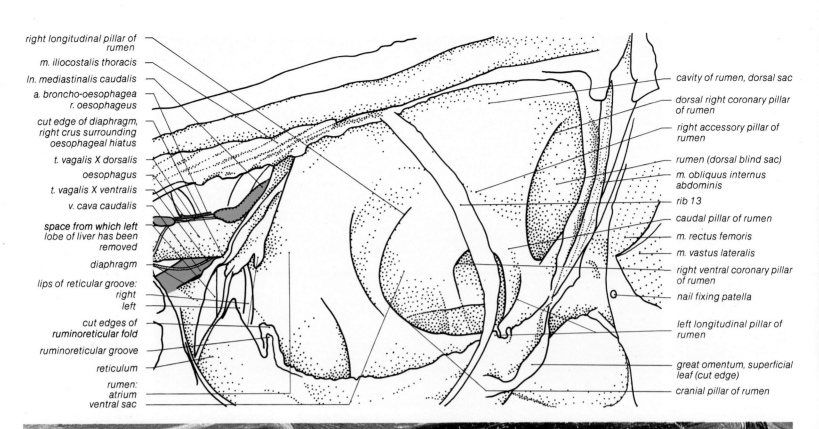

right longitudinal pillar of rumen
m. iliocostalis thoracis
ln. mediastinalis caudalis
a. broncho-oesophagea
r. oesophageus
cut edge of diaphragm, right crus surrounding oesophageal hiatus
t. vagalis X dorsalis
oesophagus
t. vagalis X ventralis
v. cava caudalis
space from which left lobe of liver has been removed
diaphragm
lips of reticular groove:
right
left
cut edges of ruminoreticular fold
ruminoreticular groove
reticulum
rumen:
atrium
ventral sac

cavity of rumen, dorsal sac
dorsal right coronary pillar of rumen
right accessory pillar of rumen
rumen (dorsal blind sac)
m. obliquus internus abdominis
rib 13
caudal pillar of rumen
m. rectus femoris
m. vastus lateralis
right ventral coronary pillar of rumen
nail fixing patella
left longitudinal pillar of rumen
great omentum, superficial leaf (cut edge)
cranial pillar of rumen

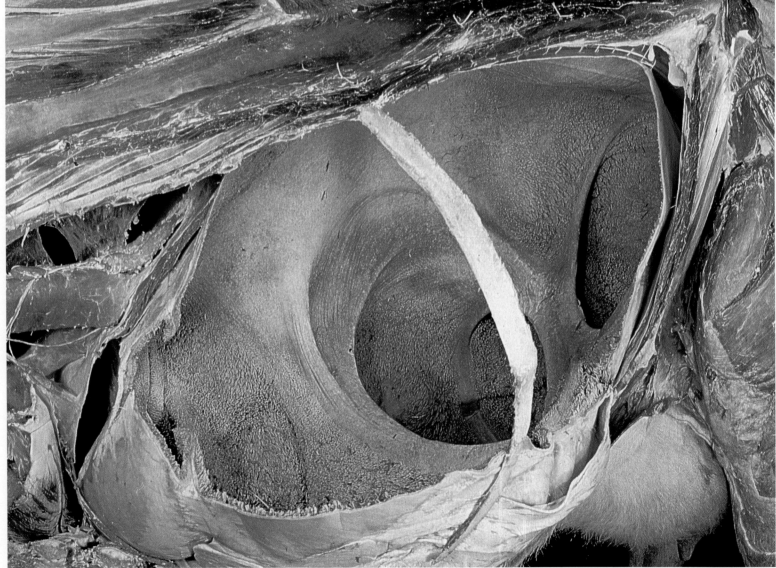

Fig. 5.21 The ruminal pillars and compartments in dorsocranial view.

The specimen is at the stage of dissection shown in fig. 5.20.

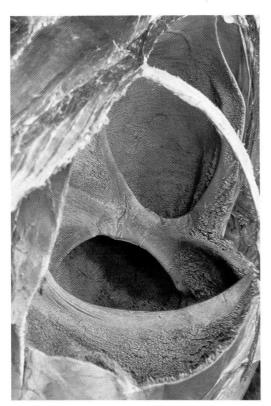

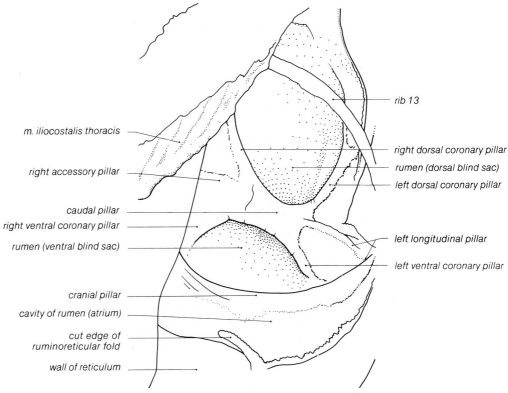

m. iliocostalis thoracis

right accessory pillar

caudal pillar

right ventral coronary pillar

rumen (ventral blind sac)

cranial pillar

cavity of rumen (atrium)

cut edge of ruminoreticular fold

wall of reticulum

rib 13

right dorsal coronary pillar

rumen (dorsal blind sac)

left dorsal coronary pillar

left longitudinal pillar

left ventral coronary pillar

Fig. 5.22 The interior of the rumen and reticulum showing the cardia and the reticular groove: caudal view.

The dissection is at a similar stage to that shown in figs. 5.20 and 5.21, but more of the cranial wall of the reticulum has been removed.

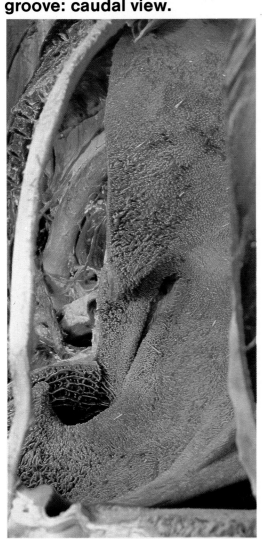

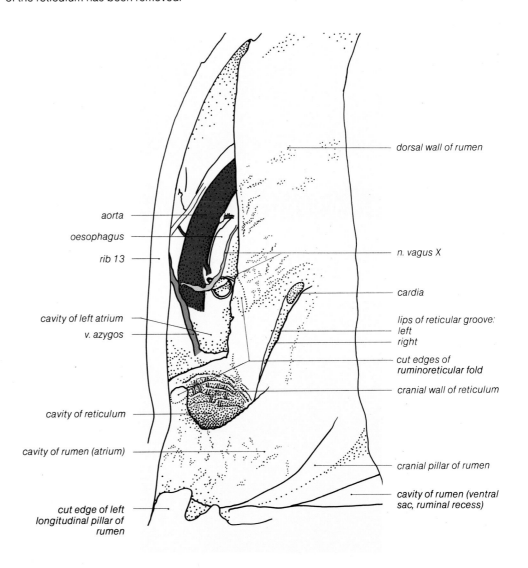

aorta

oesophagus

rib 13

cavity of left atrium

v. azygos

cavity of reticulum

cavity of rumen (atrium)

cut edge of left longitudinal pillar of rumen

dorsal wall of rumen

n. vagus X

cardia

lips of reticular groove:
left
right

cut edges of ruminoreticular fold

cranial wall of reticulum

cranial pillar of rumen

cavity of rumen (ventral sac, ruminal recess)

Fig. 5.23 The interior of the rumen and reticulum, in left lateral view.

Removal of the ventral part of the wall of the ruminal atrium and ventral sac reveals the relationships of the abomasum to the left abdominal wall, reticulum and rumen.

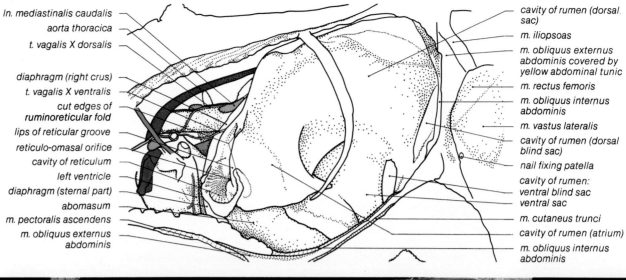

In. mediastinalis caudalis
aorta thoracica
t. vagalis X dorsalis

diaphragm (right crus)
t. vagalis X ventralis
cut edges of ruminoreticular fold
lips of reticular groove
reticulo-omasal orifice
cavity of reticulum
left ventricle
diaphragm (sternal part)
abomasum
m. pectoralis ascendens
m. obliquus externus abdominis

cavity of rumen (dorsal sac)
m. iliopsoas
m. obliquus externus abdominis covered by yellow abdominal tunic
m. rectus femoris
m. obliquus internus abdominis
m. vastus lateralis
cavity of rumen (dorsal blind sac)
nail fixing patella
cavity of rumen: ventral blind sac ventral sac
m. cutaneus trunci
cavity of rumen (atrium)
m. obliquus internus abdominis

Fig. 5.24 The abdominal viscera after removal of the dorsal and ventral ruminal sacs: left lateral view.

Part of the right longitudinal ruminal groove remains, and its attachment to the deep leaf of the great omentum is just visible.

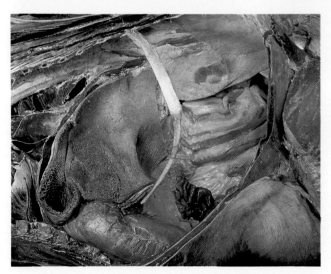

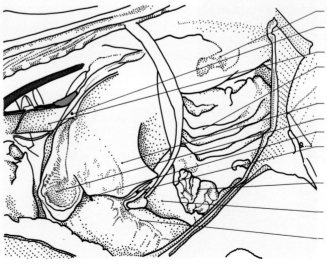

left kidney
cut edge of ruminoreticular fold
oesophagus
ascending colon (ansa spiralis in supraomental recess)
rumen (atrium)
reticulum
a. gastroepiploica sinistra
cut edge of cranial ruminal pillar with a. ruminalis sinistra
small intestine in supraomental recess
remains of deep leaf of great omentum
abomasum

Fig. 5.25 The abdominal viscera after removal of the entire rumen, in left lateral view.

The liver is related to the right surfaces of the omasum and the reticulum, but it has been removed during dissection of the right abdomen (fig. 5.31).

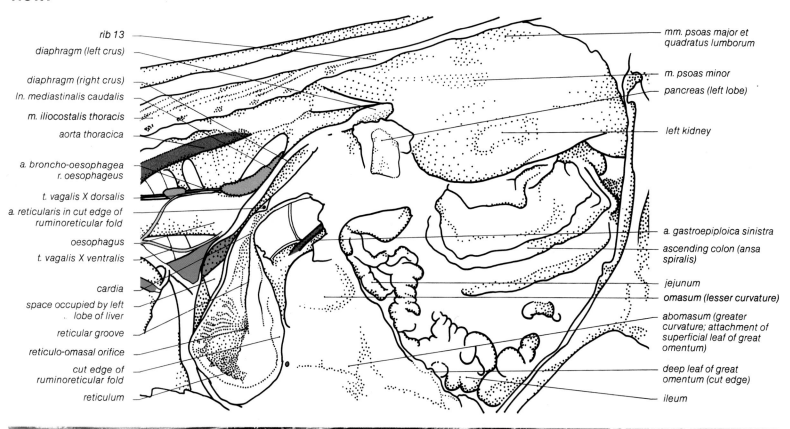

rib 13
diaphragm (left crus)

diaphragm (right crus)
ln. mediastinalis caudalis
m. iliocostalis thoracis
aorta thoracica

a. broncho-oesophagea
r. oesophageus
t. vagalis X dorsalis
a. reticularis in cut edge of ruminoreticular fold
oesophagus
t. vagalis X ventralis

cardia
space occupied by left lobe of liver
reticular groove
reticulo-omasal orifice
cut edge of ruminoreticular fold
reticulum

mm. psoas major et quadratus lumborum

m. psoas minor
pancreas (left lobe)

left kidney

a. gastroepiploica sinistra
ascending colon (ansa spiralis)

jejunum
omasum (lesser curvature)
abomasum (greater curvature; attachment of superficial leaf of great omentum)

deep leaf of great omentum (cut edge)

ileum

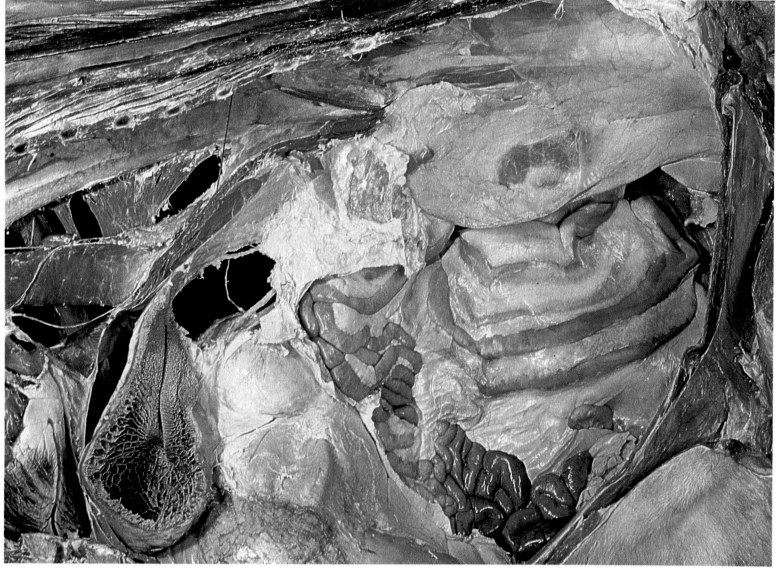

Fig. 5.26 The arteries and veins of the abdominal viscera after removal of the entire rumen: left lateral view.

The right diaphragmatic crus is held in place by a fine wire. Arrows indicate the direction of flow of ingesta in the colon. The vessels shown here are also seen in right lateral view at a slightly later stage in the dissection, in fig. 5.34.

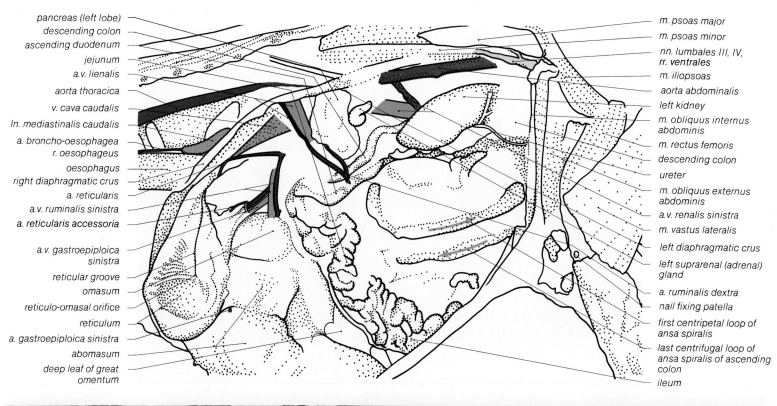

pancreas (left lobe)
descending colon
ascending duodenum
jejunum
a.v. lienalis
aorta thoracica
v. cava caudalis
ln. mediastinalis caudalis
a. broncho-oesophagea
r. oesophageus
oesophagus
right diaphragmatic crus
a. reticularis
a.v. ruminalis sinistra
a. reticularis accessoria
a.v. gastroepiploica sinistra
reticular groove
omasum
reticulo-omasal orifice
reticulum
a. gastroepiploica sinistra
abomasum
deep leaf of great omentum

m. psoas major
m. psoas minor
nn. lumbales III, IV, rr. ventrales
m. iliopsoas
aorta abdominalis
left kidney
m. obliquus internus abdominis
m. rectus femoris
descending colon
ureter
m. obliquus externus abdominis
a.v. renalis sinistra
m. vastus lateralis
left diaphragmatic crus
left suprarenal (adrenal) gland
a. ruminalis dextra
nail fixing patella
first centripetal loop of ansa spiralis
last centrifugal loop of ansa spiralis of ascending colon
ileum

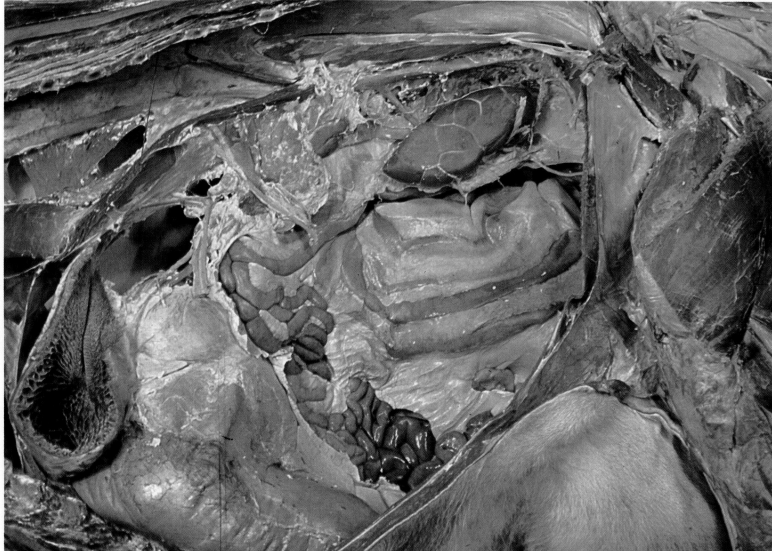

Fig. 5.27 The caecum, in left lateral view.

The small intestine has been displaced to show the unusual position of the caecum. In the adult, non-pregnant cow, this organ usually occupies a right dorsal position with its apex pointing caudally towards the pelvis as shown in fig. 5.39. However in this individual the caecal apex is ventral and points cranially towards the left. On the right side its body was situated ventrally (see fig. 5.34). This topography is reminiscent of that usually seen in the calf.

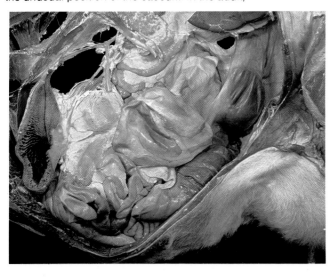

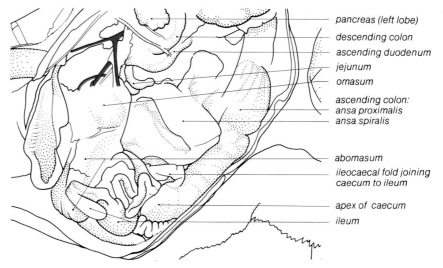

pancreas (left lobe)
descending colon
ascending duodenum
jejunum
omasum
ascending colon:
ansa proximalis
ansa spiralis

abomasum
ileocaecal fold joining
caecum to ileum

apex of caecum

ileum

Fig. 5.28 The omasoabomasal orifice and the arteries and veins of the digestive tract after removal of the entire rumen: left lateral view.

The angle of the free edge of the omasal pillar, visible in this figure, is a consequence of the rather oblique orientation of the omasum (seen in right lateral view at a later stage of dissection in fig. 5.34).

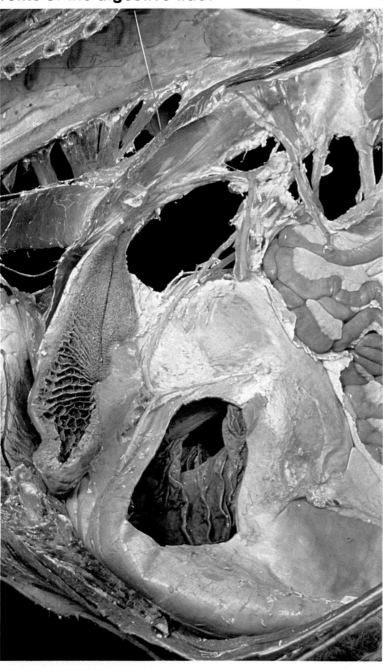

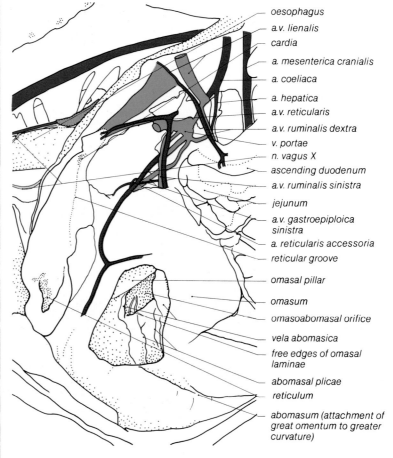

oesophagus
a.v. lienalis
cardia
a. mesenterica cranialis
a. coeliaca
a. hepatica
a.v. reticularis
a.v. ruminalis dextra
v. portae
n. vagus X
ascending duodenum
a.v. ruminalis sinistra
jejunum
a.v. gastroepiploica sinistra
a. reticularis accessoria
reticular groove

omasal pillar

omasum

omasoabomasal orifice

vela abomasica
free edges of omasal laminae

abomasal plicae
reticulum

abomasum (attachment of great omentum to greater curvature)

Fig. 5.29 The abdominal viscera lying caudal to the costal arch: right lateral view.

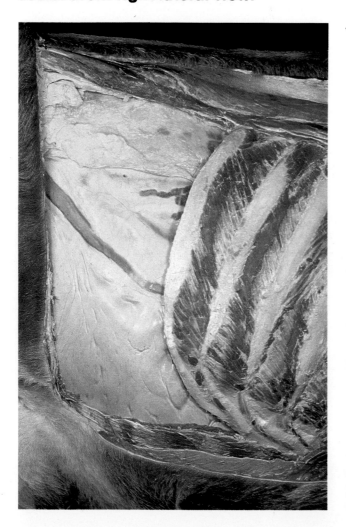

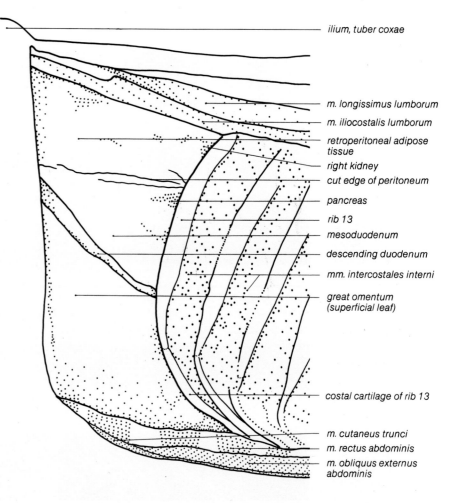

ilium, tuber coxae

m. longissimus lumborum

m. iliocostalis lumborum

retroperitoneal adipose tissue

right kidney

cut edge of peritoneum

pancreas

rib 13

mesoduodenum

descending duodenum

mm. intercostales interni

great omentum (superficial leaf)

costal cartilage of rib 13

m. cutaneus trunci

m. rectus abdominis

m. obliquus externus abdominis

Fig. 5.30 The abdominal viscera after removal of the rib cage and diaphragm: right lateral view.

No remnants were found of the falciform ligament or the round ligament (umbilical vein) of the liver; these ligaments can be seen in the calf, fig. 5.54.

The umbilical notch for the round ligament is visible in this figure.

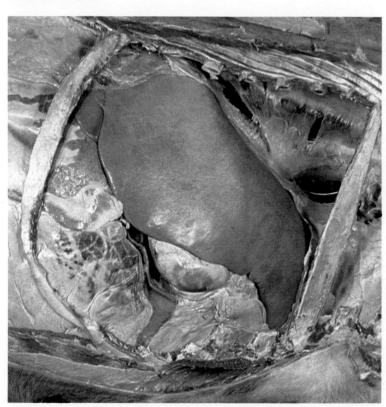

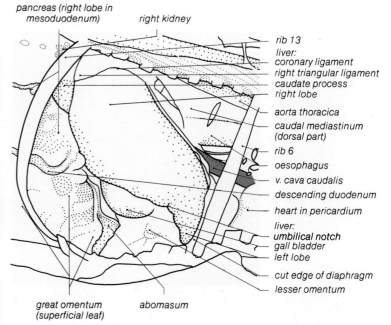

pancreas (right lobe in mesoduodenum)

right kidney

rib 13

liver:
coronary ligament
right triangular ligament
caudate process
right lobe

aorta thoracica

caudal mediastinum (dorsal part)

rib 6

oesophagus

v. cava caudalis

descending duodenum

heart in pericardium

liver:
umbilical notch
gall bladder
left lobe

cut edge of diaphragm

lesser omentum

great omentum (superficial leaf)

abomasum

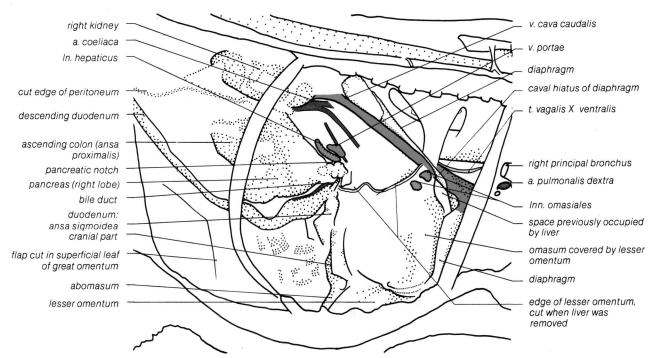

right kidney
a. coeliaca
ln. hepaticus
cut edge of peritoneum
descending duodenum
ascending colon (ansa proximalis)
pancreatic notch
pancreas (right lobe)
bile duct
duodenum: ansa sigmoidea cranial part
flap cut in superficial leaf of great omentum
abomasum
lesser omentum

v. cava caudalis
v. portae
diaphragm
caval hiatus of diaphragm
t. vagalis X ventralis
right principal bronchus
a. pulmonalis dextra
lnn. omasiales
space previously occupied by liver
omasum covered by lesser omentum
diaphragm
edge of lesser omentum, cut when liver was removed

Fig. 5.31 The abdominal viscera after removal of the liver: right lateral view.
The liver was separated from the adherent caudal vena cava, and the coronary attachment to the diaphragm is not recognisable. The attachment of the lesser omentum is preserved. The vessels severed at the hepatic porta are shown in fig. 5.33.

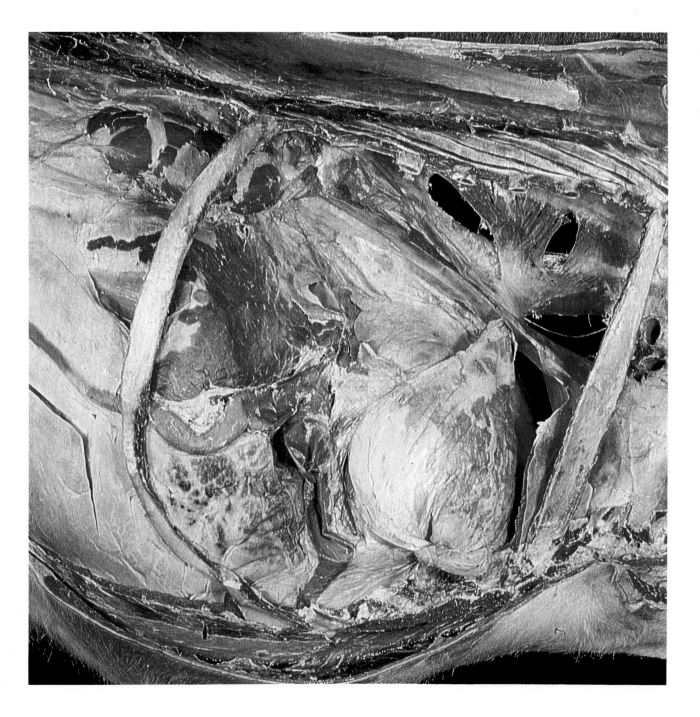

Fig. 5.32 The abdominal viscera after removal of the liver, lesser omentum and part of the great omentum: right lateral view.

The blood vessels are shown in fig. 5.33 and the large intestine is shown more completely in fig. 5.34. Arrows indicate the direction of flow of ingesta in the large intestine. The visceral surface of the liver in a foetal calf is shown in fig. 5.60.

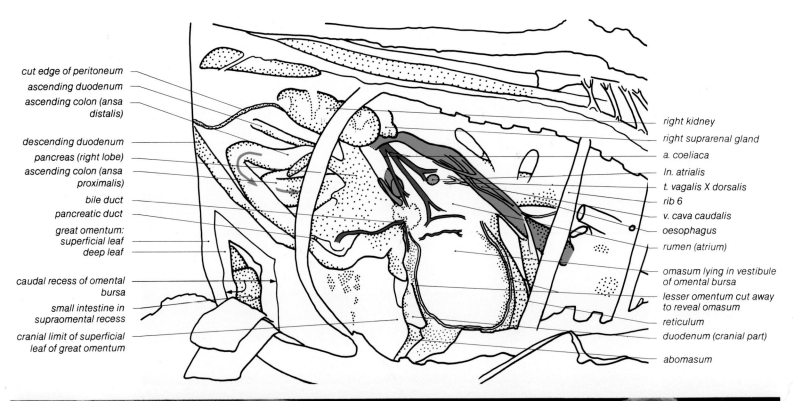

cut edge of peritoneum
ascending duodenum
ascending colon (ansa distalis)

descending duodenum
pancreas (right lobe)
ascending colon (ansa proximalis)
bile duct
pancreatic duct
great omentum:
superficial leaf
deep leaf

caudal recess of omental bursa

small intestine in supraomental recess

cranial limit of superficial leaf of great omentum

right kidney
right suprarenal gland
a. coeliaca
ln. atrialis
t. vagalis X dorsalis
rib 6
v. cava caudalis
oesophagus
rumen (atrium)
omasum lying in vestibule of omental bursa
lesser omentum cut away to reveal omasum
reticulum
duodenum (cranial part)
abomasum

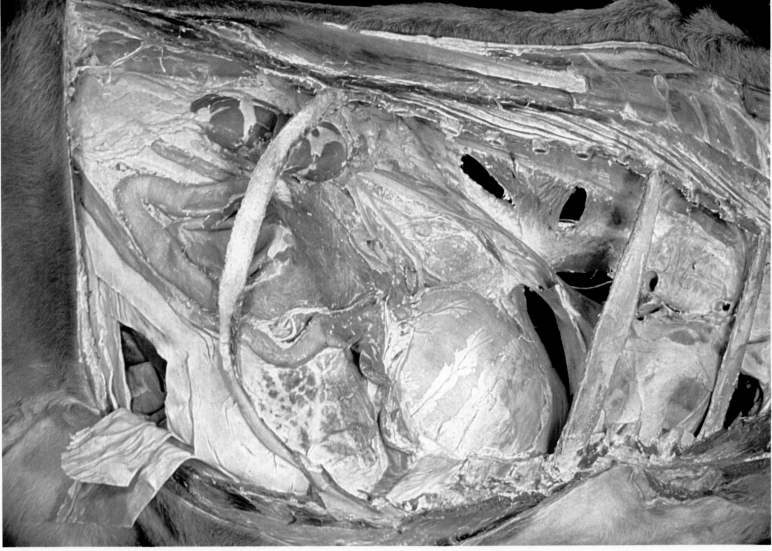

Fig. 5.33 The branches of the coeliac artery and tributaries of the hepatic portal vein, in right lateral view.

This figure shows part of the dissection from fig. 5.32. Parts of the autonomic plexi surrounding the branches of the artery are visible, but only the hepatic plexus is labelled. The autonomic nerves are shown more completely in fig. 5.57.

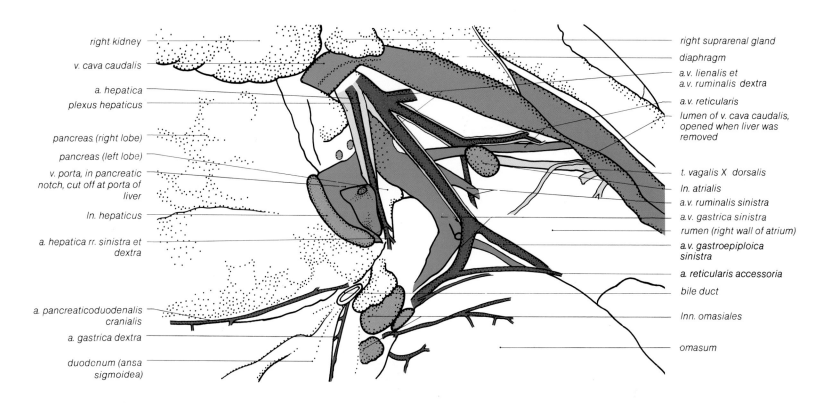

right kidney
v. cava caudalis
a. hepatica
plexus hepaticus
pancreas (right lobe)
pancreas (left lobe)
v. porta, in pancreatic notch, cut off at porta of liver
ln. hepaticus
a. hepatica rr. sinistra et dextra
a. pancreaticoduodenalis cranialis
a. gastrica dextra
duodenum (ansa sigmoidea)

right suprarenal gland
diaphragm
a.v. lienalis et a.v. ruminalis dextra
a.v. reticularis
lumen of v. cava caudalis, opened when liver was removed
t. vagalis X dorsalis
ln. atrialis
a.v. ruminalis sinistra
a.v. gastrica sinistra
rumen (right wall of atrium)
a.v. gastroepiploica sinistra
a. reticularis accessoria
bile duct
lnn. omasiales
omasum

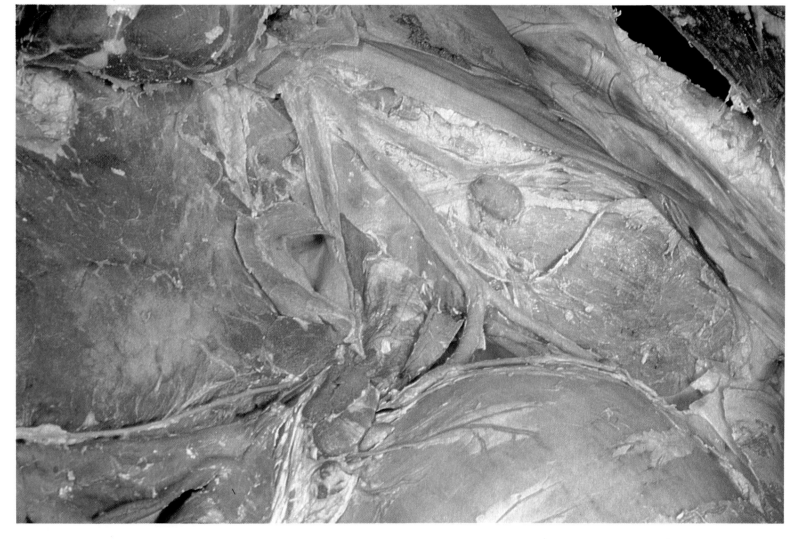

Fig. 5.34 The abdominal viscera with parts of the colon exposed and the omasum opened: right lateral view.

The entire rumen has been removed, and the dissection is at the stage shown in fig. 5.26. The caecum, usually visible in this view, is displaced ventrally so that it appears in the dissection of the left side shown in fig. 5.27. The normal topography of the caecum in adult cattle is shown in fig. 5.39. The omasal groove, normally vertical in the living animal, is oblique in this dissection, probably because the viscera tend to drop ventrally after preservation and dissection in the standing position. Arrows indicate the direction of flow of ingesta in the large intestine.

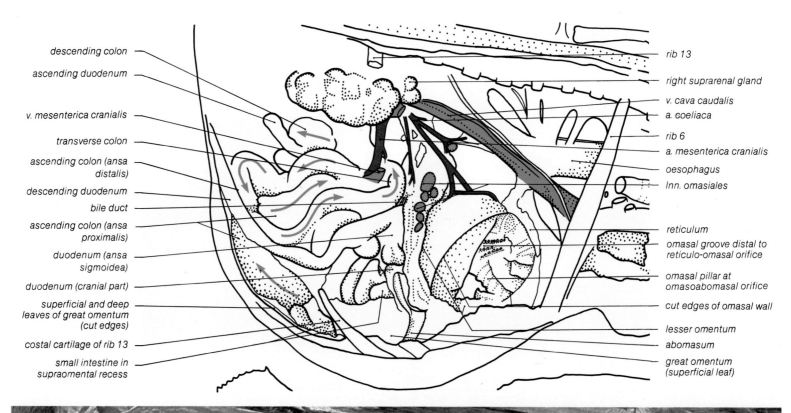

descending colon

ascending duodenum

v. mesenterica cranialis

transverse colon

ascending colon (ansa distalis)

descending duodenum

bile duct

ascending colon (ansa proximalis)

duodenum (ansa sigmoidea)

duodenum (cranial part)

superficial and deep leaves of great omentum (cut edges)

costal cartilage of rib 13

small intestine in supraomental recess

rib 13

right suprarenal gland

v. cava caudalis

a. coeliaca

rib 6

a. mesenterica cranialis

oesophagus

lnn. omasiales

reticulum

omasal groove distal to reticulo-omasal orifice

omasal pillar at omasoabomasal orifice

cut edges of omasal wall

lesser omentum

abomasum

great omentum (superficial leaf)

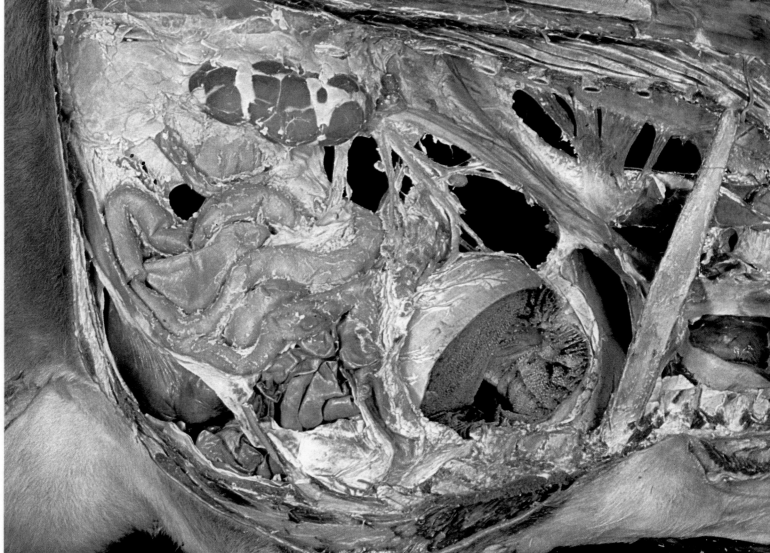

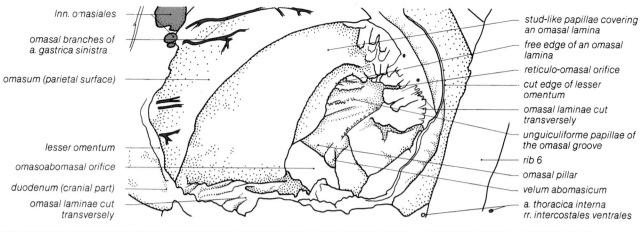

Inn. omasiales

omasal branches of a. gastrica sinistra

omasum (parietal surface)

lesser omentum

omasoabomasal orifice

duodenum (cranial part)

omasal laminae cut transversely

stud-like papillae covering an omasal lamina

free edge of an omasal lamina

reticulo-omasal orifice

cut edge of lesser omentum

omasal laminae cut transversely

unguiculiforme papillae of the omasal groove

rib 6

omasal pillar

velum abomasicum

a. thoracica interna
rr. intercostales ventrales

Fig.5.35 The interior of the omasum, in right lateral view.

This is a closer view of part of the dissection shown in fig. 5.34.

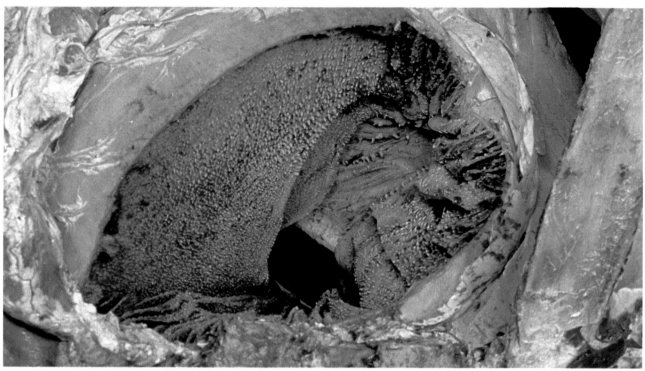

Fig.5.36 The cranial mesenteric artery and associated structures, in right lateral view.

This is a further dissection of a part of the region shown in fig. 5.34. Arrows indicate the direction of flow of ingesta within the large intestine.

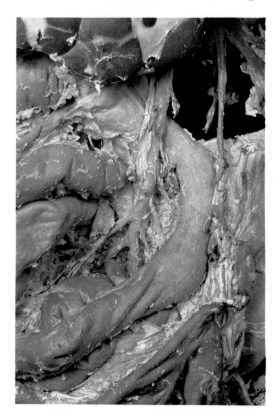

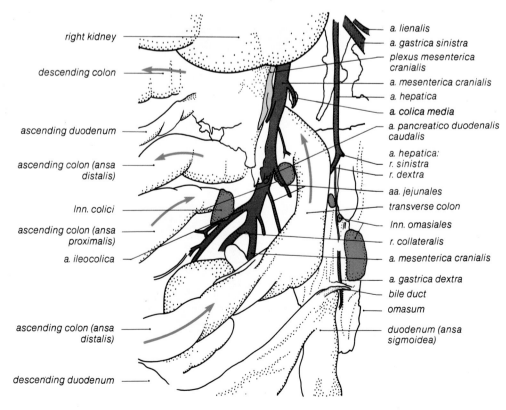

right kidney

descending colon

ascending duodenum

ascending colon (ansa distalis)

Inn. colici

ascending colon (ansa proximalis)

a. ileocolica

ascending colon (ansa distalis)

descending duodenum

a. lienalis

a. gastrica sinistra

plexus mesenterica cranialis

a. mesenterica cranialis

a. hepatica

a. colica media

a. pancreatico duodenalis caudalis

a. hepatica:
r. sinistra
r. dextra

aa. jejunales

transverse colon

Inn. omasiales

r. collateralis

a. mesenterica cranialis

a. gastrica dextra

bile duct

omasum

duodenum (ansa sigmoidea)

Fig. 5.37 The abdominal cavity of a bull calf (aged 4 months) in dorsal view.

Vertebrae, ribs, thoracic viscera and caudal vena cava have been removed. On the left side, the parietal peritoneum has been partly removed. The diaphragm remains but its lumbar attachments have been cut.

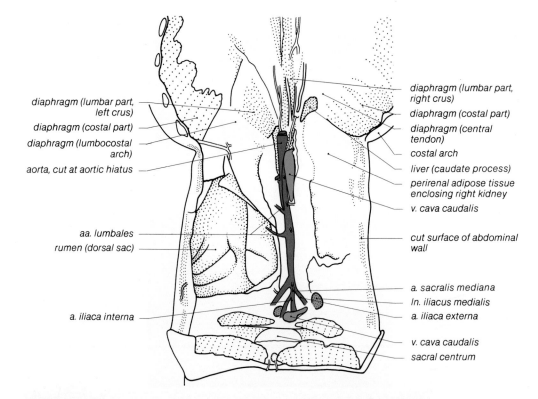

diaphragm (lumbar part, left crus)

diaphragm (costal part)

diaphragm (lumbocostal arch)

aorta, cut at aortic hiatus

aa. lumbales

rumen (dorsal sac)

a. iliaca interna

diaphragm (lumbar part, right crus)

diaphragm (costal part)

diaphragm (central tendon)

costal arch

liver (caudate process)

perirenal adipose tissue enclosing right kidney

v. cava caudalis

cut surface of abdominal wall

a. sacralis mediana

ln. iliacus medialis

a. iliaca externa

v. cava caudalis

sacral centrum

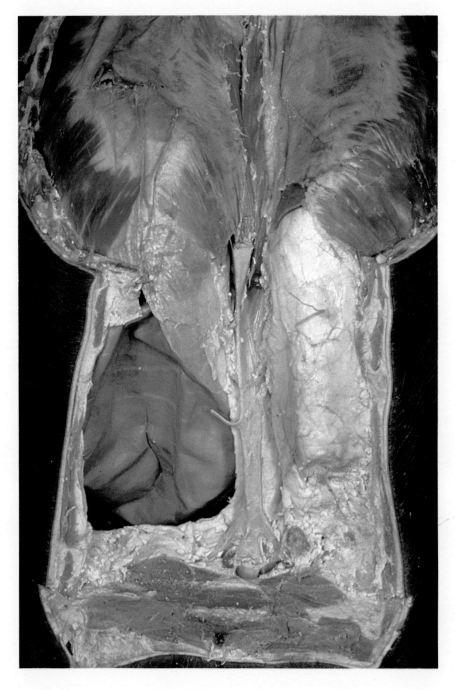

Fig. 5.38 The abdominal viscera of the 4-month calf, in dorsal view.

This figure is a further stage of the dissection shown in fig. 5.37.

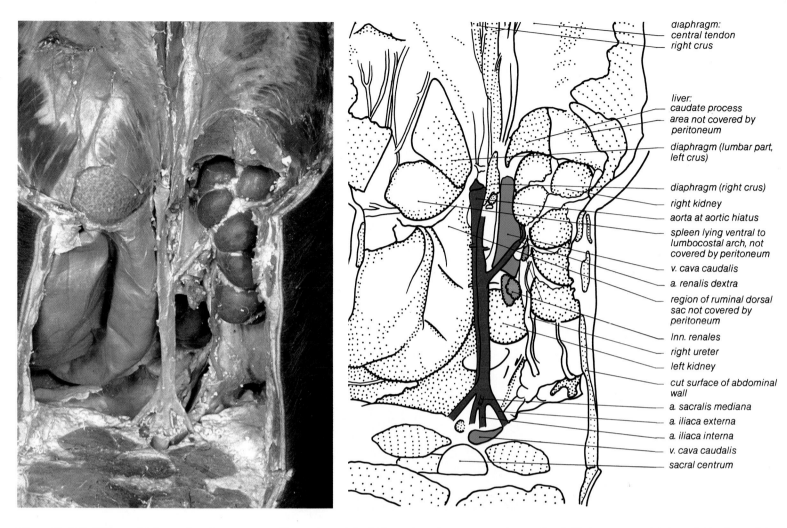

diaphragm:
central tendon
right crus

liver:
caudate process
area not covered by peritoneum

diaphragm (lumbar part, left crus)

diaphragm (right crus)

right kidney

aorta at aortic hiatus

spleen lying ventral to lumbocostal arch, not covered by peritoneum

v. cava caudalis

a. renalis dextra

region of ruminal dorsal sac not covered by peritoneum

lnn. renales

right ureter

left kidney

cut surface of abdominal wall

a. sacralis mediana

a. iliaca externa

a. iliaca interna

v. cava caudalis

sacral centrum

Fig. 5.39 The abdominal viscera lying cranial to the pelvis in the 4-month calf: dorsal view.

The aorta and the kidneys have been removed to display the intestine. The colon and duodenum have been displaced laterally to show the caecum; this should be compared with the unusual position shown in figs. 5.27 and 5.34.

Fig. 5.45 shows a cranial view of this dissection with colon and duodenum *in situ*. The sequence of these dissections of the abdomen of a 4-month calf continues with cranial views of the viscera, beginning at fig. 5.40.

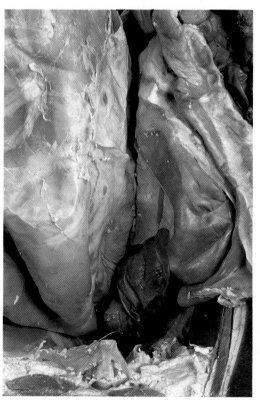

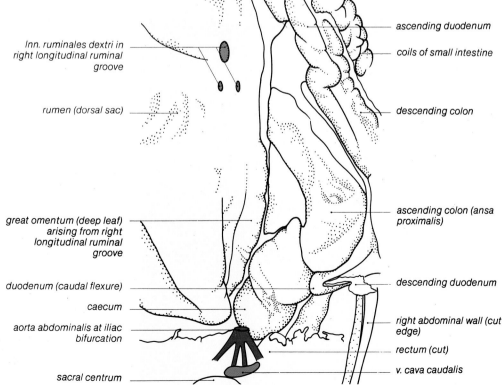

lnn. ruminales dextri in right longitudinal ruminal groove

rumen (dorsal sac)

great omentum (deep leaf) arising from right longitudinal ruminal groove

duodenum (caudal flexure)

caecum

aorta abdominalis at iliac bifurcation

sacral centrum

ascending duodenum

coils of small intestine

descending colon

ascending colon (ansa proximalis)

descending duodenum

right abdominal wall (cut edge)

rectum (cut)

v. cava caudalis

Fig. 5.40 The abdominal viscera of the 4-month calf, after removal of the diaphragm: cranial view.

Fig. 4.34 shows this specimen before removal of the diaphragm. The spleen is enlarged by barbiturate euthanasia; the approximate outline of the spleen in life is indicated by a broken blue line (compare with figs. 5.17 and 5.47).

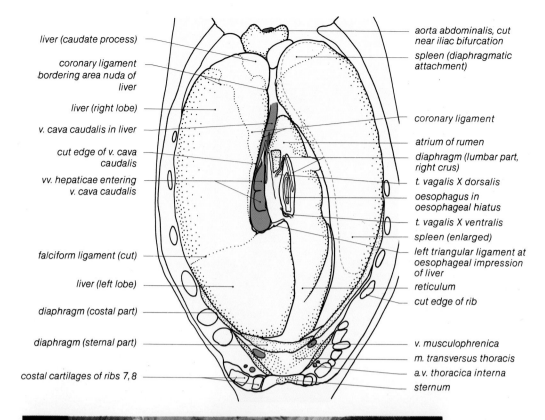

liver (caudate process)

coronary ligament bordering area nuda of liver

liver (right lobe)

v. cava caudalis in liver

cut edge of v. cava caudalis

vv. hepaticae entering v. cava caudalis

falciform ligament (cut)

liver (left lobe)

diaphragm (costal part)

diaphragm (sternal part)

costal cartilages of ribs 7, 8

aorta abdominalis, cut near iliac bifurcation

spleen (diaphragmatic attachment)

coronary ligament

atrium of rumen

diaphragm (lumbar part, right crus)

t. vagalis X dorsalis

oesophagus in oesophageal hiatus

t. vagalis X ventralis

spleen (enlarged)

left triangular ligament at oesophageal impression of liver

reticulum

cut edge of rib

v. musculophrenica

m. transversus thoracis

a.v. thoracica interna

sternum

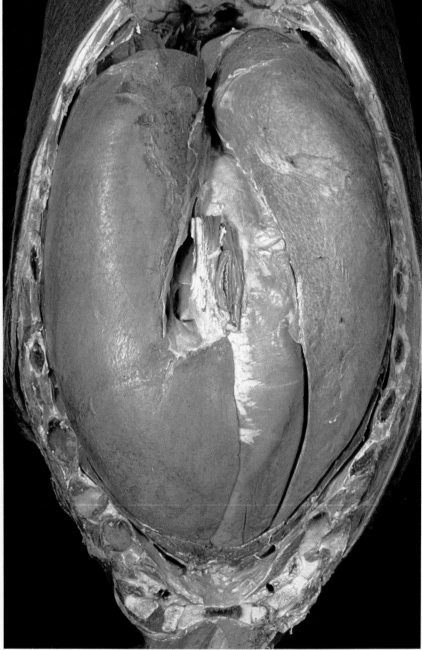

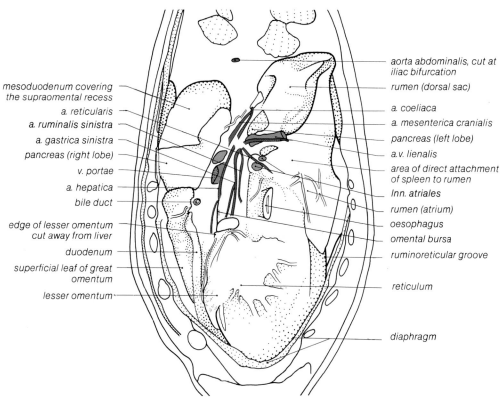

mesoduodenum covering the supraomental recess
a. reticularis
a. ruminalis sinistra
a. gastrica sinistra
pancreas (right lobe)
v. portae
a. hepatica
bile duct
edge of lesser omentum cut away from liver
duodenum
superficial leaf of great omentum
lesser omentum

aorta abdominalis, cut at iliac bifurcation
rumen (dorsal sac)
a. coeliaca
a. mesenterica cranialis
pancreas (left lobe)
a.v. lienalis
area of direct attachment of spleen to rumen
lnn. atriales
rumen (atrium)
oesophagus
omental bursa
ruminoreticular groove
reticulum

diaphragm

Fig. 5.41 The abdominal viscera of the 4-month calf after removal of the spleen, liver and kidneys: cranial view.

The omasum, shown in fig. 5.42, is too small in this young calf to be distinguished until the lesser omentum has been removed.

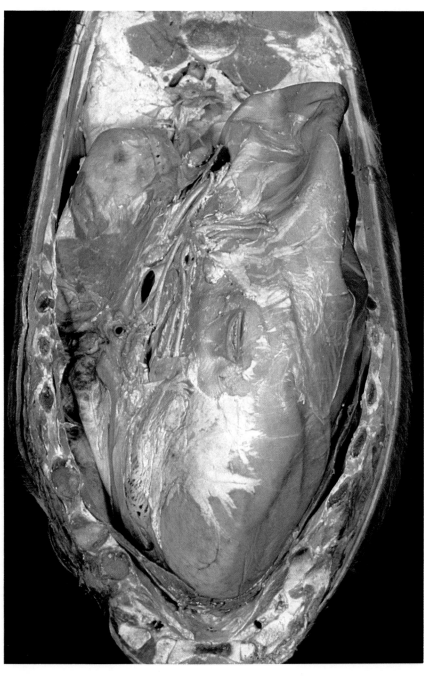

Fig. 5.42 The abdominal viscera of the 4-month calf and the distribution of the coeliac artery: right cranial view.

Removal of the lesser omentum reveals the small omasum. The cranial part of the great omentum has been removed to display the apex of the supraomental recess. The large right ruminal branch of the coeliac artery is not displayed (see figs. 5.26 and 5.53).

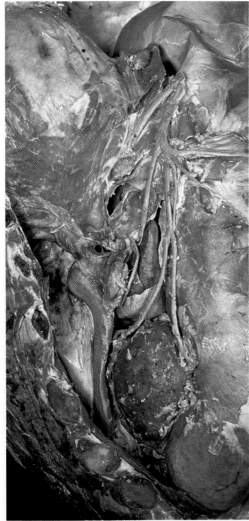
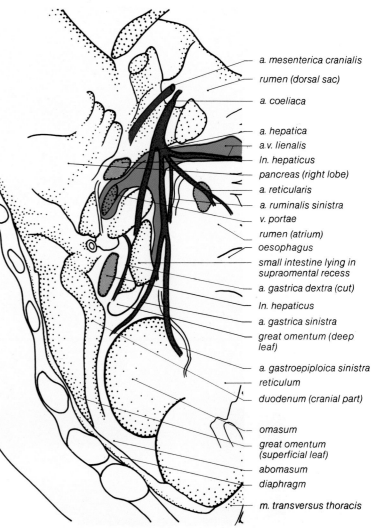

a. mesenterica cranialis
rumen (dorsal sac)
a. coeliaca
a. hepatica
a.v. lienalis
ln. hepaticus
pancreas (right lobe)
a. reticularis
a. ruminalis sinistra
v. portae
rumen (atrium)
oesophagus
small intestine lying in supraomental recess
a. gastrica dextra (cut)
ln. hepaticus
a. gastrica sinistra
great omentum (deep leaf)
a. gastroepiploica sinistra
reticulum
duodenum (cranial part)
omasum
great omentum (superficial leaf)
abomasum
diaphragm
m. transversus thoracis

Fig. 5.43 The pancreas and the caudal omental recess of the 4-month calf, in cranial view.

The caudal omental recess has been displayed by cutting the superfical leaf of the great omentum away from the duodenum and reflecting it laterally. The pancreatic duct is too far caudal to be seen (see fig. 5.32).

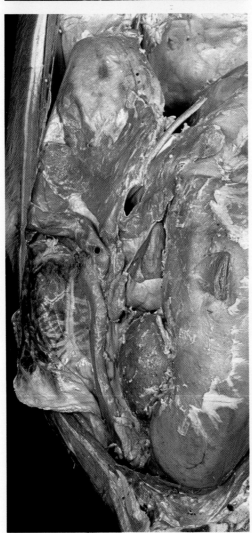
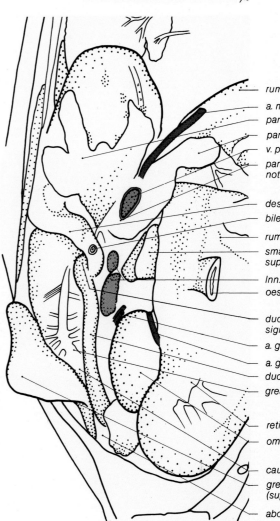

rumen (dorsal sac)
a. mesenterica cranialis
pancreas (right lobe)
pancreas (left lobe)
v. portae
pancreas (body with notch)
descending duodenum
bile duct
rumen (atrium)
small intestine in supraomental recess
lnn. hepatici
oesophagus
duodenum (ansa sigmoidea)
a. gastrica sinistra
a. gastroepiploica sinistra
duodenum (cranial part)
great omentum (deep leaf)
reticulum
omasum
caudal omental recess
great omentum (superficial leaf)
abomasum

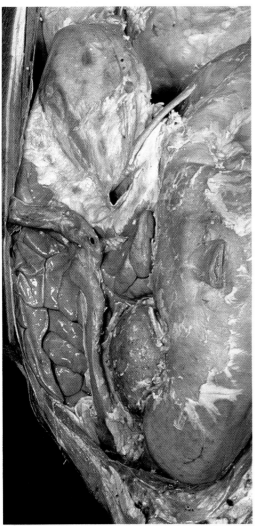

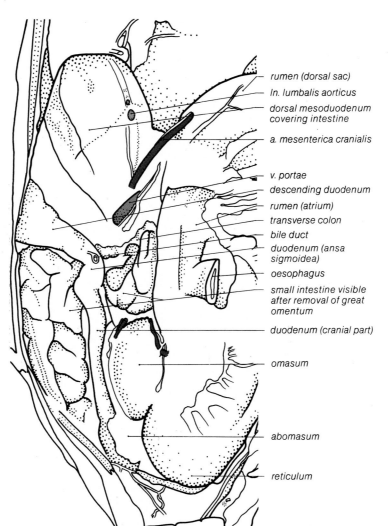

Fig. 5.44 The abdominal viscera of the 4-month calf after removal of the great omentum and pancreas: cranial view.
The lateral and cranial walls of the supraomental recess have been removed to expose the intestines, but the caudal roof of the recess, formed by the mesoduodenum, remains intact.

rumen (dorsal sac)
ln. lumbalis aorticus
dorsal mesoduodenum covering intestine
a. mesenterica cranialis
v. portae
descending duodenum
rumen (atrium)
transverse colon
bile duct
duodenum (ansa sigmoidea)
oesophagus
small intestine visible after removal of great omentum
duodenum (cranial part)
omasum
abomasum
reticulum

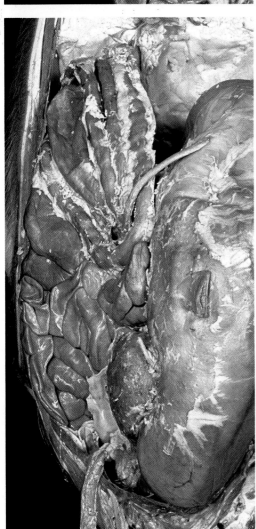

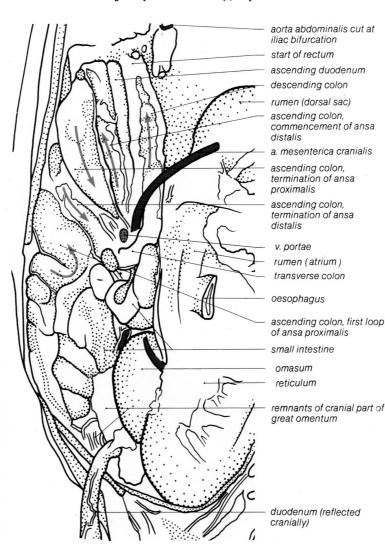

Fig. 5.45 The intestine within the supraomental recess of the 4-month calf, in cranial view.
Removal of the mesoduodenum and descending duodenum has exposed the large intestine lying dorsally in the supraomental recess of the peritoneal cavity. Blue arrows indicate the direction of flow of ingesta in the various parts of the colon. Compare with the dorsal view (fig. 5.39) and with the lateral view of the adult cow (fig. 5.34).

aorta abdominalis cut at iliac bifurcation
start of rectum
ascending duodenum
descending colon
rumen (dorsal sac)
ascending colon, commencement of ansa distalis
a. mesenterica cranialis
ascending colon, termination of ansa proximalis
ascending colon, termination of ansa distalis
v. portae
rumen (atrium)
transverse colon
oesophagus
ascending colon, first loop of ansa proximalis
small intestine
omasum
reticulum
remnants of cranial part of great omentum
duodenum (reflected cranially)

Fig. 5.46 The abdominal viscera caudal to the diaphragm, in the 1-week bull calf: left lateral view.

The spleen is enlarged; in life it does not extend caudal to the last rib.

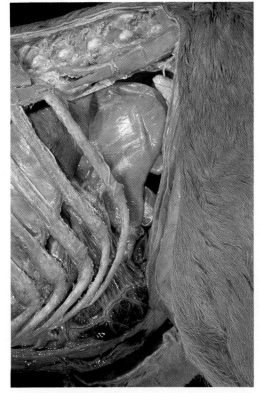

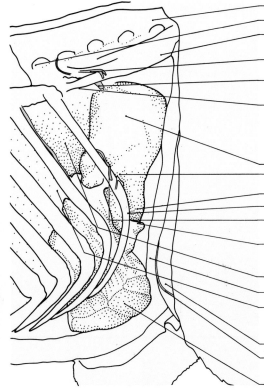

m. longissimus (cut)
mammillary process of L1
m. iliocostalis
n. lumbalis I:
r. cutaneus lateralis dorsalis
r. ventralis
cut edge of m. transversus abdominis, transversus fascia, and parietal peritoneum
rumen:
dorsal sac
left dorsal coronary groove
dorsal blind sac
rib 13
n. costoabdominalis (Th XIII)
attachment of superficial leaf of great omentum to rumen (caudal groove)
spleen (enlarged)
abdominal wall
diaphragm (costal part showing limits of costal attachments)
position of stifle joint
n. cutaneus femoris lateralis (L III, IV)
omental bursa (with fluid)

Fig. 5.47 The abdominal viscera in the 1-week calf, after removal of the rib cage: left lateral view.

The diaphragm and the caudal lobe of the left lung have also been removed. The spleen is enlarged after barbiturate euthanasia; this obscures most of the abdominal cavity cranial to the costal arch. This figure should be compared with fig. 5.17, but it should be noted that the adult cow was put down with chloral hydrate and does not show splenic enlargement.

aorta thoracica
scapular cartilage
dorsocaudal mediastinum
ln. mediastinalis caudalis
oesophagus
right crus of diaphragm
t. vagalis X . ventralis
n phrenicus
rumen (atrium)
reticulum
left lung (cranial lobe)
rib 6
position of olecranon

rumen (dorsal sac)
spleen (normal outline)
spleen (enlarged)
left kidney
t. vagalis X . dorsalis
accessory lobe of right lung (covered by mediastinum)
small intestine lying caudal to the supraomental recess
abomasum
omental bursa (filled with preserving fluid)

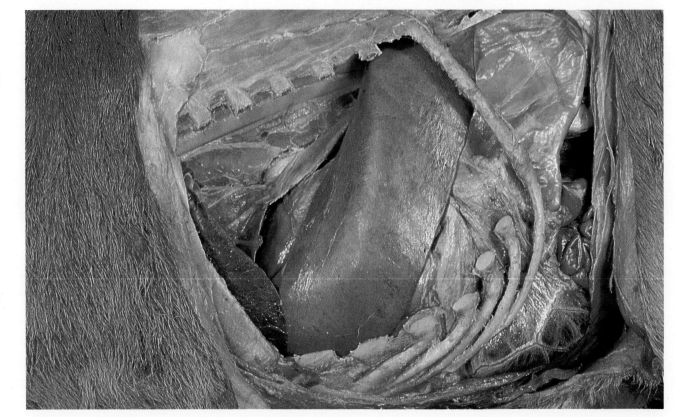

Fig. 5.48 The oesophageal hiatus of the diaphragm and associated structures of the thorax and abdomen in the 1-week calf: left lateral view.

The hiatus has been exposed by reflecting the crura of the diaphragm with a glass rod (compare with fig. 5.47).

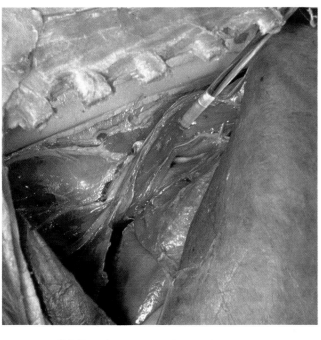
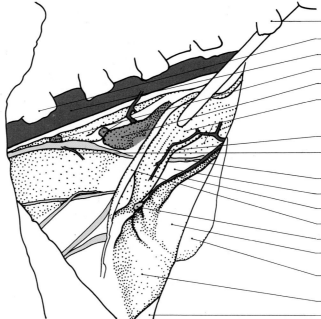

- rib 12
- rib 8
- aorta thoracica
- lnn. haemales
- ln. mediastinalis caudalis
- right crus of diaphragm surrounding the oesophageal hiatus
- a. reticularis r. phrenicus
- a. broncho-oesophagea r. oesophageus
- t. vagalis X dorsalis
- position of cardia
- a. reticularis
- diaphragm (cut edge)
- t. vagalis X ventralis
- rumen (atrium)
- area of splenic attachment to diaphragm
- reticulum
- abomasum

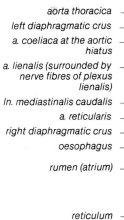
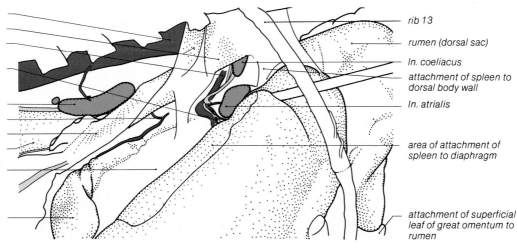

- aorta thoracica
- left diaphragmatic crus
- a. coeliaca at the aortic hiatus
- a. lienalis (surrounded by nerve fibres of plexus lienalis)
- ln. mediastinalis caudalis
- a. reticularis
- right diaphragmatic crus
- oesophagus
- rumen (atrium)
- reticulum

- rib 13
- rumen (dorsal sac)
- ln. coeliacus
- attachment of spleen to dorsal body wall
- ln. atrialis
- area of attachment of spleen to diaphragm
- attachment of superficial leaf of great omentum to rumen

Fig. 5.49 The aortic hiatus of the diaphragm and associated structures in the 1-week calf: left lateral view.

The hiatus has been exposed by depressing the spleen with a glass rod, (compare with fig. 5.47).

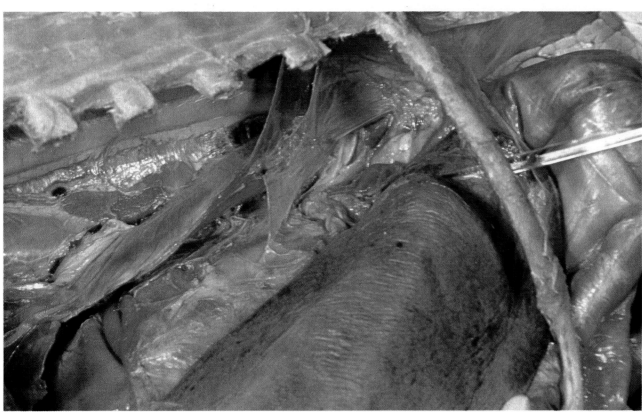

5.33

Fig. 5.50 The abdominal viscera in the 1-week calf after removal of the spleen: left lateral view.

The dorsal sac of the rumen has been reflected laterally to reveal the left kidney and the intestine within, and caudal to, the supraomental peritoneal recess.

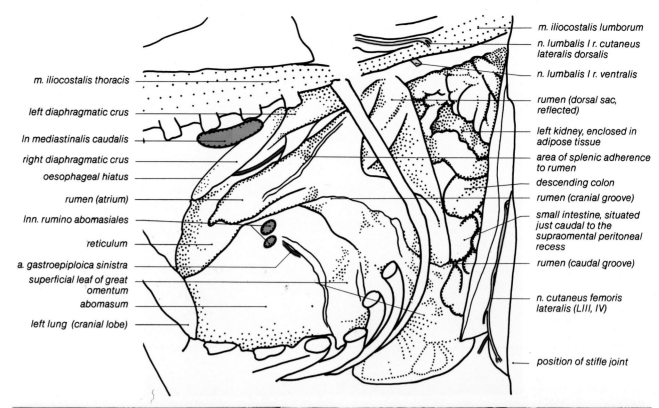

m. iliocostalis thoracis

left diaphragmatic crus

ln mediastinalis caudalis

right diaphragmatic crus

oesophageal hiatus

rumen (atrium)

lnn. rumino abomasiales

reticulum

a. gastroepiploica sinistra

superficial leaf of great omentum

abomasum

left lung (cranial lobe)

m. iliocostalis lumborum

n. lumbalis I r. cutaneus lateralis dorsalis

n. lumbalis I r. ventralis

rumen (dorsal sac, reflected)

left kidney, enclosed in adipose tissue

area of splenic adherence to rumen

descending colon

rumen (cranial groove)

small intestine, situated just caudal to the supraomental peritoneal recess

rumen (caudal groove)

n. cutaneus femoris lateralis (LIII, IV)

position of stifle joint

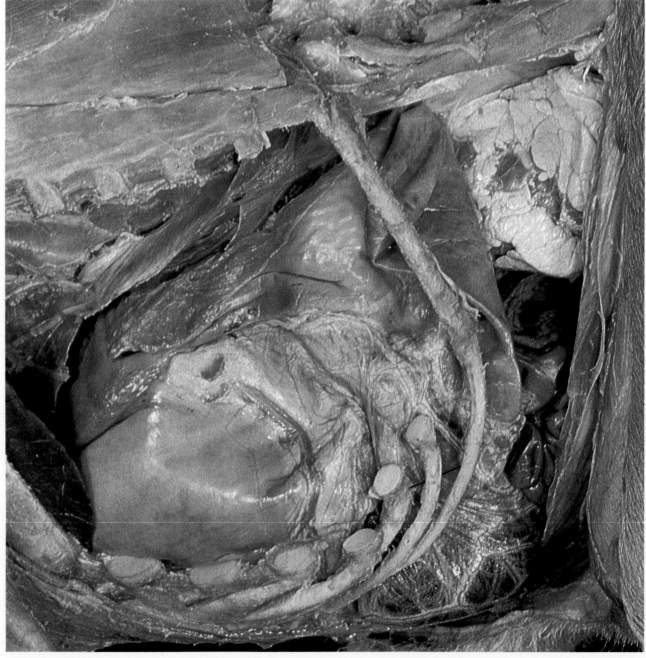

5.34

Fig. 5.51 The aortic hiatus and associated structures in the 1-week calf after removal of the spleen: left lateral view.

A deeper dissection of this region is shown in fig. 5.53.

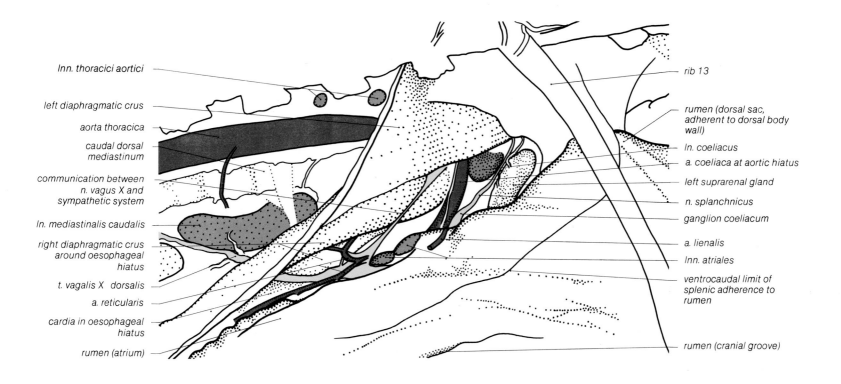

Inn. thoracici aortici

left diaphragmatic crus

aorta thoracica

caudal dorsal mediastinum

communication between n. vagus X and sympathetic system

ln. mediastinalis caudalis

right diaphragmatic crus around oesophageal hiatus

t. vagalis X dorsalis

a. reticularis

cardia in oesophageal hiatus

rumen (atrium)

rib 13

rumen (dorsal sac, adherent to dorsal body wall)

ln. coeliacus

a. coeliaca at aortic hiatus

left suprarenal gland

n. splanchnicus

ganglion coeliacum

a. lienalis

lnn. atriales

ventrocaudal limit of splenic adherence to rumen

rumen (cranial groove)

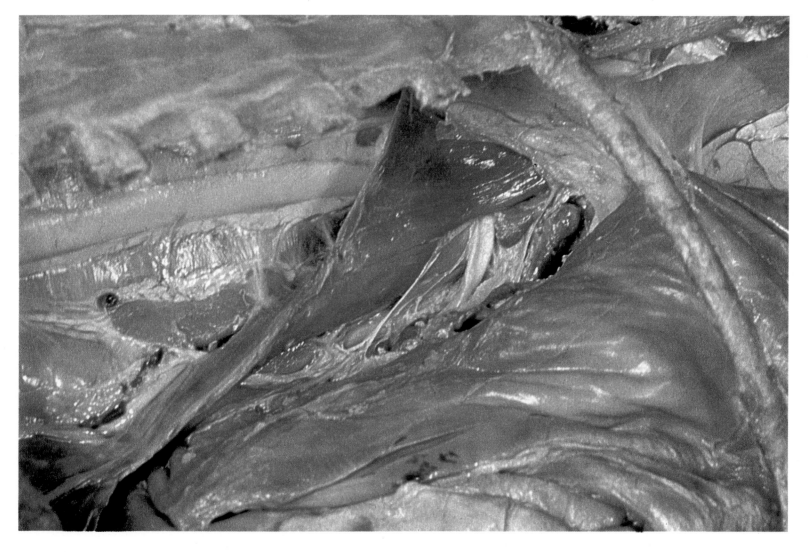

5.35

Fig. 5.52 The interior of the reticulum and the dorsal ruminal sac in the 1-week calf: left lateral view.

This calf had been milk-fed, with access to hay and straw.

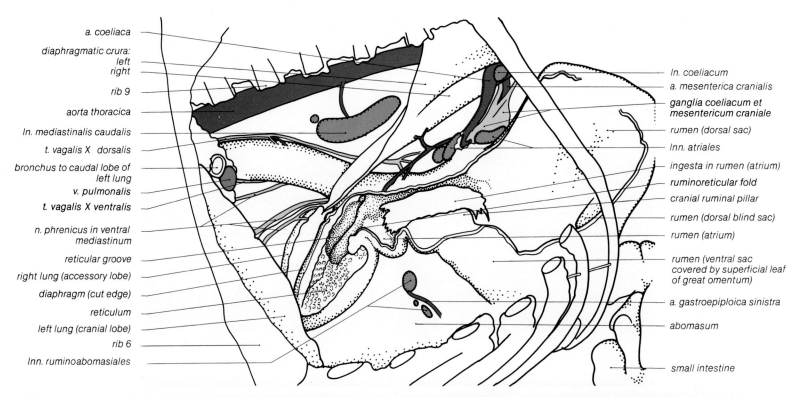

a. coeliaca

diaphragmatic crura:
left
right

rib 9

aorta thoracica

ln. mediastinalis caudalis

t. vagalis X dorsalis

bronchus to caudal lobe of left lung

v. pulmonalis

t. vagalis X ventralis

n. phrenicus in ventral mediastinum

reticular groove

right lung (accessory lobe)

diaphragm (cut edge)

reticulum

left lung (cranial lobe)

rib 6

lnn. ruminoabomasiales

ln. coeliacum

a. mesenterica cranialis

ganglia coeliacum et mesentericum craniale

rumen (dorsal sac)

lnn. atriales

ingesta in rumen (atrium)

ruminoreticular fold

cranial ruminal pillar

rumen (dorsal blind sac)

rumen (atrium)

rumen (ventral sac covered by superficial leaf of great omentum)

a. gastroepiploica sinistra

abomasum

small intestine

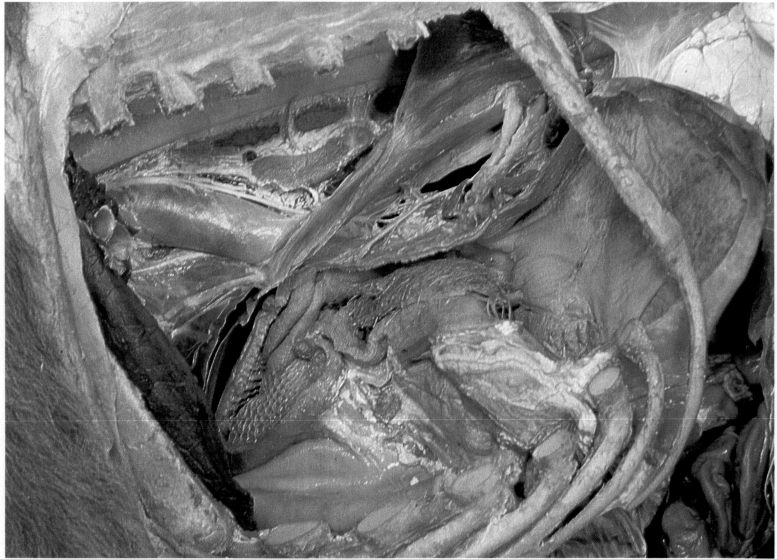

Fig. 5.53 Nerves, blood vessels and lymph nodes of the aortic and oesophageal hiatuses in the 1-week calf: left lateral view.

This is a closer view of a part of the dissection shown in fig. 5.52. A more superficial view of this region, prior to removal of the spleen, is shown in fig. 5.49.

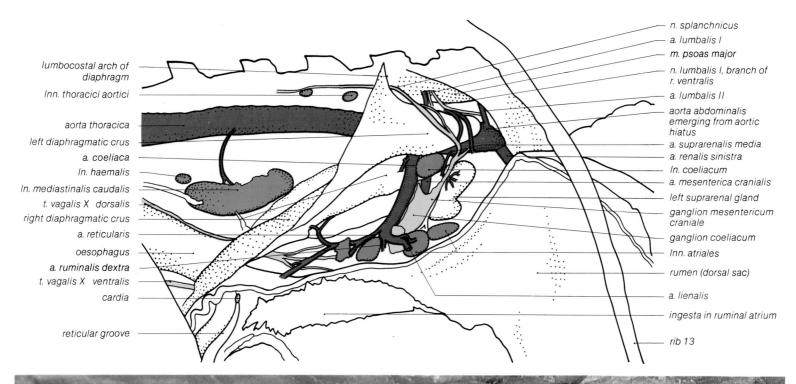

lumbocostal arch of diaphragm
Inn. thoracici aortici
aorta thoracica
left diaphragmatic crus
a. coeliaca
In. haemalis
In. mediastinalis caudalis
t. vagalis X dorsalis
right diaphragmatic crus
a. reticularis
oesophagus
a. ruminalis dextra
t. vagalis X ventralis
cardia
reticular groove

n. splanchnicus
a. lumbalis I
m. psoas major
n. lumbalis I, branch of r. ventralis
a. lumbalis II
aorta abdominalis emerging from aortic hiatus
a. suprarenalis media
a. renalis sinistra
In. coeliacum
a. mesenterica cranialis
left suprarenal gland
ganglion mesentericum craniale
ganglion coeliacum
Inn. atriales
rumen (dorsal sac)
a. lienalis
ingesta in ruminal atrium
rib 13

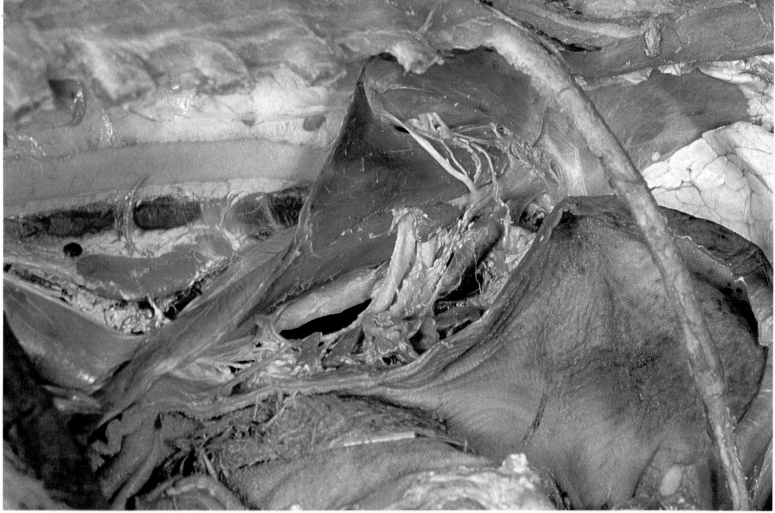

**Fig. 5.54
Superficial
abdominal
viscera of the
1-week calf,
in right lateral
view.**

The abdominal wall,
ribs, diaphragm and
caudal lobe of the right
lung have been
removed. Compare this
figure with the similar
dissection of the cow
(fig. 5.30).

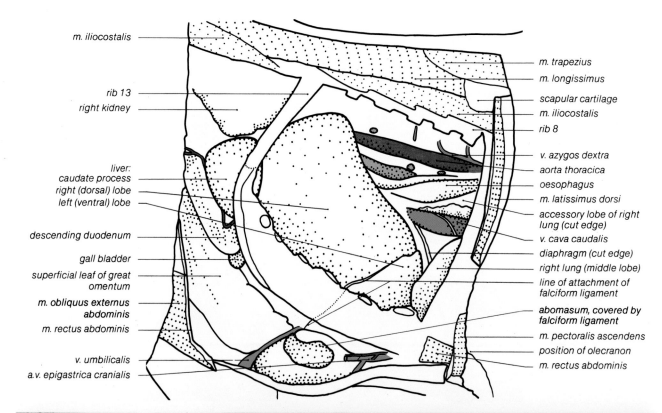

m. iliocostalis

rib 13

right kidney

liver:
caudate process
right (dorsal) lobe
left (ventral) lobe

descending duodenum

gall bladder

superficial leaf of great
omentum

m. obliquus externus
abdominis

m. rectus abdominis

v. umbilicalis

a.v. epigastrica cranialis

m. trapezius

m. longissimus

scapular cartilage

m. iliocostalis

rib 8

v. azygos dextra

aorta thoracica

oesophagus

m. latissimus dorsi

accessory lobe of right
lung (cut edge)

v. cava caudalis

diaphragm (cut edge)

right lung (middle lobe)

line of attachment of
falciform ligament

abomasum, covered by
falciform ligament

m. pectoralis ascendens

position of olecranon

m. rectus abdominis

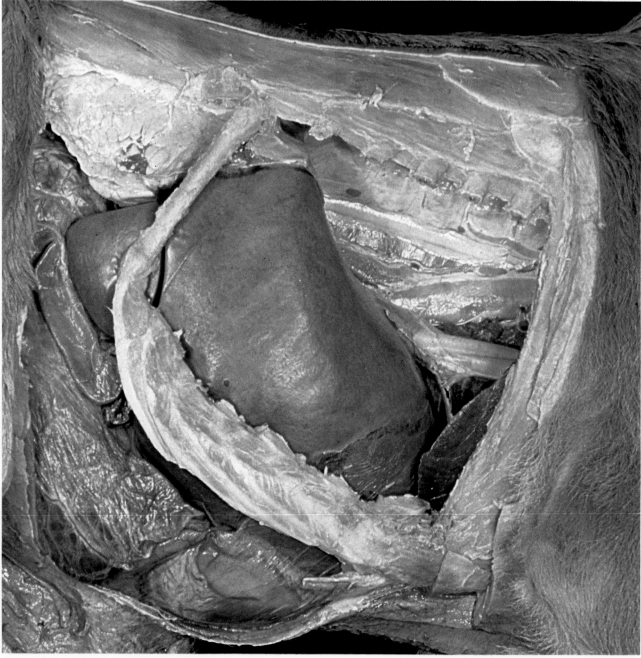

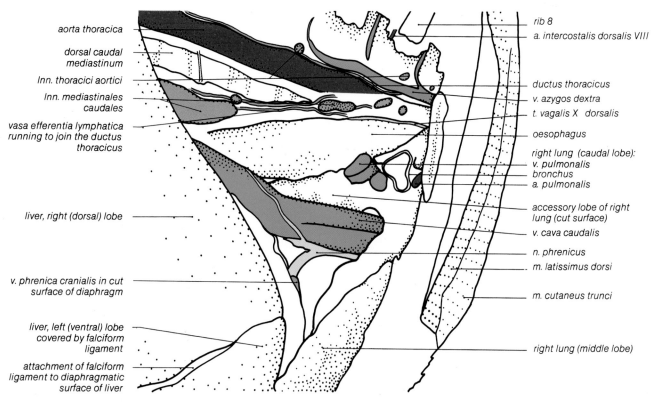

aorta thoracica

dorsal caudal mediastinum

Inn. thoracici aortici

Inn. mediastinales caudales

vasa efferentia lymphatica running to join the ductus thoracicus

liver, right (dorsal) lobe

v. phrenica cranialis in cut surface of diaphragm

liver, left (ventral) lobe covered by falciform ligament

attachment of falciform ligament to diaphragmatic surface of liver

rib 8

a. intercostalis dorsalis VIII

ductus thoracicus

v. azygos dextra

t. vagalis X dorsalis

oesophagus

right lung (caudal lobe):
v. pulmonalis
bronchus
a. pulmonalis

accessory lobe of right lung (cut surface)

v. cava caudalis

n. phrenicus

m. latissimus dorsi

m. cutaneus trunci

right lung (middle lobe)

Fig. 5.55 Vessels, lymph nodes and nerves of the caudal mediastinum in the 1-week calf: right lateral view.

This is a closer view of a part of the dissection shown in fig. 5.54.

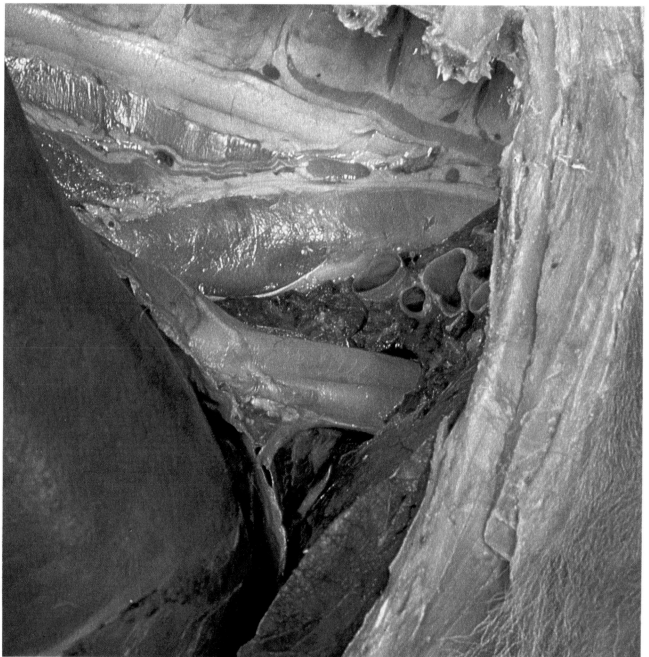

Fig. 5.56 The abdominal viscera and mesenteries after removal of the liver in the 1-week calf: right lateral view.

The arrow marks the position of the epiploic foramen, through which the lesser peritoneal sac (omental bursa) communicates with the greater peritoneal sac. Fig. 5.57 shows a further stage in the dissection. The visceral surface of the liver in a foetal calf is shown in fig. 5.60.

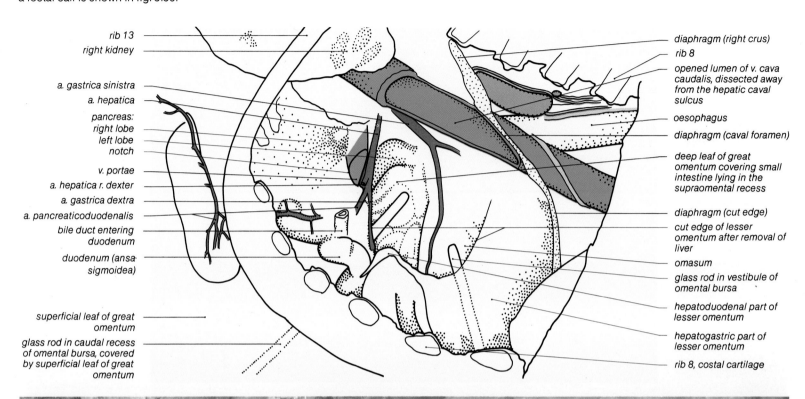

rib 13
right kidney

a. gastrica sinistra
a. hepatica

pancreas:
right lobe
left lobe
notch

v. portae
a. hepatica r. dexter
a. gastrica dextra
a. pancreaticoduodenalis
bile duct entering duodenum

duodenum (ansa sigmoidea)

superficial leaf of great omentum

glass rod in caudal recess of omental bursa, covered by superficial leaf of great omentum

diaphragm (right crus)
rib 8
opened lumen of v. cava caudalis, dissected away from the hepatic caval sulcus

oesophagus
diaphragm (caval foramen)

deep leaf of great omentum covering small intestine lying in the supraomental recess

diaphragm (cut edge)
cut edge of lesser omentum after removal of liver

omasum
glass rod in vestibule of omental bursa

hepatoduodenal part of lesser omentum

hepatogastric part of lesser omentum

rib 8, costal cartilage

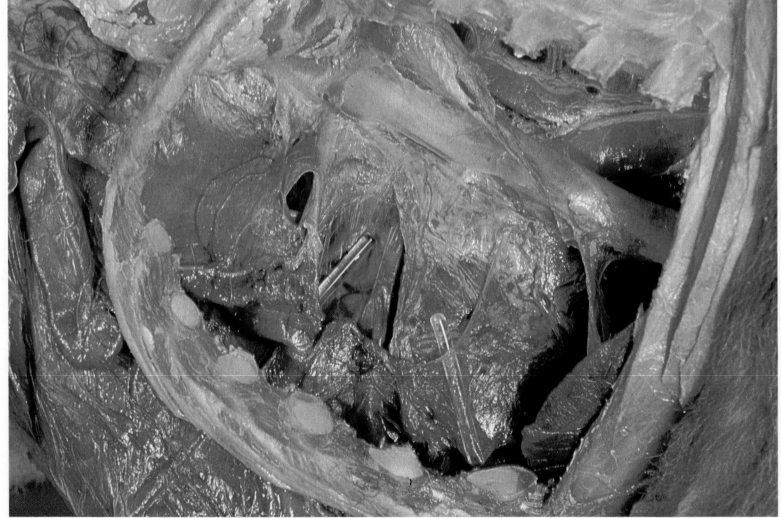

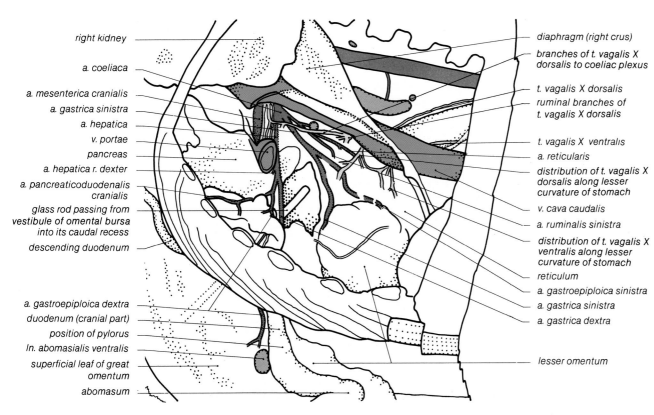

right kidney
a. coeliaca
a. mesenterica cranialis
a. gastrica sinistra
a. hepatica
v. portae
pancreas
a. hepatica r. dexter
a. pancreaticoduodenalis cranialis
glass rod passing from vestibule of omental bursa into its caudal recess
descending duodenum

a. gastroepiploica dextra
duodenum (cranial part)
position of pylorus
ln. abomasialis ventralis
superficial leaf of great omentum
abomasum

diaphragm (right crus)
branches of t. vagalis X dorsalis to coeliac plexus
t. vagalis X dorsalis
ruminal branches of t. vagalis X dorsalis
t. vagalis X ventralis
a. reticularis
distribution of t. vagalis X dorsalis along lesser curvature of stomach
v. cava caudalis
a. ruminalis sinistra
distribution of t. vagalis X ventralis along lesser curvature of stomach
reticulum
a. gastroepiploica sinistra
a. gastrica sinistra
a. gastrica dextra

lesser omentum

Fig. 5.57 Arteries and nerves of the stomach in the 1-week calf: right lateral view.
The abomasum has been displaced ventrally.

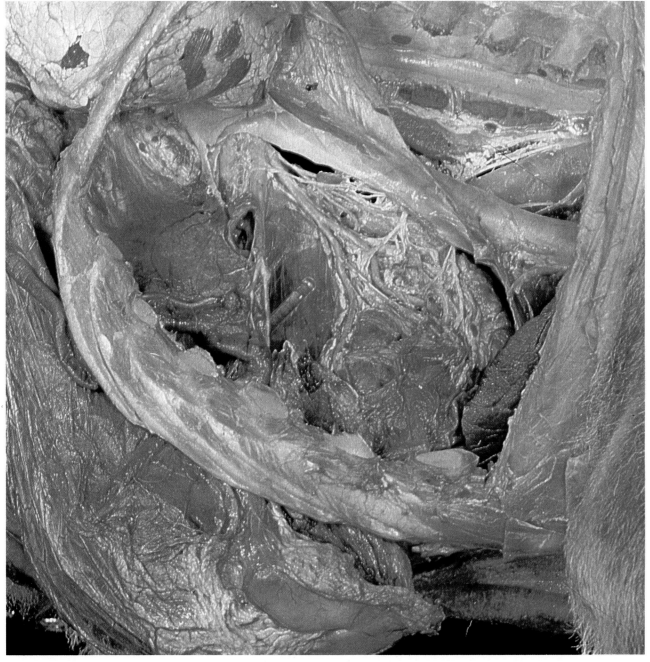

Fig. 5.58 Viscera and blood vessels of thorax and abdomen in a female bovine foetus (aged about 230 days), in left lateral view.

The left lung and all of the abdominal viscera except liver, kidneys and urinary bladder have been removed. Note the relative sizes of left and right ventricles, and compare with those seen in the adult cow (fig.4.17). Further details are shown in figs. 5.59 and 5.60.

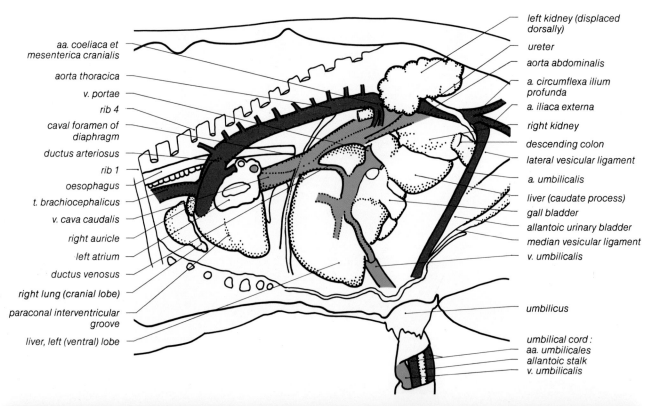

aa. coeliaca et mesenterica cranialis
aorta thoracica
v. portae
rib 4
caval foramen of diaphragm
ductus arteriosus
rib 1
oesophagus
t. brachiocephalicus
v. cava caudalis
right auricle
left atrium
ductus venosus
right lung (cranial lobe)
paraconal interventricular groove
liver, left (ventral) lobe

left kidney (displaced dorsally)
ureter
aorta abdominalis
a. circumflexa ilium profunda
a. iliaca externa
right kidney
descending colon
lateral vesicular ligament
a. umbilicalis
liver (caudate process)
gall bladder
allantoic urinary bladder
median vesicular ligament
v. umbilicalis
umbilicus
umbilical cord:
aa. umbilicales
allantoic stalk
v. umbilicalis

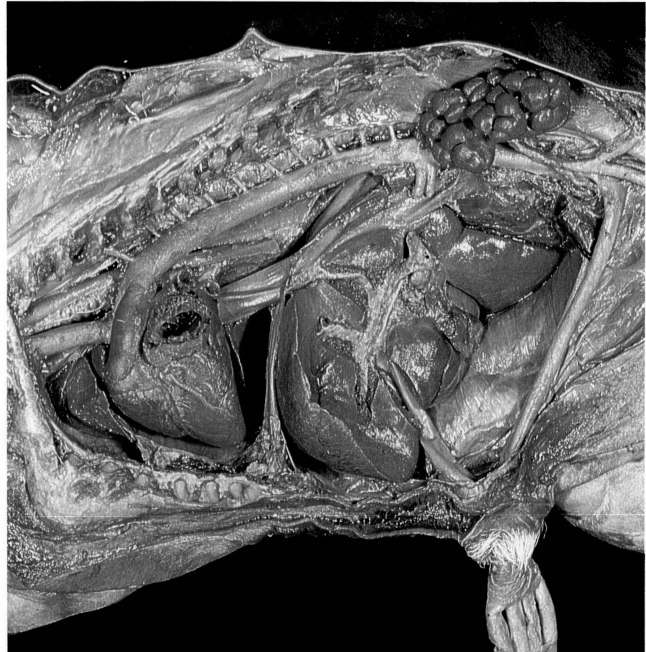

Fig.5.59 The base of the foetal heart to show components of the foetal circulation: left lateral view.

The tubular foramen ovale has been filled with a plug of cotton wool to show the rather irregular orifice leading into the left atrium from the caudal vena cava. This orifice undergoes anatomical closure 2 or 3 weeks after birth.

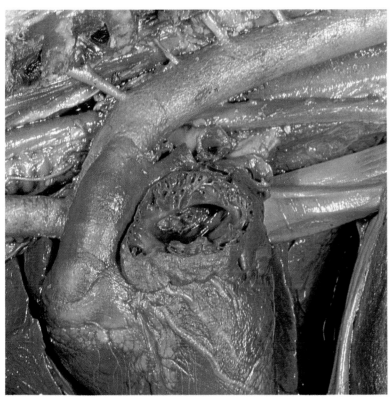

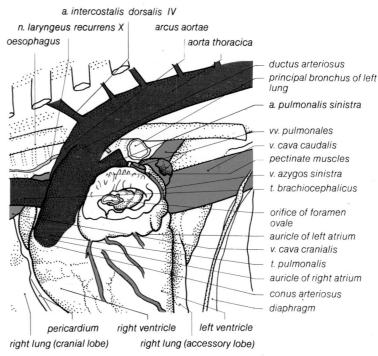

a. intercostalis dorsalis IV
n. laryngeus recurrens X
oesophagus
arcus aortae
aorta thoracica
ductus arteriosus
principal bronchus of left lung
a. pulmonalis sinistra
vv. pulmonales
v. cava caudalis
pectinate muscles
v. azygos sinistra
t. brachiocephalicus
orifice of foramen ovale
auricle of left atrium
v. cava cranialis
t. pulmonalis
auricle of right atrium
conus arteriosus
diaphragm
pericardium right ventricle left ventricle
right lung (cranial lobe) right lung (accessory lobe)

Fig.5.60 The visceral surface of the foetal liver to show the connections between umbilical, portal and caudal veins: left lateral view.

The veins have been dissected out from the liver parenchyma. In the ruminants, the ductus venosus persists until birth.

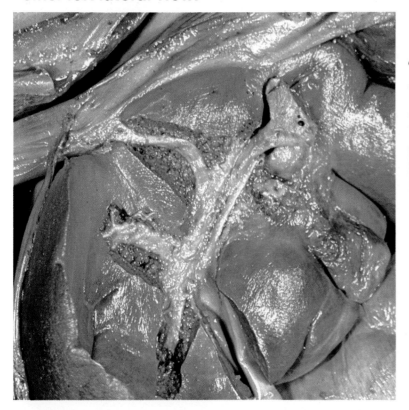

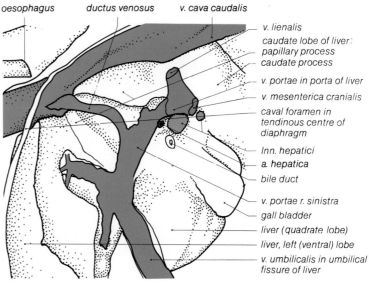

oesophagus ductus venosus v. cava caudalis
v. lienalis
caudate lobe of liver:
papillary process
caudate process
v. portae in porta of liver
v. mesenterica cranialis
caval foramen in tendinous centre of diaphragm
lnn. hepatici
a. hepatica
bile duct
v. portae r. sinistra
gall bladder
liver (quadrate lobe)
liver, left (ventral) lobe
v. umbilicalis in umbilical fissure of liver

Fig. 5.61 Abdominal viscera of a billy goat, aged 6 months, in left lateral view.

The abdominal and thoracic walls, diaphragm and caudal lobe of the left lung have all been removed. The position of this animal during embalming is described in the legend to fig. 5.65.

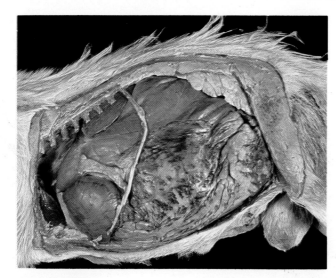

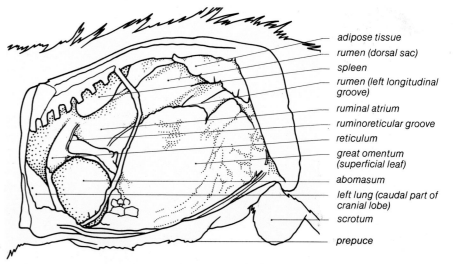

adipose tissue
rumen (dorsal sac)
spleen
rumen (left longitudinal groove)
ruminal atrium
ruminoreticular groove
reticulum
great omentum (superficial leaf)
abomasum
left lung (caudal part of cranial lobe)
scrotum
prepuce

Fig. 5.62 Abdominal viscera of the goat after removal of the great omentum: left lateral view.

The superficial leaf of the great omentum has been removed to display the full extent of the rumen.

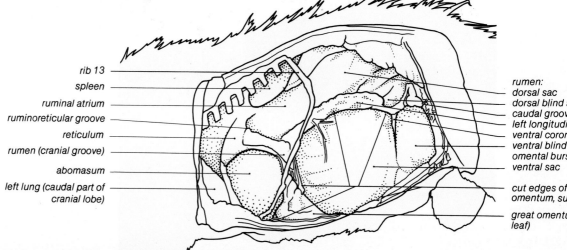

rib 13
spleen
ruminal atrium
ruminoreticular groove
reticulum
rumen (cranial groove)
abomasum
left lung (caudal part of cranial lobe)

rumen:
dorsal sac
dorsal blind sac
caudal groove
left longitudinal groove
ventral coronary groove
ventral blind sac lying in omental bursa
ventral sac

cut edges of great omentum, superficial leaf

great omentum, (deep leaf)

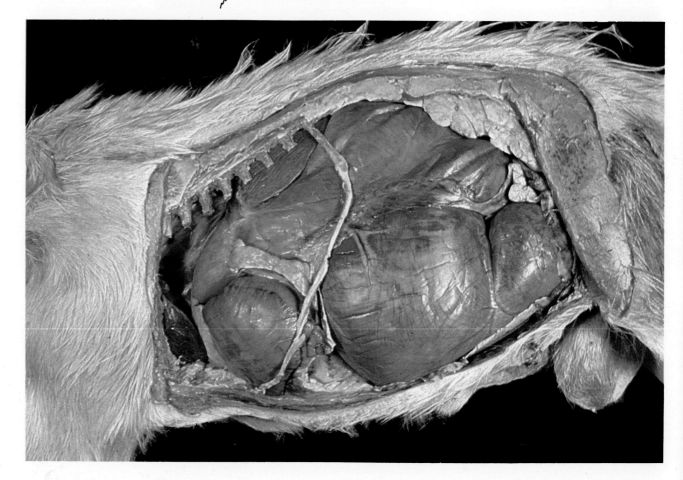

Fig. 5.63 Abdominal viscera of the goat, in right lateral view.

The dissection carried out on the left side (fig. 5.61) showed the attachment of the superficial leaf of the great omentum to the stomach. This dissection shows its attachments on the right side.

The dotted blue line shows where the superficial leaf was cut and removed at the next dissection, in fig. 5.64.

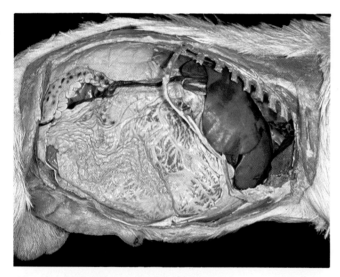

adipose tissue covering dorsal mesoduodenum

descending colon
duodenum (caudal flexure)
liver (caudate process)
descending duodenum
duodenum (cranial part)
rumen (dorsal sac)
great omentum (caudal border)
rib 7
liver (right lobe)
umbilical notch of the liver
gall bladder
great omentum (superficial leaf attaching dorsally to duodenum)
liver (left lobe)
costal arch

Fig. 5.64 The omental bursa of the goat, in right lateral view.

Removal of the superficial leaf of the great omentum has opened up the entire caudal recess of the omental bursa, which lies between superficial and deep omental leaves.

The dotted blue line shows where the deep leaf was cut and removed at the next dissection, in fig. 5.65.

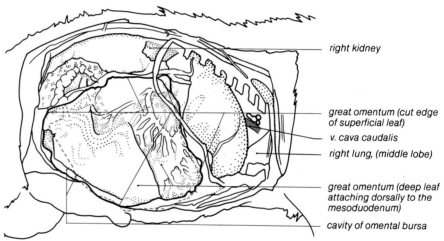

right kidney

great omentum (cut edge of superficial leaf)
v. cava caudalis
right lung, (middle lobe)

great omentum (deep leaf attaching dorsally to the mesoduodenum)

cavity of omental bursa

Fig.5.65 Abdominal viscera of the goat, showing the supraomental peritoneal recess and the great omentum: right lateral view.

This goat was embalmed while lying on its left side with the hind quarters elevated. The intestinal mass within the supraomental peritoneal recess has been displaced cranially. The apex of the caecum, which usually lies near the pelvic inlet has also been displaced as is shown by the arrow. Compare this figure with the dissection of the left side of the adult cow (fig. 5.27).

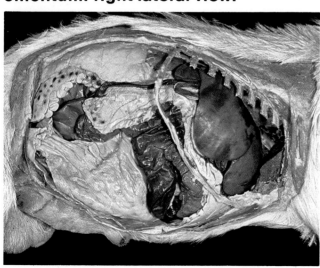

rumen (caudal groove)

great omentum (cut edge of deep leaf)

ascending colon (ansa proximalis)
great omentum: deep leaf, cut edge near attachment to mesoduodenum

great omentum (cut edge of superficial leaf)

supraomental peritoneal recess contains:
ileum
caecum

great omentum: deep leaf arising from right longitudinal ruminal groove, forming left wall of supraomental recess
cut edge of deep leaf
cut edge of superficial leaf

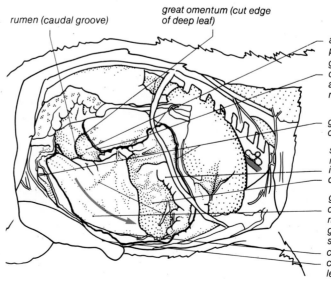

5.45

6 The Hindlimb

Fig. 6.1 Surface features of the pelvic regions, in left lateral view.

The palpable features have been shaved.

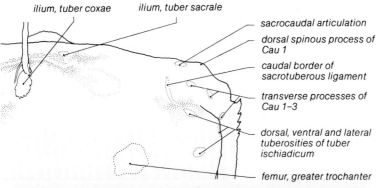

ilium, tuber coxae — ilium, tuber sacrale

sacrocaudal articulation
dorsal spinous process of Cau 1
caudal border of sacrotuberous ligament
transverse processes of Cau 1–3
dorsal, ventral and lateral tuberosities of tuber ischiadicum
femur, greater trochanter

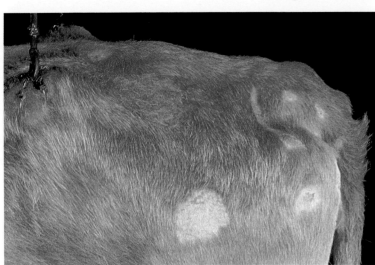

Fig. 6.2 Bones of the pelvic regions, in left lateral view.

The bony features shaved in fig. 6.1 have been coloured red. The tail has been mounted too low in this skeleton.

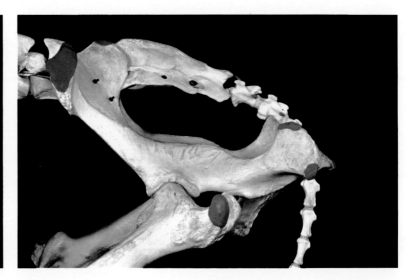

Fig. 6.3 Surface features of the hindlimb, in left lateral view (1).

The palpable features have been shaved. The patella is marked by an incision through which it was nailed to the femoral trochlea to fix the stifle joint.

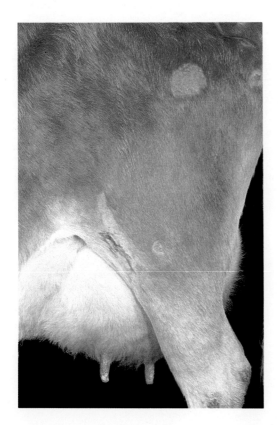

caudal border of sacrotuberous ligament

dorsal and lateral tuberosities of tuber ischiadicum
femur, greater trochanter
femoral region
femur, tuberculum of trochlea
patella
tibia, lateral condyle
tibia, extensor sulcus
patellar ligaments, lateral and intermediate
tibial tuberosity
tibial crest
crural region
calcaneus, tuberosity
tarsal region

udder   fibula, lateral malleolus

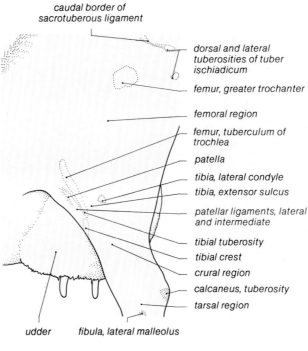

Fig. 6.4 Bones of the pelvic, femoral, crural and tarsal regions, in left lateral view.

The features shaved in fig. 6.3 have been coloured red except for the tuberculum of the femoral trochlea. The right stifle joint is superimposed on that of the left limb. The relative positions of patella and tuberculum vary with movements of the joint.

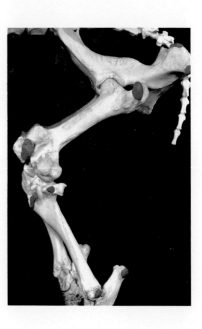

Fig. 6.5 Surface features of the hindlimb, in left lateral view (2).

The palpable features have been shaved. The patella is marked by an incision.

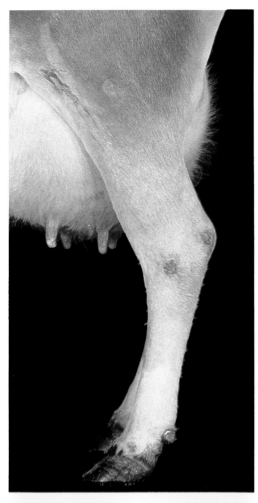

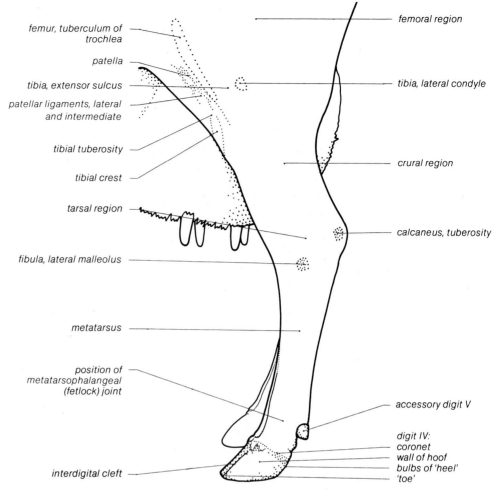

femur, tuberculum of trochlea

patella

tibia, extensor sulcus

patellar ligaments, lateral and intermediate

tibial tuberosity

tibial crest

tarsal region

fibula, lateral malleolus

metatarsus

position of metatarsophalangeal (fetlock) joint

interdigital cleft

femoral region

tibia, lateral condyle

crural region

calcaneus, tuberosity

accessory digit V

digit IV:
coronet
wall of hoof
bulbs of 'heel'
'toe'

Fig. 6.6 Bones of the femoral, crural, tarsal, metatarsal and digital regions, in left lateral view.

The features shaved in fig. 6.5 have been coloured red except for the tuberculum of the trochlear of the femur. Further details of the bones of the pes are given in figs. 7.10 – 7.12.

Fig. 6.7 Superficial muscles of the pelvis and hindlimb, in left lateral view.

The deep gluteal fascia and the fascia latae have been removed. A window has been excised in the deep crural fascia. The cutaneous nerves are shown in fig. 6.27.

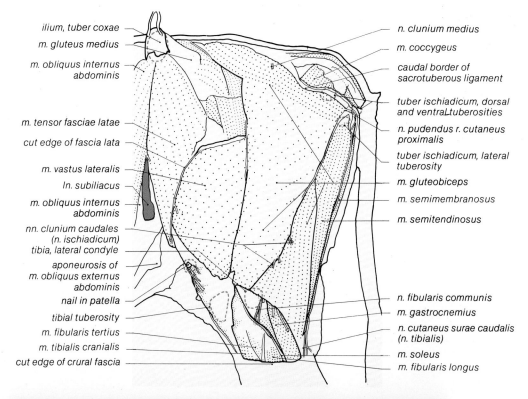

ilium, tuber coxae
m. gluteus medius
m. obliquus internus abdominis
m. tensor fasciae latae
cut edge of fascia lata
m. vastus lateralis
ln. subiliacus
m. obliquus internus abdominis
nn. clunium caudales (n. ischiadicum)
tibia, lateral condyle
aponeurosis of m. obliquus externus abdominis
nail in patella
tibial tuberosity
m. fibularis tertius
m. tibialis cranialis
cut edge of crural fascia

n. clunium medius
m. coccygeus
caudal border of sacrotuberous ligament
tuber ischiadicum, dorsal and ventral tuberosities
n. pudendus r. cutaneus proximalis
tuber ischiadicum, lateral tuberosity
m. gluteobiceps
m. semimembranosus
m. semitendinosus
n. fibularis communis
m. gastrocnemius
n. cutaneus surae caudalis (n. tibialis)
m. soleus
m. fibularis longus

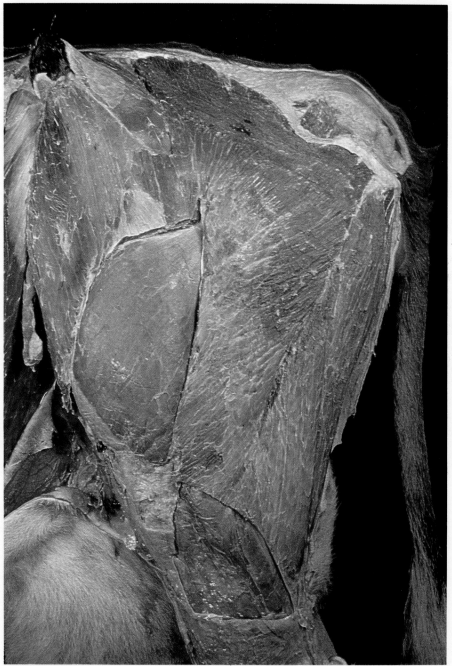

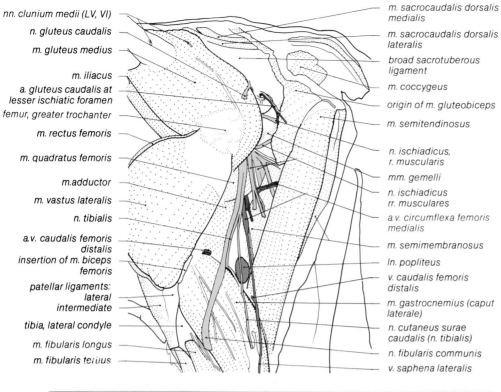

nn. clunium medii (LV, VI)
n. gluteus caudalis
m. gluteus medius
m. iliacus
a. gluteus caudalis at
lesser ischiatic foramen
femur, greater trochanter
m. rectus femoris
m. quadratus femoris
m.adductor
m. vastus lateralis
n. tibialis
a.v. caudalis femoris
distalis
insertion of m. biceps
femoris
patellar ligaments:
lateral
intermediate
tibia, lateral condyle
m. fibularis longus
m. fibularis tertius

m. sacrocaudalis dorsalis
medialis
m. sacrocaudalis dorsalis
lateralis
broad sacrotuberous
ligament
m. coccygeus
origin of m. gluteobiceps
m. semitendinosus
n. ischiadicus,
r. muscularis
mm. gemelli
n. ischiadicus
rr. musculares
a.v. circumflexa femoris
medialis
m. semimembranosus
ln. popliteus
v. caudalis femoris
distalis
m. gastrocnemius (caput
laterale)
n. cutaneus surae
caudalis (n. tibialis)
n. fibularis communis
v. saphena lateralis

Fig. 6.8 Deeper structures of the gluteal and femoral regions, in left lateral view.

Removal of the gluteobiceps and tensor fasciae latae muscles exposes the vessels and nerves in the lateral femoral region.

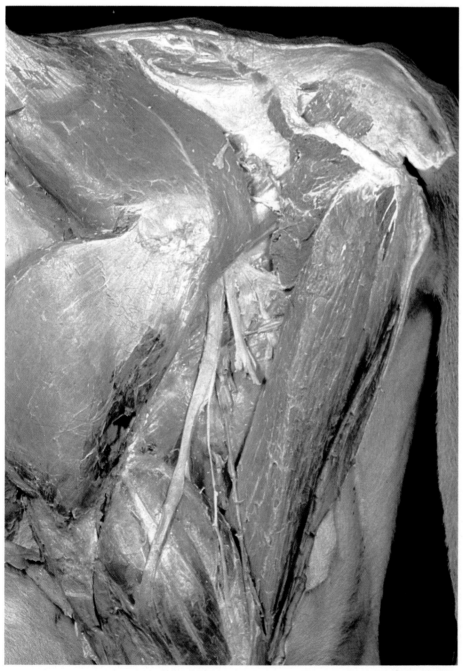

Fig. 6.9 The ischiatic and gluteal nerves, in left lateral view.

Removal of the gluteobiceps and middle gluteal muscles exposes the course of the ischiatic nerve from the greater ischiatic foramen to its termination. The semitendinosus muscle has also been removed.

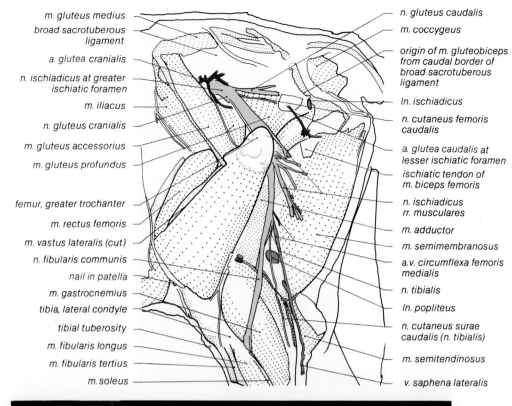

m. gluteus medius
broad sacrotuberous ligament
a. glutea cranialis
n. ischiadicus at greater ischiatic foramen
m. iliacus
n. gluteus cranialis
m. gluteus accessorius
m. gluteus profundus
femur, greater trochanter
m. rectus femoris
m. vastus lateralis (cut)
n. fibularis communis
nail in patella
m. gastrocnemius
tibia, lateral condyle
tibial tuberosity
m. fibularis longus
m. fibularis tertius
m. soleus

n. gluteus caudalis
m. coccygeus
origin of m. gluteobiceps from caudal border of broad sacrotuberous ligament
ln. ischiadicus
n. cutaneus femoris caudalis
a. glutea caudalis at lesser ischiatic foramen
ischiatic tendon of m. biceps femoris
n. ischiadicus rr. musculares
m. adductor
m. semimembranosus
a.v. circumflexa femoris medialis
n. tibialis
ln. popliteus
n. cutaneus surae caudalis (n. tibialis)
m. semitendinosus
v. saphena lateralis

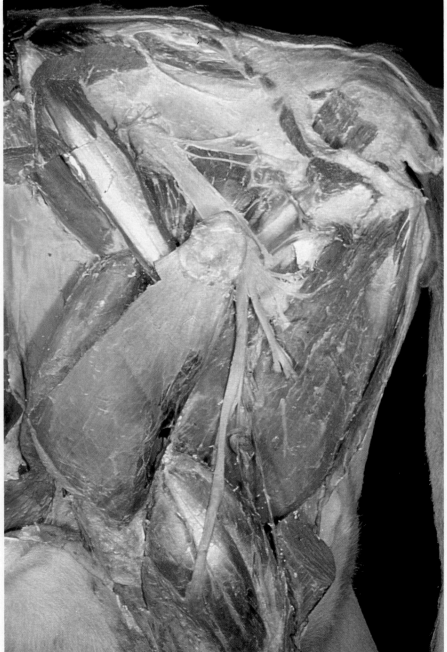

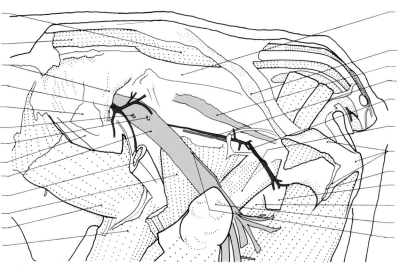

m. sacrocaudalis dorsalis lateralis
m. longissimus lumborum
body of sacrum
a. glutea cranialis
sacrum, auricular surface
n. gluteus cranialis
n. gluteus caudalis
wing of sacrum
n. ischiadicus
shaft of ilium
m. gluteus profundus
m. iliacus
m. rectus femoris

broad sacrotuberous ligament
m. gluteobiceps (origin)
n. pudendus
a.v. iliaca interna
a. glutea caudalis at lesser ischiatic foramen
mm. gemelli
tuber ischiadicum
m. semitendinosus (origin)
m. biceps femoris
m. quadratus femoris
femur, greater trochanter
n. cutaneus femoris caudalis (displaced ventrally)

Fig. 6.10 The sacroiliac articulation and deep structures of the gluteal region, in left lateral view.

The wing of the ilium has been removed to show the sacroiliac joint. The broad sacro-tuberous ligament has also been partly removed.

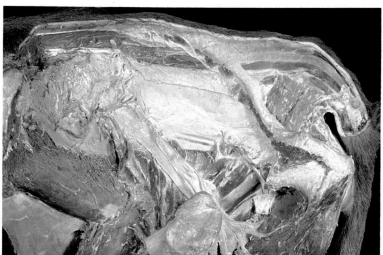

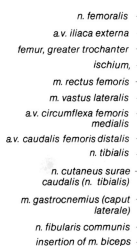

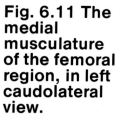

n. femoralis
a.v. iliaca externa
femur, greater trochanter
ischium,
m. rectus femoris
m. vastus lateralis
a.v. circumflexa femoris medialis
a.v. caudalis femoris distalis
n. tibialis
n. cutaneus surae caudalis (n. tibialis)
m. gastrocnemius (caput laterale)
n. fibularis communis
insertion of m. biceps femoris

m. semimembranosus
n. pudendus r. cutaneus distalis
m. biceps femoris
m. quadratus femoris
m. adductor
m. semimembranosus (origin from pelvic symphysis)
m. gracilis
n. ischiadicus rr. musculares
m. semimembranosus
m. semitendinosus
n. ischiadicus (reflected)

Fig. 6.11 The medial musculature of the femoral region, in left caudolateral view.

The dissection is at a slightly later stage than that shown in figs. 6.9 and 6.10. The semi-membranosus muscle has been transected and displaced ventrally to reveal the adductor and gracilis muscles. The transected ischiatic nerve (see fig. 6.12) is reflected ventrally.

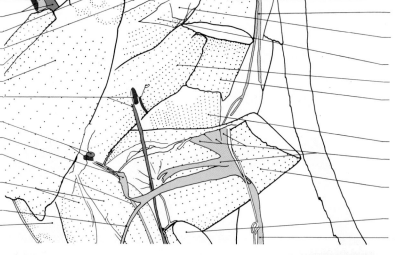

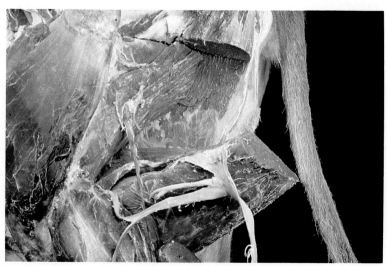

Fig. 6.12

Fig. 6.12
Nerves of the hindlimb, in left lateral view.

The iliopsoas muscle and the iliac fascia have been removed to display the vessels and nerves running immediately cranial to and medial to the ilium. The sciatic nerve has been transected and its spinal origins have been displayed.

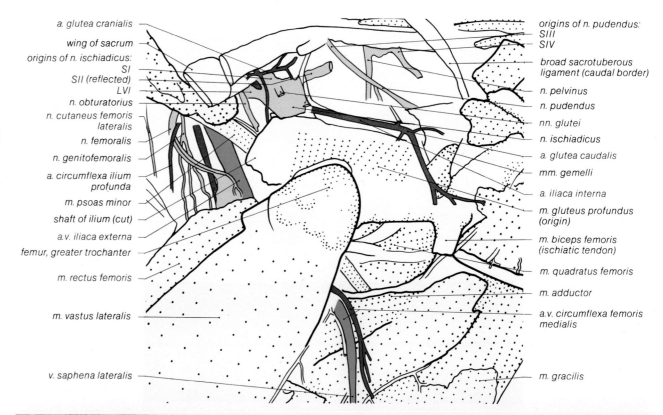

a. glutea cranialis

wing of sacrum

origins of n. ischiadicus:
SI
SII (reflected)
LVI

n. obturatorius

n. cutaneus femoris lateralis

n. femoralis

n. genitofemoralis

a. circumflexa ilium profunda

m. psoas minor

shaft of ilium (cut)

a.v. iliaca externa

femur, greater trochanter

m. rectus femoris

m. vastus lateralis

v. saphena lateralis

origins of n. pudendus:
SIII
SIV

broad sacrotuberous ligament (caudal border)

n. pelvinus

n. pudendus

nn. glutei

n. ischiadicus

a. glutea caudalis

mm. gemelli

a. iliaca interna

m. gluteus profundus (origin)

m. biceps femoris (ischiatic tendon)

m. quadratus femoris

m. adductor

a.v. circumflexa femoris medialis

m. gracilis

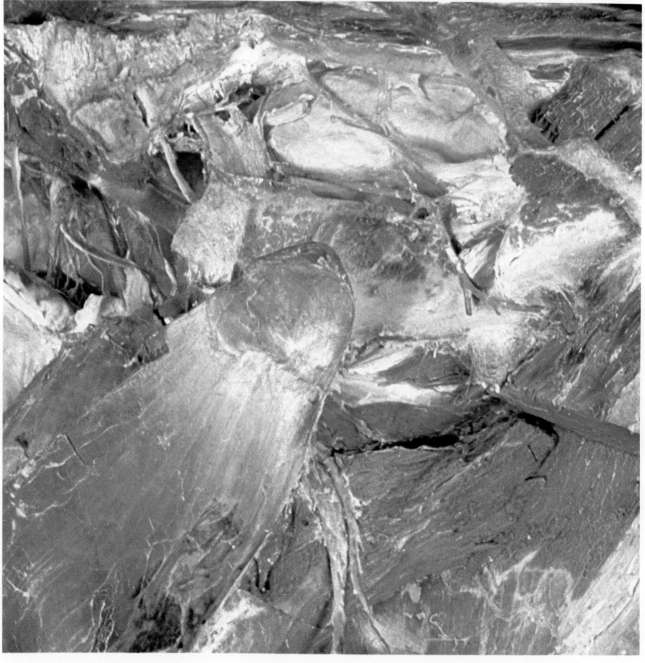

Fig. 6.13 Superficial structures of the hindlimb, in left lateral view.

The leg has been removed from the body. The contributions of the hamstring muscles and crural fascia to the common calcaneal tendon are shown in figs. 6.20 and 6.28. The term 'fibular' is used throughout in preference to 'peroneal'.

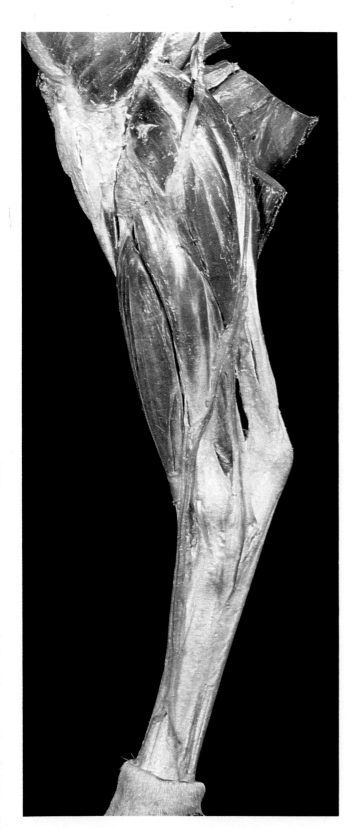

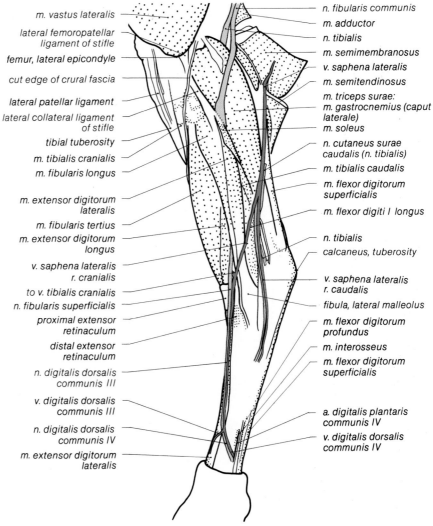

m. vastus lateralis

lateral femoropatellar ligament of stifle

femur, lateral epicondyle

cut edge of crural fascia

lateral patellar ligament

lateral collateral ligament of stifle

tibial tuberosity

m. tibialis cranialis

m. fibularis longus

m. extensor digitorum lateralis

m. fibularis tertius

m. extensor digitorum longus

v. saphena lateralis r. cranialis

to v. tibialis cranialis

n. fibularis superficialis

proximal extensor retinaculum

distal extensor retinaculum

n. digitalis dorsalis communis III

v. digitalis dorsalis communis III

n. digitalis dorsalis communis IV

m. extensor digitorum lateralis

n. fibularis communis

m. adductor

n. tibialis

m. semimembranosus

v. saphena lateralis

m. semitendinosus

m. triceps surae:
m. gastrocnemius (caput laterale)
m. soleus

n. cutaneus surae caudalis (n. tibialis)

m. tibialis caudalis

m. flexor digitorum superficialis

m. flexor digiti I longus

n. tibialis

calcaneus, tuberosity

v. saphena lateralis r. caudalis

fibula, lateral malleolus

m. flexor digitorum profundus

m. interosseus

m. flexor digitorum superficialis

a. digitalis plantaris communis IV

v. digitalis dorsalis communis IV

Fig. 6.14 Superficial structures of the hindlimb, in caudolateral view.

Removal of the third fibular and long digital extensor muscles exposes the cranial tibial muscle. Further dorsal views are shown in figs. 6.16 and 6.21.

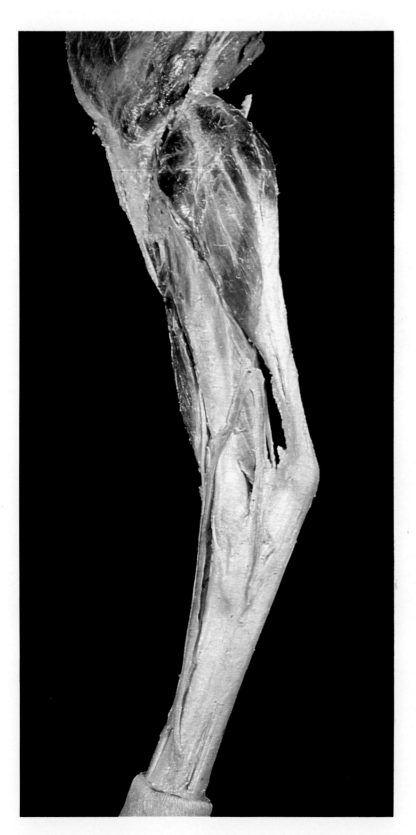

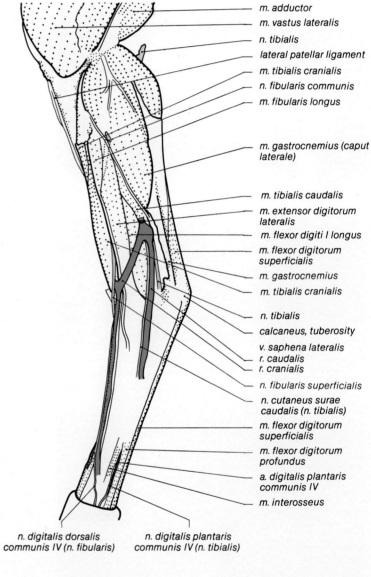

m. adductor
m. vastus lateralis
n. tibialis
lateral patellar ligament
m. tibialis cranialis
n. fibularis communis
m. fibularis longus

m. gastrocnemius (caput laterale)

m. tibialis caudalis
m. extensor digitorum lateralis
m. flexor digiti I longus
m. flexor digitorum superficialis
m. gastrocnemius
m. tibialis cranialis

n. tibialis
calcaneus, tuberosity
v. saphena lateralis
r. caudalis
r. cranialis
n. fibularis superficialis
n. cutaneus surae caudalis (n. tibialis)
m. flexor digitorum superficialis
m. flexor digitorum profundus
a. digitalis plantaris communis IV
m. interosseus

n. digitalis dorsalis communis IV (n. fibularis)   n. digitalis plantaris communis IV (n. tibialis)

Fig. 6.15 Deeper structures of the hock, in dorsal view.

Removal of the third fibular and long digital extensor muscles exposes the cranial tibial muscle. Further dorsal views are shown in figs. 6.16 and 6.21.

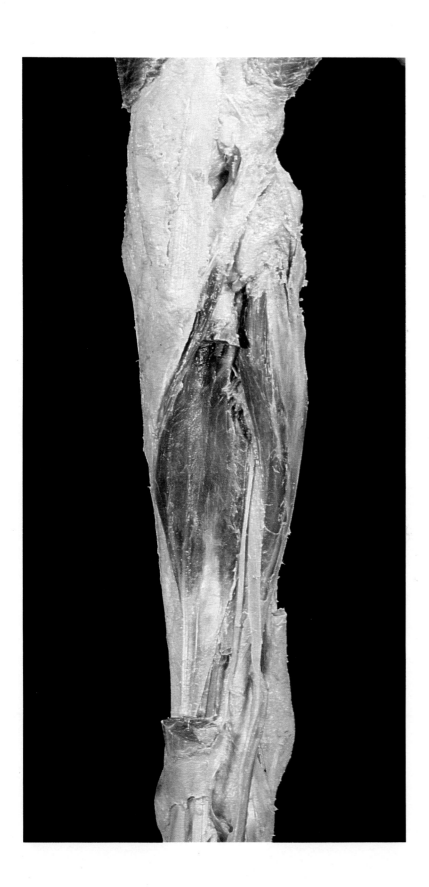

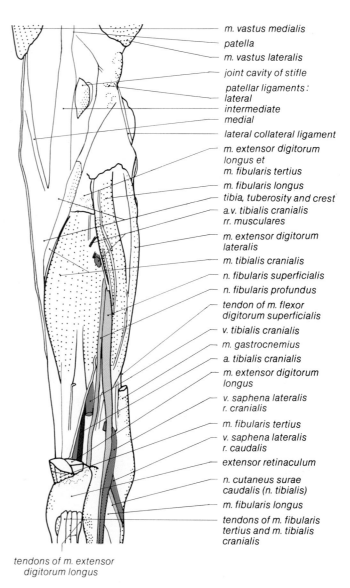

m. vastus medialis
patella
m. vastus lateralis
joint cavity of stifle
patellar ligaments:
lateral
intermediate
medial
lateral collateral ligament
m. extensor digitorum longus et m. fibularis tertius
m. fibularis longus
tibia, tuberosity and crest
a.v. tibialis cranialis rr. musculares
m. extensor digitorum lateralis
m. tibialis cranialis
n. fibularis superficialis
n. fibularis profundus
tendon of m. flexor digitorum superficialis
v. tibialis cranialis
m. gastrocnemius
a. tibialis cranialis
m. extensor digitorum longus
v. saphena lateralis r. cranialis
m. fibularis tertius
v. saphena lateralis r. caudalis
extensor retinaculum
n. cutaneus surae caudalis (n. tibialis)
m. fibularis longus
tendons of m. fibularis tertius and m. tibialis cranialis

tendons of m. extensor digitorum longus

Fig. 6.16 Structures of the hindlimb, in dorsal view.

Further details of the more distal part of this dissection are shown in fig.6.21.

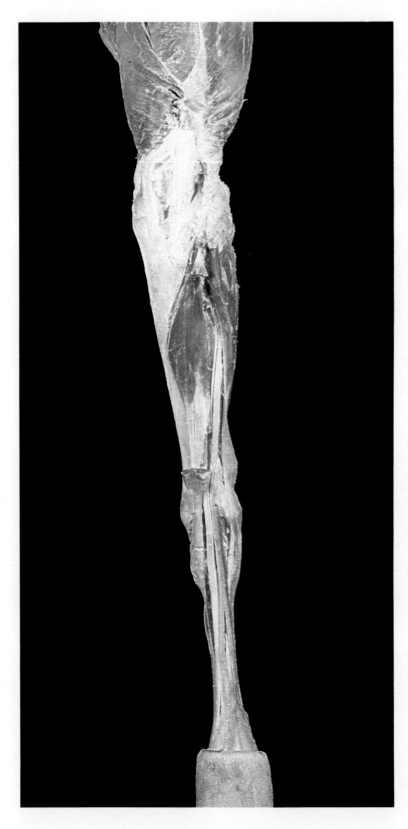

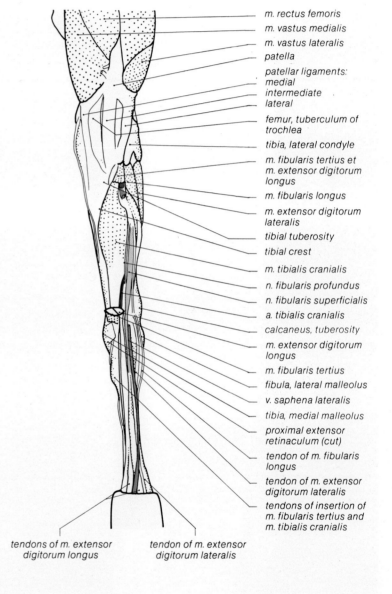

m. rectus femoris
m. vastus medialis
m. vastus lateralis
patella
patellar ligaments:
medial
intermediate
lateral
femur, tuberculum of trochlea
tibia, lateral condyle
m. fibularis tertius et m. extensor digitorum longus
m. fibularis longus
m. extensor digitorum lateralis
tibial tuberosity
tibial crest
m. tibialis cranialis
n. fibularis profundus
n. fibularis superficialis
a. tibialis cranialis
calcaneus, tuberosity
m. extensor digitorum longus
m. fibularis tertius
fibula, lateral malleolus
v. saphena lateralis
tibia, medial malleolus
proximal extensor retinaculum (cut)
tendon of m. fibularis longus
tendon of m. extensor digitorum lateralis
tendons of insertion of m. fibularis tertius and m. tibialis cranialis

tendons of m. extensor digitorum longus

tendon of m. extensor digitorum lateralis

Fig. 6.17 Structures of the hindlimb, in medial view (1)

After removal of the limb from the trunk, the broad gracilis muscle has been cut away. The medial plantar artery, which extends as far as the digits, has been cut short at the hock.

The specimen is at the same stage of dissection as that shown in Fig. 6.13.

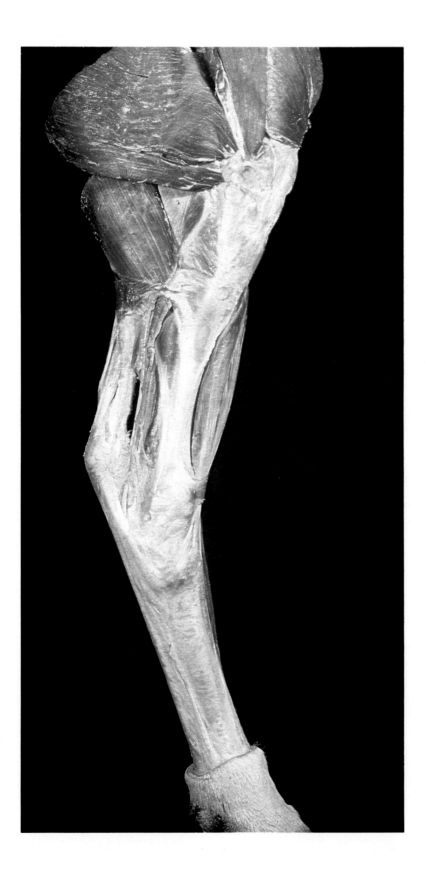

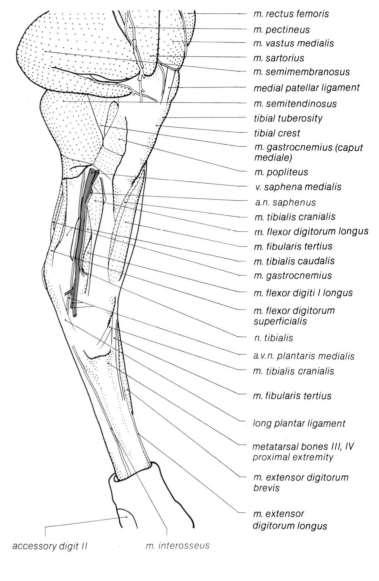

m. rectus femoris
m. pectineus
m. vastus medialis
m. sartorius
m. semimembranosus
medial patellar ligament
m. semitendinosus
tibial tuberosity
tibial crest
m. gastrocnemius (caput mediale)
m. popliteus
v. saphena medialis
a.n. saphenus
m. tibialis cranialis
m. flexor digitorum longus
m. fibularis tertius
m. tibialis caudalis
m. gastrocnemius
m. flexor digiti I longus
m. flexor digitorum superficialis
n. tibialis
a.v.n. plantaris medialis
m. tibialis cranialis
m. fibularis tertius
long plantar ligament
metatarsal bones III, IV proximal extremity
m. extensor digitorum brevis
m. extensor digitorum longus

accessory digit II   m. interosseus

Fig. 6.18 Structures of the hindlimb, in medial view (2).

The sartorius and semitendinosus muscles have been removed. Removal of the superficial medial saphenous structures exposes more clearly the course of the tibial nerve.

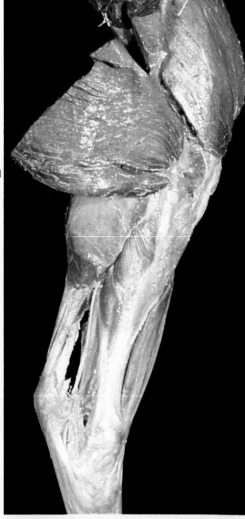

m. pectineus
m. rectus femoris
m. adductor
m. vastus medialis

a. femoralis

m. semimembranosus
medial patellar ligament
capsule of stifle joint
medial collateral ligament of stifle
tibial tuberosity
m. gastrocnemius (caput mediale)
m. popliteus
m. fibularis tertius
m. tibialis cranialis
m. gastrocnemius
m. flexor digitorum superficialis
n. tibialis
m. tibialis caudalis
m. flexor digitorum longus
crural fascia
m. flexor digiti I longus
n. plantaris medialis
extensor retinaculum
a. plantaris medialis
long plantar ligament
tendon of m. peroneus tertius
tendon of m. tibialis cranialis

Fig. 6.19 Structures of the hindlimb, in medial view (3).

The medial gastrocnemius and third fibular muscles have now been removed.

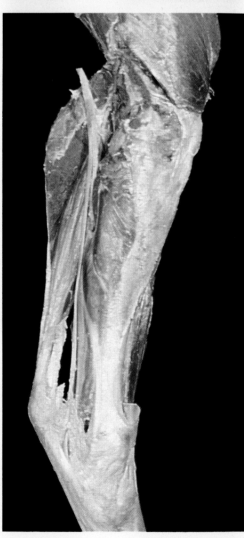

m. adductor
a. poplitea
a. caudalis femoris
n. tibialis
m. gastrocnemius (origin of caput mediale)
m. semimembranosus
m. gastrocneumius, caput laterale
m. flexor digitorum superficialis
femur, medial condyle
medial collateral ligament of stifle
m. popliteus
m. flexor digitorum longus
m. gastrocnemius (caput mediale)
m. flexor digiti I longus
m. tibialis caudalis
m. flexor digitorum superficialis
crural fascia
v. saphena medialis
a. plantaris medialis
long plantar ligament
n. plantaris medialis
m. tibialis cranialis
m. fibularis tertius
m. extensor digitorum communis
m. extensor digitorum brevis

Fig. 6.20 Deep structures of the hindlimb, in medial view.

The stage of dissection is that shown in figs. 6.22 and 6.16. Removal of the heads of the gastrocnemius muscle reveals the tendinous structure of the superficial digital flexor muscle.

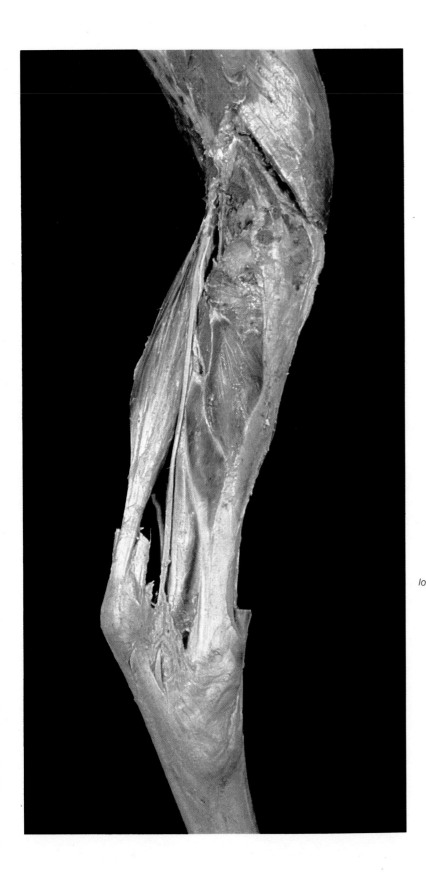

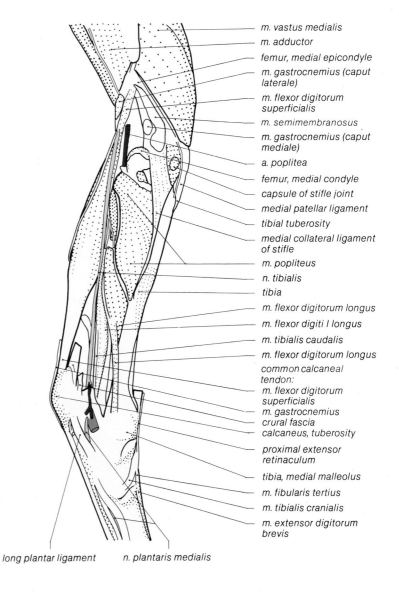

m. vastus medialis

m. adductor

femur, medial epicondyle

m. gastrocnemius (caput laterale)

m. flexor digitorum superficialis

m. semimembranosus

m. gastrocnemius (caput mediale)

a. poplitea

femur, medial condyle

capsule of stifle joint

medial patellar ligament

tibial tuberosity

medial collateral ligament of stifle

m. popliteus

n. tibialis

tibia

m. flexor digitorum longus

m. flexor digiti I longus

m. tibialis caudalis

m. flexor digitorum longus

common calcaneal tendon:
m. flexor digitorum superficialis
m. gastrocnemius
crural fascia
calcaneus, tuberosity

proximal extensor retinaculum

tibia, medial malleolus

m. fibularis tertius

m. tibialis cranialis

m. extensor digitorum brevis

long plantar ligament   n. plantaris medialis

Fig. 6.21 Structures of the hock and metatarsus: (1), dorsal view.

This is a closer view of a part of the dissection shown in fig. 6.16. Figs. 6.21–6.26 show features of the pes, but the structures of the digits (manus and pes) are dealt with in chapter 7.

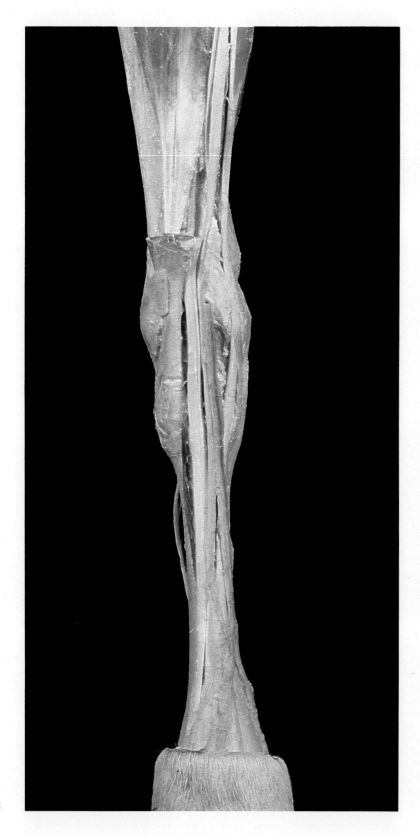

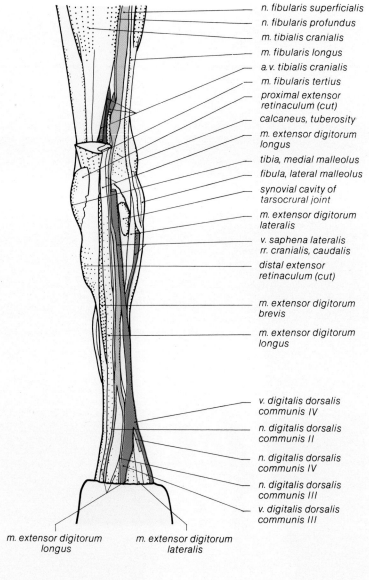

n. fibularis superficialis
n. fibularis profundus
m. tibialis cranialis
m. fibularis longus
a.v. tibialis cranialis
m. fibularis tertius
proximal extensor retinaculum (cut)
calcaneus, tuberosity
m. extensor digitorum longus
tibia, medial malleolus
fibula, lateral malleolus
synovial cavity of tarsocrural joint
m. extensor digitorum lateralis
v. saphena lateralis rr. cranialis, caudalis
distal extensor retinaculum (cut)

m. extensor digitorum brevis

m. extensor digitorum longus

v. digitalis dorsalis communis IV
n. digitalis dorsalis communis II
n. digitalis dorsalis communis IV
n. digitalis dorsalis communis III
v. digitalis dorsalis communis III

m. extensor digitorum longus   m. extensor digitorum lateralis

Fig. 6.22 Structures of the hock and metatarsus: (2), left lateral view.

The third fibular and long extensor muscles have been removed and the superficial flexor exposed by removal of the gastrocnemius muscle.

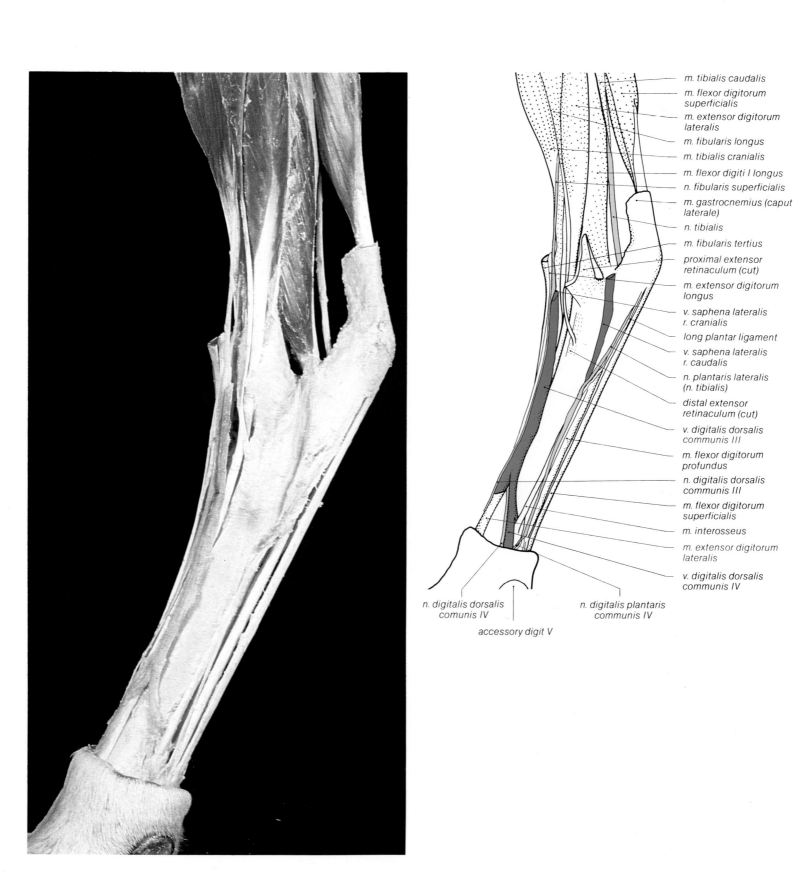

m. tibialis caudalis
m. flexor digitorum superficialis
m. extensor digitorum lateralis
m. fibularis longus
m. tibialis cranialis
m. flexor digiti I longus
n. fibularis superficialis
m. gastrocnemius (caput laterale)
n. tibialis
m. fibularis tertius
proximal extensor retinaculum (cut)
m. extensor digitorum longus
v. saphena lateralis r. cranialis
long plantar ligament
v. saphena lateralis r. caudalis
n. plantaris lateralis (n. tibialis)
distal extensor retinaculum (cut)
v. digitalis dorsalis communis III
m. flexor digitorum profundus
n. digitalis dorsalis communis III
m. flexor digitorum superficialis
m. interosseus
m. extensor digitorum lateralis
v. digitalis dorsalis communis IV

n. digitalis dorsalis comunis IV

n. digitalis plantaris communis IV

accessory digit V

Fig. 6.23 Structures of the hock and metatarsus: (3), medial view.

Dorsal and lateral views of the specimen at this stage of the dissection are shown in figs. 6.21 and 6.22. The tarsal canal has been exposed by transecting the flexor retinaculum, and the course of the medial plantar nerve by removing part of the long plantar ligament.

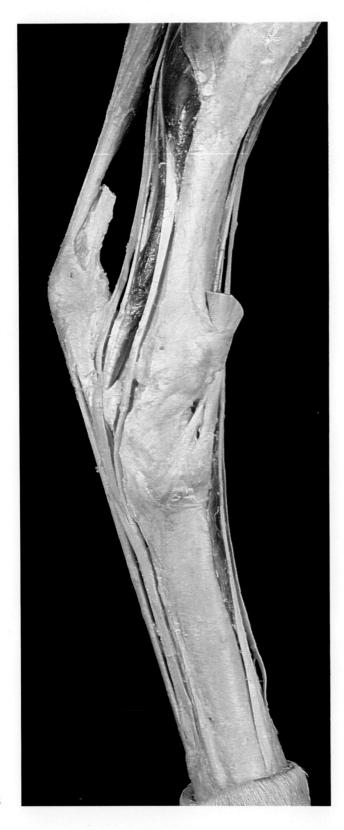

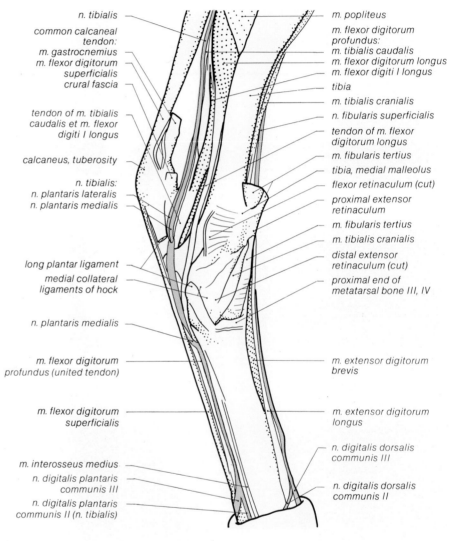

n. tibialis

common calcaneal tendon:
m. gastrocnemius
m. flexor digitorum superficialis
crural fascia

tendon of m. tibialis caudalis et m. flexor digiti I longus

calcaneus, tuberosity

n. tibialis:
n. plantaris lateralis
n. plantaris medialis

long plantar ligament
medial collateral ligaments of hock

n. plantaris medialis

m. flexor digitorum profundus (united tendon)

m. flexor digitorum superficialis

m. interosseus medius
n. digitalis plantaris communis III
n. digitalis plantaris communis II (n. tibialis)

m. popliteus
m. flexor digitorum profundus:
m. tibialis caudalis
m. flexor digitorum longus
m. flexor digiti I longus
tibia
m. tibialis cranialis
n. fibularis superficialis
tendon of m. flexor digitorum longus
m. fibularis tertius
tibia, medial malleolus
flexor retinaculum (cut)
proximal extensor retinaculum
m. fibularis tertius
m. tibialis cranialis
distal extensor retinaculum (cut)
proximal end of metatarsal bone III, IV

m. extensor digitorum brevis

m. extensor digitorum longus

n. digitalis dorsalis communis III

n. digitalis dorsalis communis II

Fig. 6.24 Vessels and nerves of the hock and metatarsus, in dorsolateral view.

The tendons of the common digital extensor and cranial tibial muscle have been displaced medially to reveal the cranial tibial vessels and the deep fibular nerve. The superficial digital flexor muscle has been removed.

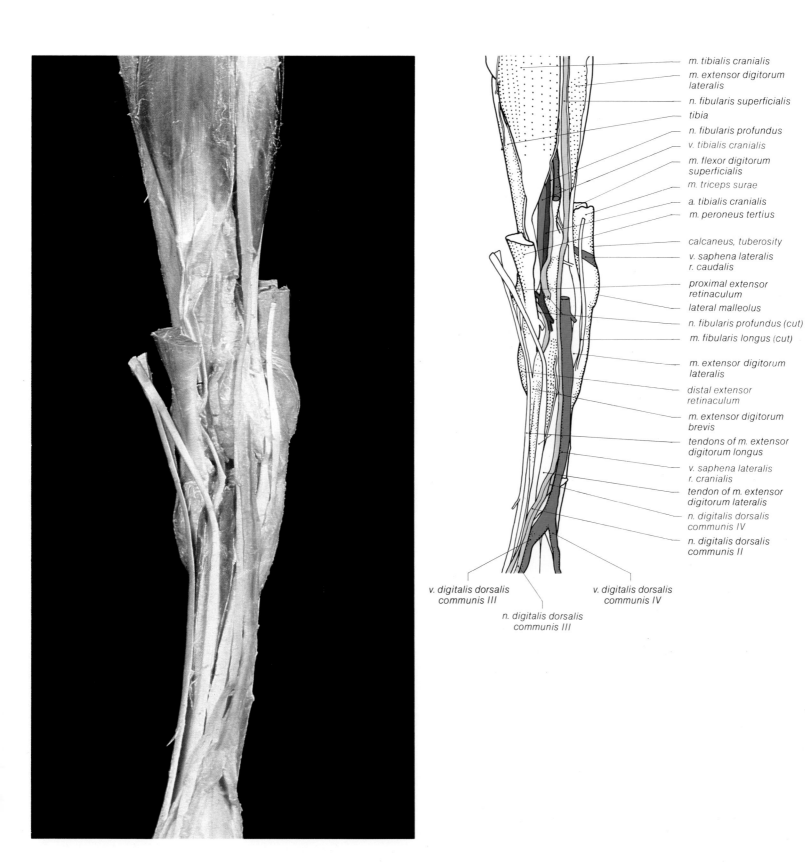

m. tibialis cranialis

m. extensor digitorum lateralis

n. fibularis superficialis

tibia

n. fibularis profundus

v. tibialis cranialis

m. flexor digitorum superficialis

m. triceps surae

a. tibialis cranialis

m. peroneus tertius

calcaneus, tuberosity

v. saphena lateralis r. caudalis

proximal extensor retinaculum

lateral malleolus

n. fibularis profundus (cut)

m. fibularis longus (cut)

m. extensor digitorum lateralis

distal extensor retinaculum

m. extensor digitorum brevis

tendons of m. extensor digitorum longus

v. saphena lateralis r. cranialis

tendon of m. extensor digitorum lateralis

n. digitalis dorsalis communis IV

n. digitalis dorsalis communis II

v. digitalis dorsalis communis III

v. digitalis dorsalis communis IV

n. digitalis dorsalis communis III

Fig. 6.25 Caudal muscles of the tibia, in dorsocaudal view.

The superficial digital flexor muscle has been removed to display the deep digital flexor and the popliteus muscles. On the medial side, the tendon of the long digital flexor muscle has been exposed as shown in fig. 6.23.

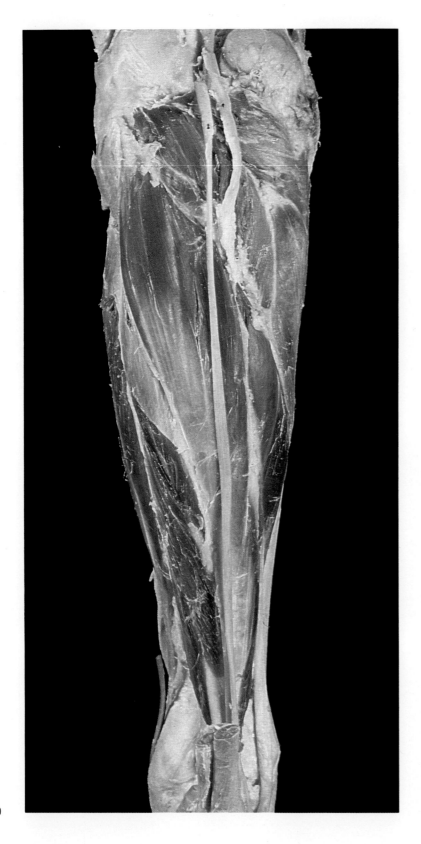

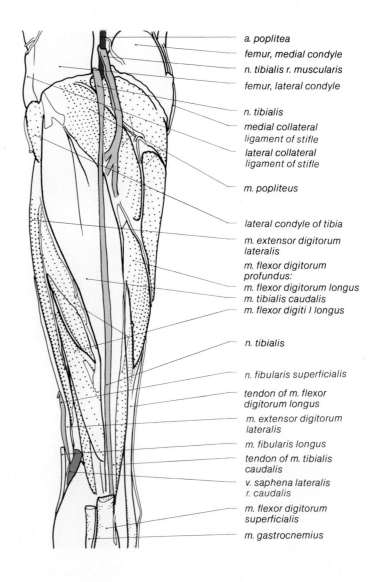

a. poplitea

femur, medial condyle

n. tibialis r. muscularis

femur, lateral condyle

n. tibialis

medial collateral ligament of stifle

lateral collateral ligament of stifle

m. popliteus

lateral condyle of tibia

m. extensor digitorum lateralis

m. flexor digitorum profundus:
m. flexor digitorum longus
m. tibialis caudalis
m. flexor digiti I longus

n. tibialis

n. fibularis superficialis

tendon of m. flexor digitorum longus

m. extensor digitorum lateralis

m. fibularis longus

tendon of m. tibialis caudalis

v. saphena lateralis r. caudalis

m. flexor digitorum superficialis

m. gastrocnemius

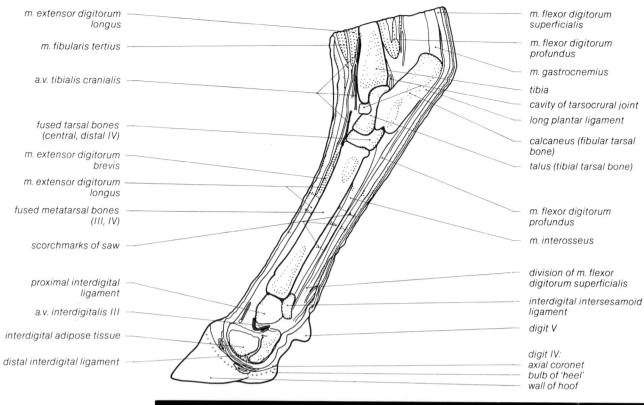

m. extensor digitorum longus

m. fibularis tertius

a.v. tibialis cranialis

fused tarsal bones (central, distal IV)

m. extensor digitorum brevis

m. extensor digitorum longus

fused metatarsal bones (III, IV)

scorchmarks of saw

proximal interdigital ligament

a.v. interdigitalis III

interdigital adipose tissue

distal interdigital ligament

m. flexor digitorum superficialis

m. flexor digitorum profundus

m. gastrocnemius

tibia

cavity of tarsocrural joint

long plantar ligament

calcaneus (fibular tarsal bone)

talus (tibial tarsal bone)

m. flexor digitorum profundus

m. interosseus

division of m. flexor digitorum superficialis

interdigital intersesamoid ligament

digit V

digit IV:
axial coronet
bulb of 'heel'
wall of hoof

Fig. 6.26 Median section through the right pes: medial view.
The plane of sectioning in the digital region is shown in fig. 7.14. In the metatarsus, the bending of the saw cut in order to pass through the axial plane of the tarsus has scorched the specimen. The digital region of the medial side of this specimen is shown in fig. 7.28.

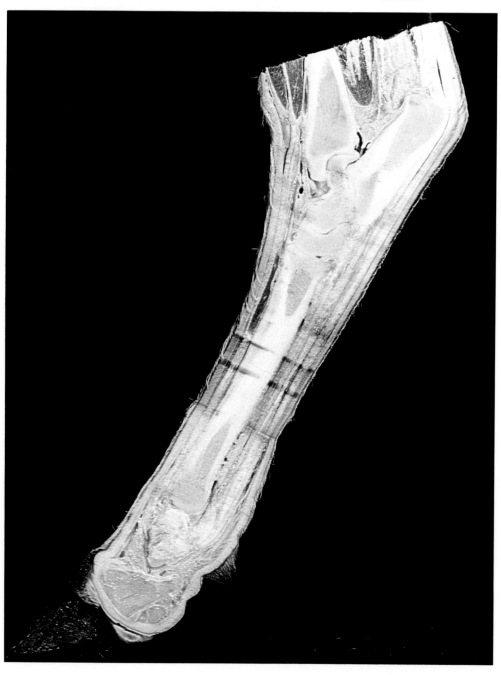

Fig. 6.27 Superficial nerves and muscles of the pelvic and femoral regions of a 1-week bull calf: left lateral view.

Figs. 6.27 – 6.29 show dissections of these regions in a calf in which the hindlimb was rather flexed at embalming. The nerves and blood vessels in the superficial fascia of the hindlimb are shown in detail in figs. 7.33–7.36.

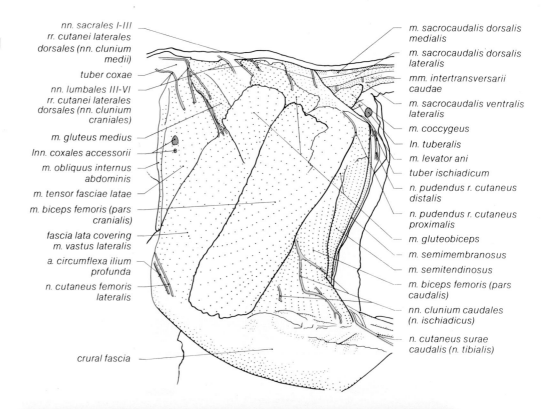

nn. sacrales I-III
rr. cutanei laterales dorsales (nn. clunium medii)
tuber coxae
nn. lumbales III-VI rr. cutanei laterales dorsales (nn. clunium craniales)
m. gluteus medius
lnn. coxales accessorii
m. obliquus internus abdominis
m. tensor fasciae latae
m. biceps femoris (pars cranialis)
fascia lata covering m. vastus lateralis
a. circumflexa ilium profunda
n. cutaneus femoris lateralis
crural fascia

m. sacrocaudalis dorsalis medialis
m. sacrocaudalis dorsalis lateralis
mm. intertransversarii caudae
m. sacrocaudalis ventralis lateralis
m. coccygeus
ln. tuberalis
m. levator ani
tuber ischiadicum
n. pudendus r. cutaneus distalis
n. pudendus r. cutaneus proximalis
m. gluteobiceps
m. semimembranosus
m. semitendinosus
m. biceps femoris (pars caudalis)
nn. clunium caudales (n. ischiadicus)
n. cutaneus surae caudalis (n. tibialis)

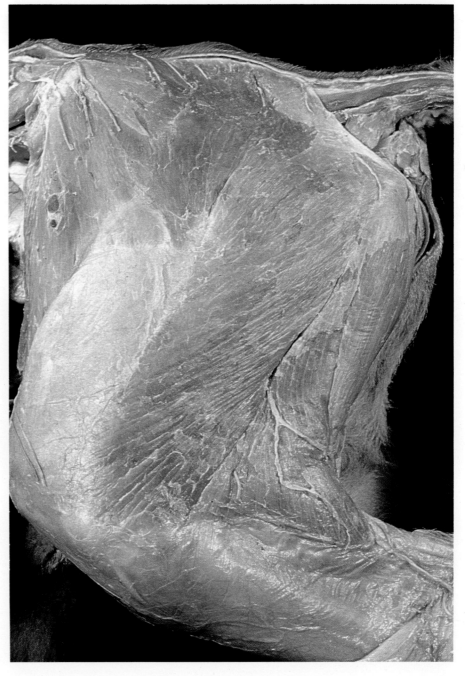

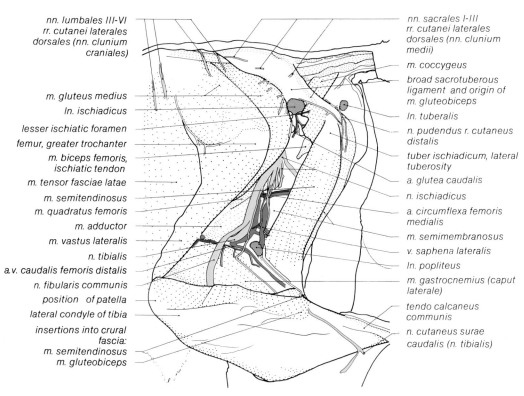

nn. lumbales III-VI
rr. cutanei laterales
dorsales (nn. clunium
craniales)

m. gluteus medius

ln. ischiadicus

lesser ischiatic foramen
femur, greater trochanter
m. biceps femoris,
ischiatic tendon
m. tensor fasciae latae
m. semitendinosus
m. quadratus femoris
m. adductor
m. vastus lateralis
n. tibialis
a.v. caudalis femoris distalis
n. fibularis communis
position of patella
lateral condyle of tibia
insertions into crural
fascia:
m. semitendinosus
m. gluteobiceps

nn. sacrales I-III
rr. cutanei laterales
dorsales (nn. clunium
medii)

m. coccygeus

broad sacrotuberous
ligament and origin of
m. gluteobiceps

ln. tuberalis

n. pudendus r. cutaneus
distalis

tuber ischiadicum, lateral
tuberosity

a. glutea caudalis

n. ischiadicus

a. circumflexa femoris
medialis

m. semimembranosus

v. saphena lateralis

ln. popliteus

m. gastrocnemius (caput
laterale)

tendo calcaneus
communis

n. cutaneus surae
caudalis (n. tibialis)

Fig. 6.28 Pelvic and femoral regions of the calf to show the tibial and fibular nerves, in left lateral view.

The gluteobiceps muscle has been removed. The middle gluteal muscle still hides the main part of the sciatic nerve. The lesser ischiatic foramen is visible.

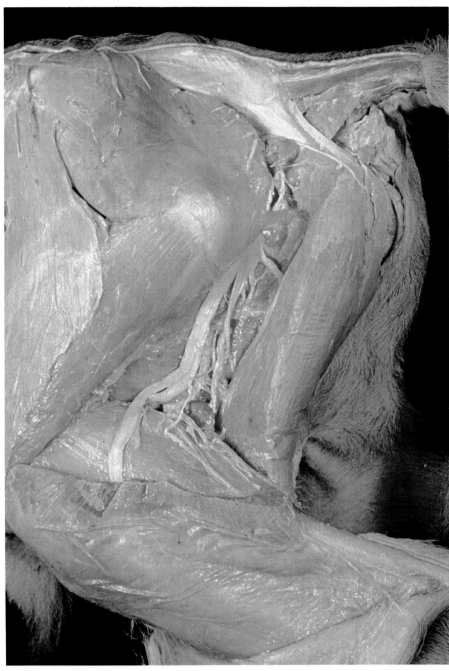

6.23

Fig. 6.29 The ischiatic and gluteal nerves of the calf, in left lateral view.

Removal of the middle gluteal muscle exposes the structures emerging from the greater ischiatic foramen. Fig. 6.30 shows the structures lying medial to the tensor muscle of the fascia lata.

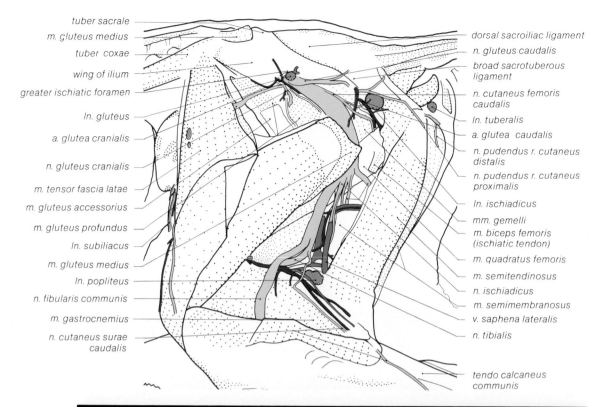

tuber sacrale
m. gluteus medius
tuber coxae
wing of ilium
greater ischiatic foramen
ln. gluteus
a. glutea cranialis
n. gluteus cranialis
m. tensor fascia latae
m. gluteus accessorius
m. gluteus profundus
ln. subiliacus
m. gluteus medius
ln. popliteus
n. fibularis communis
m. gastrocnemius
n. cutaneus surae caudalis

dorsal sacroiliac ligament
n. gluteus caudalis
broad sacrotuberous ligament
n. cutaneus femoris caudalis
ln. tuberalis
a. glutea caudalis
n. pudendus r. cutaneus distalis
n. pudendus r. cutaneus proximalis
ln. ischiadicus
mm. gemelli
m. biceps femoris (ischiatic tendon)
m. quadratus femoris
m. semitendinosus
n. ischiadicus
m. semimembranosus
v. saphena lateralis
n. tibialis
tendo calcaneus communis

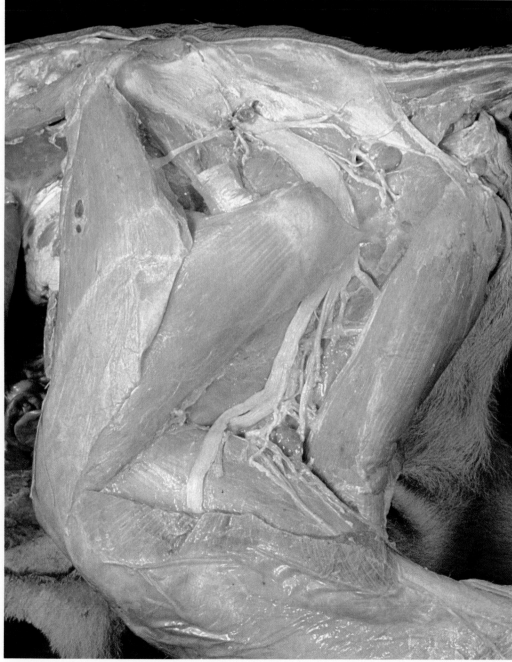

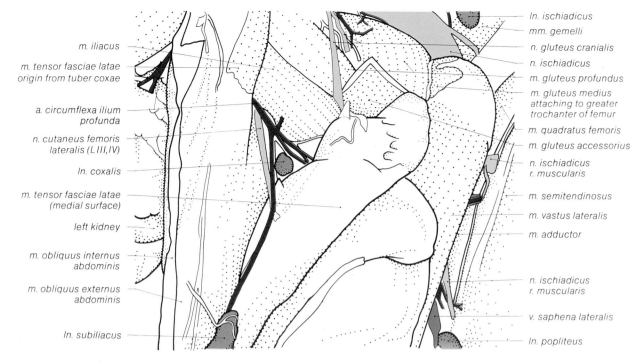

m. iliacus

m. tensor fasciae latae
origin from tuber coxae

a. circumflexa ilium
profunda

n. cutaneus femoris
lateralis (L III, IV)

ln. coxalis

m. tensor fasciae latae
(medial surface)

left kidney

m. obliquus internus
abdominis

m. obliquus externus
abdominis

ln. subiliacus

ln. ischiadicus

mm. gemelli

n. gluteus cranialis

n. ischiadicus

m. gluteus profundus

m. gluteus medius
attaching to greater
trochanter of femur

m. quadratus femoris

m. gluteus accessorius

n. ischiadicus
r. muscularis

m. semitendinosus

m. vastus lateralis

m. adductor

n. ischiadicus
r. muscularis

v. saphena lateralis

ln. popliteus

**Fig. 6.30
Structures
lying medial to
the tensor
muscle of the
fascia lata of
the calf:
craniolateral
view.**
The origin of the
muscle from the tuber
coxae has been cut
and the muscle has
been reflected
ventrally onto the
vastus muscles.

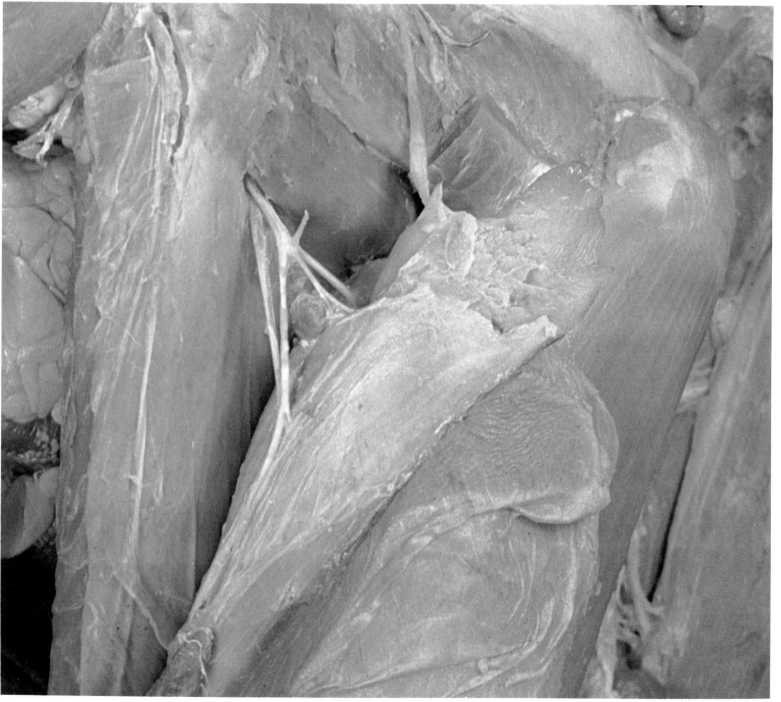

7 The Foot

Fig. 7.1 Surface features of the left carpus, in craniolateral view.
The palpable position of the radiocarpal joint has been shaved. The constituent bones can be seen in fig. 7.4. The dorsum of the carpus is directed somewhat laterally in normal level standing, and the medial surface of the carpus is markedly convex.

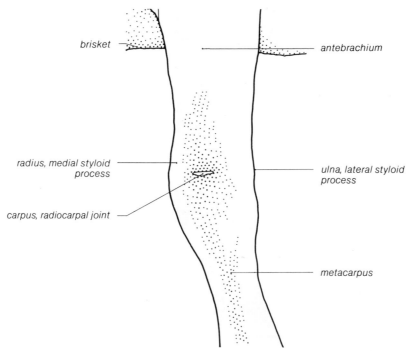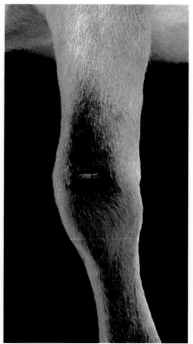

brisket

antebrachium

radius, medial styloid process

ulna, lateral styloid process

carpus, radiocarpal joint

metacarpus

Fig. 7.2 Surface features of the left manus, in lateral view.
Two palpable features have been shaved. The bones can be seen in fig. 7.5. The lateral rotation of the "toe", mentioned in fig. 7.7, reveals the interdigital cleft from a lateral view in normal level standing.

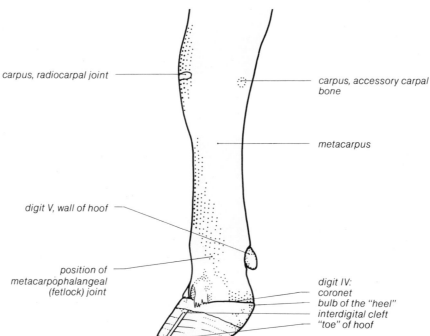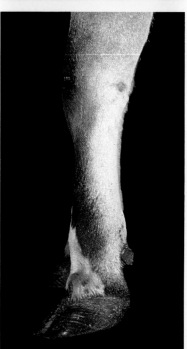

carpus, radiocarpal joint

carpus, accessory carpal bone

metacarpus

digit V, wall of hoof

position of metacarpophalangeal (fetlock) joint

digit IV:
coronet
bulb of the "heel"
interdigital cleft
"toe" of hoof

Fig. 7.3 Surface features of the left manus, in caudolateral view.
One palpable feature has been shaved. The bones can be seen in fig.7.6. A palmar view of the hoof is shown in fig. 7.20.

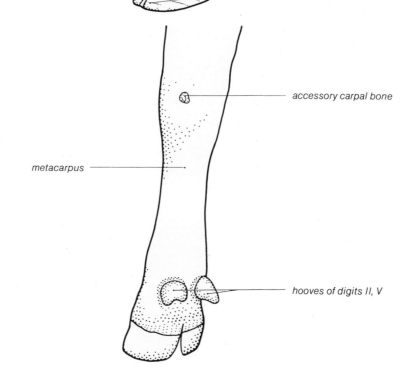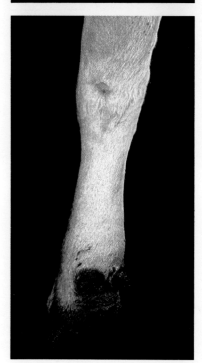

accessory carpal bone

metacarpus

hooves of digits II, V

7.2

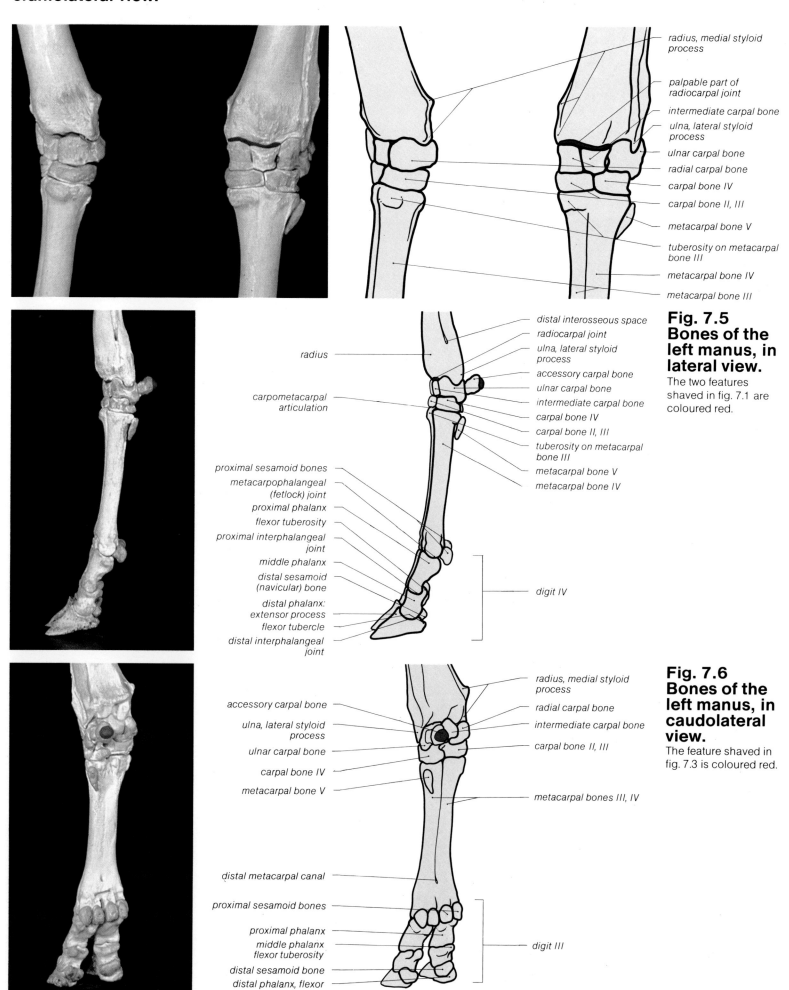

Fig. 7.4 Bones of the left and right carpus, in left craniolateral view.

One palpable feature shown in fig. 7.1 has been coloured red. The bones of the digits are shown in craniolateral view in fig. 7.10.

radius, medial styloid process

palpable part of radiocarpal joint

intermediate carpal bone

ulna, lateral styloid process

ulnar carpal bone

radial carpal bone

carpal bone IV

carpal bone II, III

metacarpal bone V

tuberosity on metacarpal bone III

metacarpal bone IV

metacarpal bone III

Fig. 7.5 Bones of the left manus, in lateral view.

The two features shaved in fig. 7.1 are coloured red.

distal interosseous space

radiocarpal joint

ulna, lateral styloid process

accessory carpal bone

ulnar carpal bone

intermediate carpal bone

carpal bone IV

carpal bone II, III

tuberosity on metacarpal bone III

metacarpal bone V

metacarpal bone IV

radius

carpometacarpal articulation

proximal sesamoid bones

metacarpophalangeal (fetlock) joint

proximal phalanx

flexor tuberosity

proximal interphalangeal joint

middle phalanx

distal sesamoid (navicular) bone

distal phalanx: extensor process

flexor tubercle

distal interphalangeal joint

digit IV

Fig. 7.6 Bones of the left manus, in caudolateral view.

The feature shaved in fig. 7.3 is coloured red.

radius, medial styloid process

radial carpal bone

intermediate carpal bone

carpal bone II, III

accessory carpal bone

ulna, lateral styloid process

ulnar carpal bone

carpal bone IV

metacarpal bone V

metacarpal bones III, IV

distal metacarpal canal

proximal sesamoid bones

proximal phalanx

middle phalanx

flexor tuberosity

distal sesamoid bone

distal phalanx, flexor tubercle

digit III

Fig. 7.7 Surface features of the hindlimbs, in left craniolateral view.

The position of the pes in normal level standing, and the action of the foot during locomotion, are variable. When the udder is large, the limb is abducted and the "toes" of the hooves tend to be rotated laterally at all stages of the step. The bones are shown in fig. 7.10

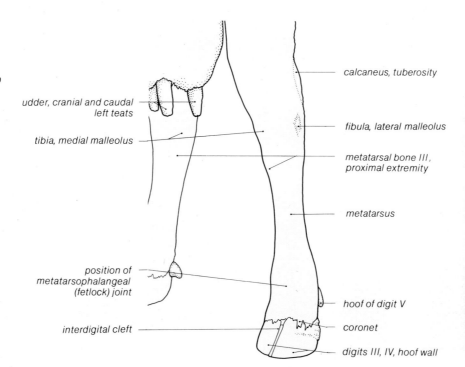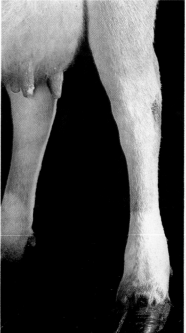

udder, cranial and caudal left teats

tibia, medial malleolus

position of metatarsophalangeal (fetlock) joint

interdigital cleft

calcaneus, tuberosity

fibula, lateral malleolus

metatarsal bone III, proximal extremity

metatarsus

hoof of digit V

coronet

digits III, IV, hoof wall

Fig. 7.8 Surface features of the left pes, in lateral view.

Two palpable features have been shaved. The bones can be seen in fig. 7.11. Compare the angle of the main digits (dorsum of the hoof wall) with that seen in the forelimb (fig.7.2).

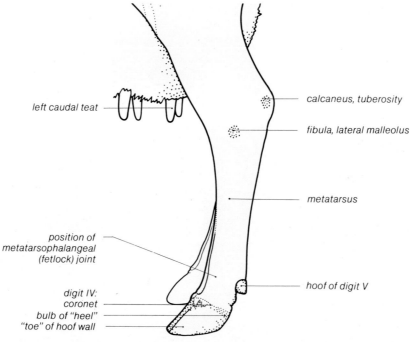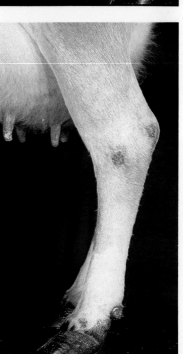

left caudal teat

position of metatarsophalangeal (fetlock) joint

digit IV: coronet
bulb of "heel"
"toe" of hoof wall

calcaneus, tuberosity

fibula, lateral malleolus

metatarsus

hoof of digit V

Fig. 7.9 Surface features of the left pes, in caudal view.

Two palpable features have been shaved. The bones can be seen in fig. 7.12.

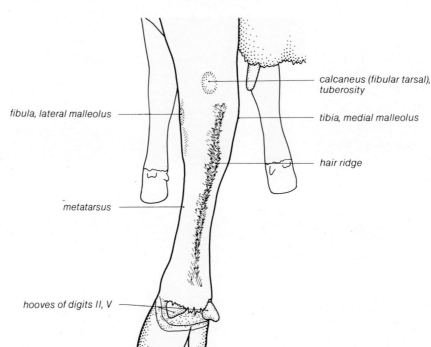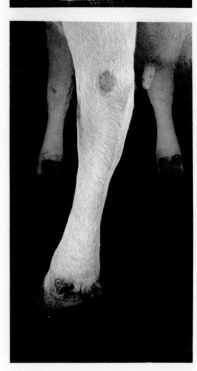

fibula, lateral malleolus

metatarsus

hooves of digits II, V

calcaneus (fibular tarsal), tuberosity

tibia, medial malleolus

hair ridge

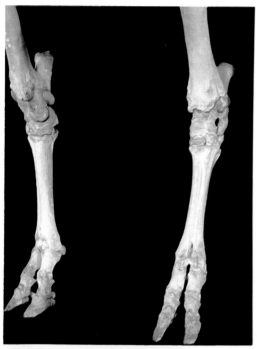
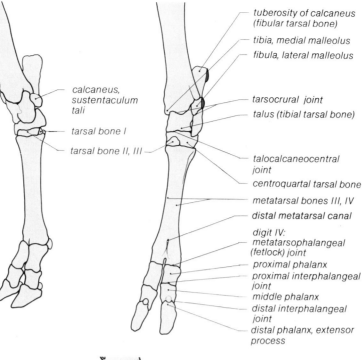

tuberosity of calcaneus (fibular tarsal bone)
tibia, medial malleolus
fibula, lateral malleolus

calcaneus, sustentaculum tali

tarsocrural joint
talus (tibial tarsal bone)

tarsal bone I
tarsal bone II, III

talocalcaneocentral joint
centroquartal tarsal bone
metatarsal bones III, IV
distal metatarsal canal
digit IV:
metatarsophalangeal (fetlock) joint
proximal phalanx
proximal interphalangeal joint
middle phalanx
distal interphalangeal joint
distal phalanx, extensor process

Fig. 7.10
Bones of the left and right pes, in left craniolateral view.

The two features shaved in fig. 7.7 are coloured red. In life, the solar surface of the distal phalanx lies horizontal in level standing (see fig. 7.17). The talus is also called the astragalus or, more aptly, the tibial tarsal bone.

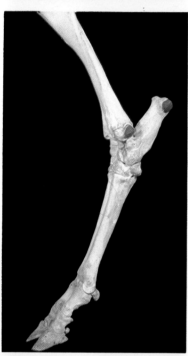
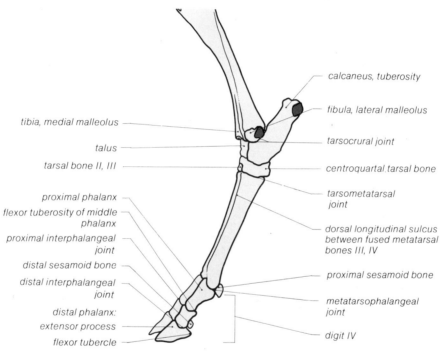

calcaneus, tuberosity

fibula, lateral malleolus

tibia, medial malleolus

talus

tarsocrural joint

tarsal bone II, III

centroquartal tarsal bone

proximal phalanx
flexor tuberosity of middle phalanx
proximal interphalangeal joint

tarsometatarsal joint

distal sesamoid bone

dorsal longitudinal sulcus between fused metatarsal bones III, IV

distal interphalangeal joint

proximal sesamoid bone

distal phalanx:
extensor process

metatarsophalangeal joint

flexor tubercle

digit IV

Fig. 7.11
Bones of the left pes, in lateral view.

The two features shaved in fig. 7.7 are coloured red. The calcaneus is more aptly called the fibular tarsal bone.

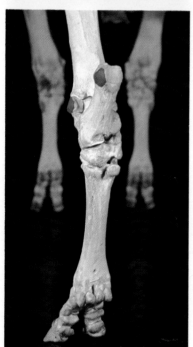
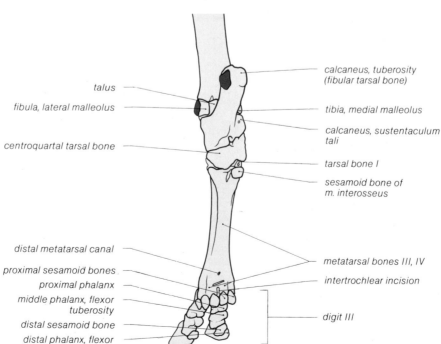

talus

fibula, lateral malleolus

centroquartal tarsal bone

calcaneus, tuberosity (fibular tarsal bone)

tibia, medial malleolus

calcaneus, sustentaculum tali

tarsal bone I

sesamoid bone of m. interosseus

distal metatarsal canal
proximal sesamoid bones
proximal phalanx
middle phalanx, flexor tuberosity
distal sesamoid bone
distal phalanx, flexor tubercle

metatarsal bones III, IV

intertrochlear incision

digit III

Fig. 7.12
Bones of the left pes, in caudal view.

The features shaved in fig. 7.9 are coloured red.

Fig. 7.13 Digital region of the right pes, in lateral view.

The angle of the dorsum of the hoof wall should be compared with that of the manus (compare with fig. 7.17). The axial line of the coronet has been traced onto this drawing from fig. 7.15.

The periople is continuous with the bulb of the heel, and there are good reasons for considering them as specialised parts of one structure.

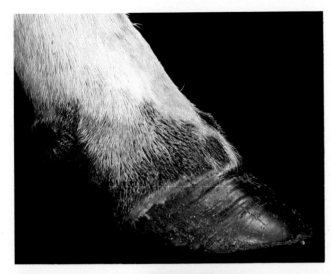

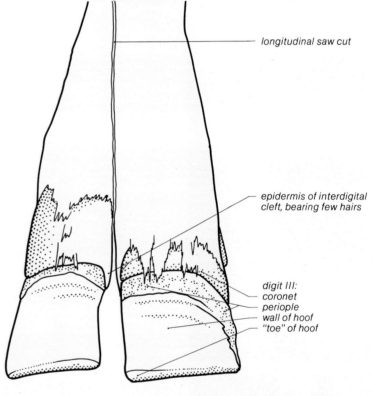

level of metatarsophalangeal (fetlock) joint

digit V:
wall of hoof

digit IV:
abaxial line of coronet
periople
abaxial part of hoof wall
axial line of coronet
junction between wall and bulb
"toe" of hoof

bulb of "heel" (torus digitalis)

Fig. 7.14 Digital region of the right pes, in cranial view.

The saw cut made to display the axial structures of the digit (see fig. 7.15) is also shown.

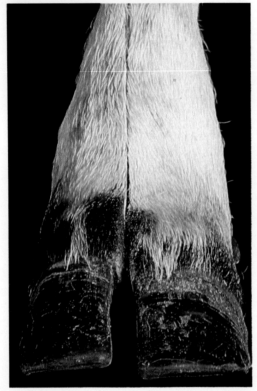

longitudinal saw cut

epidermis of interdigital cleft, bearing few hairs

digit III:
coronet
periople
wall of hoof
"toe" of hoof

Fig. 7.15 The interdigital region of the right pes, in lateral view.

The interdigital cleft has been revealed by sectioning as shown in fig. 7.14. The medial half of the sectioned limb (containing the third digit) is viewed from the lateral aspect. The deeper structures are fully labelled in fig. 7.28.

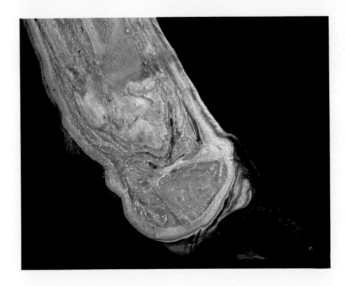

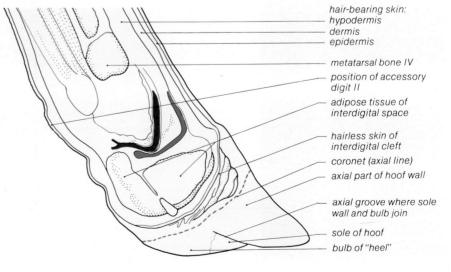

hair-bearing skin:
hypodermis
dermis
epidermis

metatarsal bone IV

position of accessory digit II

adipose tissue of interdigital space

hairless skin of interdigital cleft

coronet (axial line)

axial part of hoof wall

axial groove where sole wall and bulb join

sole of hoof

bulb of "heel"

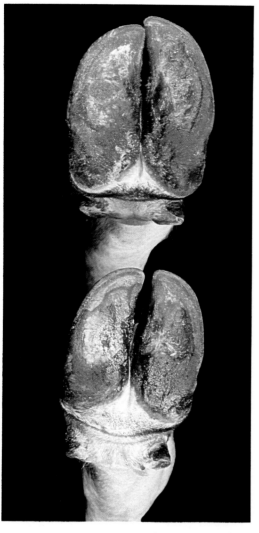

digit III of forelimb:

— "toe" of larger, medial hoof

parts of hoof wall:
— abaxial
— axial

— white zone

— termination of hoof wall

— approximate position of distal sesamoid bone

— interdigital cleft

digit II of forelimb:
parts of hoof wall
— axial
— abaxial

— metacarpus

digit III of hind limb:

— white zone

— sole of hoof

— axial groove

— junction between sole and bulb

— bulb of "heel"

— hairless skin of interdigital cleft

— coronet at "heel"

— digit II of hindlimb, sole of hoof

— metatarsus

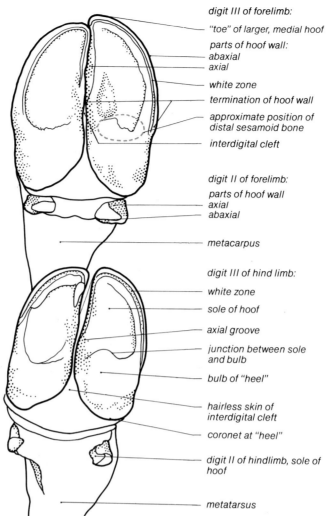

Fig. 7.16 Solar surfaces of the hooves of the right manus and pes.

The limbs were fixed while the cow was in the standing position. During maximum weight bearing, in life, the main digits are splayed apart more than in these feet, and the fetlock drops so that the accessory digits may touch the ground. The feet were scrubbed and dried, but not trimmed. Note that the so-called "white zone" is, in fact, darker than the sole and wall. Its salient characteristic is that it is laminar in structure.

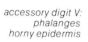

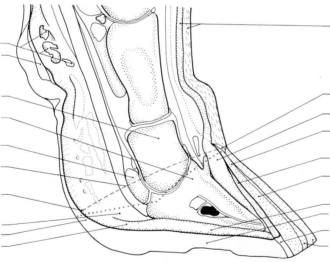

accessory digit V:
phalanges
horny epidermis

middle phalanx

distal phalanx

distal sesamoid bone

m. flexor digitorum profundus

coronet of "heel"

bulb:
digital cushion
horny epidermis
corium

— hair-bearing skin

— periople

— coronary corium of wall

— horny epidermis of coronary region

— laminae of wall

— horny epidermis of wall

sole:
— corium
— horny epidermis

— horn of white zone

— "toes" of hooves of digits III, IV

Fig. 7.17 The hoof of the right manus, in sagittal section.

This figure is a lateral view of the fourth digit of the right manus and is a close-up of fig. 3.24. The deeper structures are dealt with in fig. 7.27. The plane of sectioning is shown in fig. 3.23. The dotted and broken blue lines show the position of the coronet on the axial and abaxial aspects of the digit (see also figs. 7.13 and 7.15). Note that the deepest layer of the wall of the hoof is white.

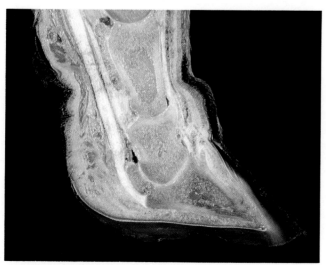

Fig. 7.18 Superficial digital structures of the left manus: (1), dorsal view.

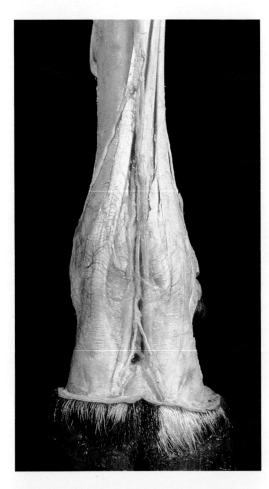

The superficial structures of the metacarpal region of the manus are shown in an earlier dissection (figs. 3.18 – 3.21). The relationships of the vessels and nerves of the manus to those of the more proximal regions of the limb are shown in the dissection of a calf limb (figs. 7.29 – 7.32).

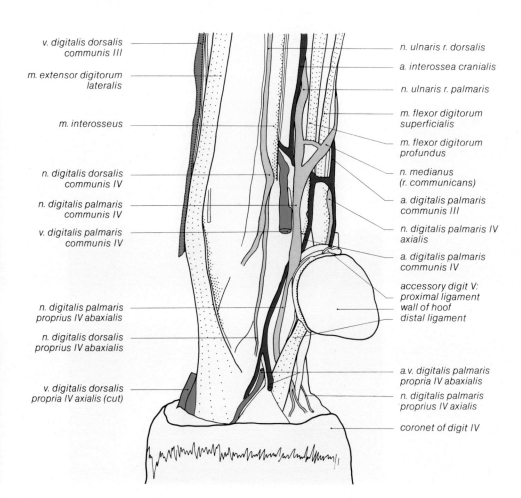

v. cephalica accessoria

m. extensor digitorum communis

metacarpal bone (III, IV)

n. digitalis dorsalis communis II

a. metacarpea dorsalis III

aa. digitales dorsales propriae III, IV axiales

vv. digitales dorsales propriae III, IV axiales

interdigital cleft

digit IV

m. extensor digitorum lateralis

n. radialis r. superficialis (n. cutaneus antebrachii lateralis)

n. digitalis dorsalis communis III

v. digitalis dorsalis communis III (cut)

nn. digitales dorsales propriae III, IV axiales

m. interosseus (suspensory ligament)

v. interdigitalis III (cut stump)

digit III

Fig. 7.19 Superficial digital structures of the left manus: (2), lateral view.

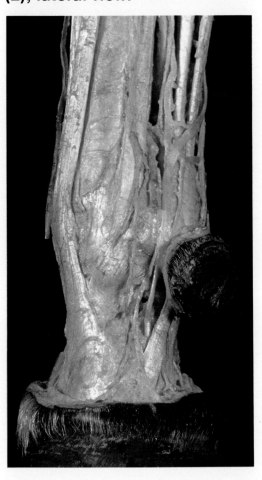

Figs. 3.19 and 7.30 (right forelimb of a calf) should also be consulted.

v. digitalis dorsalis communis III

m. extensor digitorum lateralis

m. interosseus

n. digitalis dorsalis communis IV

n. digitalis palmaris communis IV

v. digitalis palmaris communis IV

n. digitalis palmaris proprius IV abaxialis

n. digitalis dorsalis proprius IV abaxialis

v. digitalis dorsalis propria IV axialis (cut)

n. ulnaris r. dorsalis

a. interossea cranialis

n. ulnaris r. palmaris

m. flexor digitorum superficialis

m. flexor digitorum profundus

n. medianus (r. communicans)

a. digitalis palmaris communis III

n. digitalis palmaris IV axialis

a. digitalis palmaris communis IV

accessory digit V: proximal ligament wall of hoof distal ligament

a.v. digitalis palmaris propria IV abaxialis

n. digitalis palmaris proprius IV axialis

coronet of digit IV

Fig. 7.20 Superficial digital structures of the left manus: (3), palmar view.

Figs. 3.20 and 7.31 (right forelimb of a calf) should also be consulted. The axial palmar digital nerve IV was not given off from the ulnar nerve in this specimen, but it arose with the axial palmar digital nerve III from the median nerve.

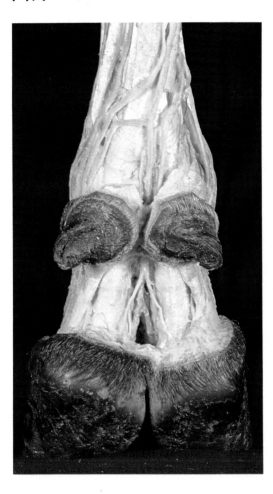

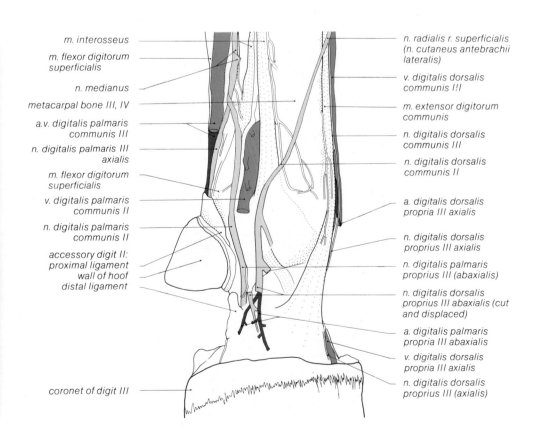

n. ulnaris r. dorsalis
n. ulnaris r. palmaris
n. medianus r. communicans
m. interosseus
communication with a. interossea cranialis
n. digitalis palmaris communis IV
n. digitalis dorsalis communis IV
a.v. digitalis palmaris communis IV
n. digitalis palmaris IV axialis
a. digitalis palmaris propria IV abaxialis
v. digitalis palmaris communis III (cut)
n. digitalis palmaris proprius IV axialis
n. digitalis palmaris proprius IV abaxialis
a.v. digitalis palmaris propria IV axialis

m. flexor digitorum superficialis
n. medianus
a.v. digitalis palmaris communis III
n. digitalis palmaris communis II
n. digitalis palmaris III axialis
v. digitalis palmaris communis II
accessory digit II: proximal ligament
coronet
bulb of "heel"
sole of hoof
"toe" of hoof wall
distal ligament
v. interdigitalis III (cut)
n. digitalis palmaris proprius III abaxialis
n. digitalis palmaris proprius III axialis
a. digitalis palmaris propria III abaxialis
a.v. digitalis palmaris propria III axialis
digit III: interdigital cleft
coronet
wall of hoof
bulb of "heel"

Fig. 7.21 Superficial digital structures of the left manus: (4), medial view.

Figs. 3.21 and 7.32 (right forelimb of a calf) should also be consulted.

m. interosseus
m. flexor digitorum superficialis
n. medianus
metacarpal bone III, IV
a.v. digitalis palmaris communis III
n. digitalis palmaris III axialis
m. flexor digitorum superficialis
v. digitalis palmaris communis II
n. digitalis palmaris communis II
accessory digit II: proximal ligament
wall of hoof
distal ligament
coronet of digit III

n. radialis r. superficialis (n. cutaneus antebrachii lateralis)
v. digitalis dorsalis communis I!I
m. extensor digitorum communis
n. digitalis dorsalis communis III
n. digitalis dorsalis communis II
a. digitalis dorsalis propria III axialis
n. digitalis dorsalis proprius III axialis
n. digitalis palmaris proprius III (abaxialis)
n. digitalis dorsalis proprius III abaxialis (cut and displaced)
a. digitalis palmaris propria III abaxialis
v. digitalis dorsalis propria III axialis
n. digitalis dorsalis proprius III (axialis)

Fig. 7.22 Digital muscles and ligaments of the left manus: (1), dorsal view.

Figs. 7.22 – 7.26 show the deeper structures of the manus after removal of the nerves and vessels. The shining tendons of the common digital extensor muscle are enclosed by tendon sheaths. The dorsal surfaces of the fetlock joint capsules also reveal where they are overlain by the synovial bursae of the so-called "proper" extensor tendons of digits III and IV.

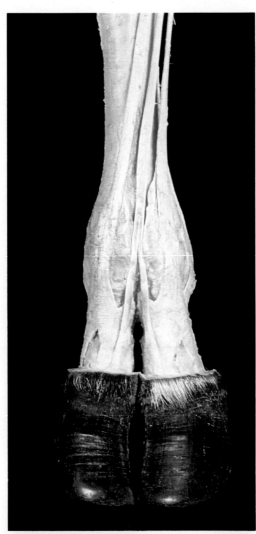

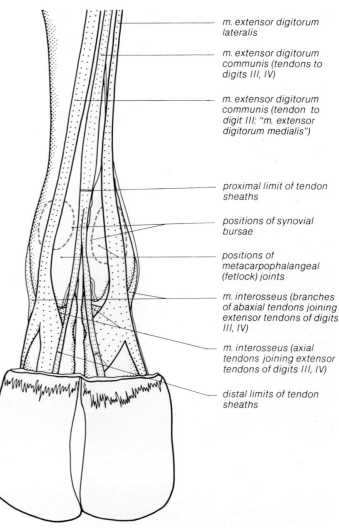

m. extensor digitorum lateralis

m. extensor digitorum communis (tendons to digits III, IV)

m. extensor digitorum communis (tendon to digit III: "m. extensor digitorum medialis")

proximal limit of tendon sheaths

positions of synovial bursae

positions of metacarpophalangeal (fetlock) joints

m. interosseus (branches of abaxial tendons joining extensor tendons of digits III, IV)

m. interosseus (axial tendons joining extensor tendons of digits III, IV)

distal limits of tendon sheaths

Fig. 7.23 Digital muscles and ligaments of the left manus: (2), lateral view.

The deep palmar fascia has been removed to reveal the flexor muscles except where its fibres are arranged transversely to form the annular ligaments of the digit. The ligaments of the accessory digit, which are parts of the deep palmar fascia, have been almost completely removed.

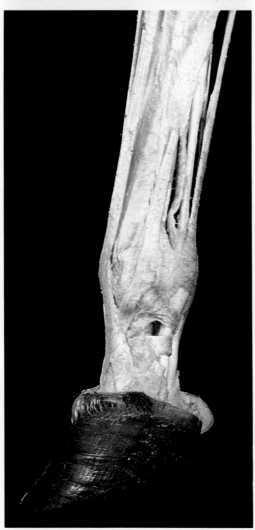

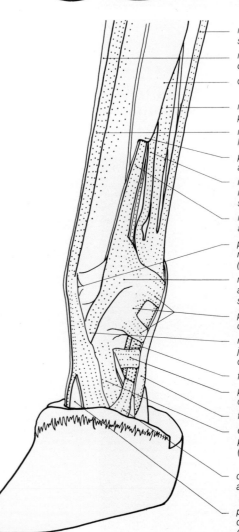

m. flexor digitorum superficialis

m. extensor digitorum communis

deep fascia (cut)

m. flexor digitorum profundus

m. extensor digitorum lateralis

proximal ligament of accessory digit V (cut)

m. interosseus (tendon to m. flexor digitorum superficialis)

m. interosseus (lateral abaxial tendon)

position of metacarpophalangeal (fetlock) joint

m. interosseus, attachment to proximal sesamoid bone of digit IV

palmar annular ligament of fetlock

m. interosseus (tendon joining m. extensor digitorum lateralis)

flexor tendons of digit IV

palmar annular ligament of proximal phalanx

flexor tendons of digit III

collateral ligament, proximal interphalangeal (pastern) joint

distal ligament of accessory digit V (cut)

position of dorsal part of distal interphalangeal (coffin) joint capsule

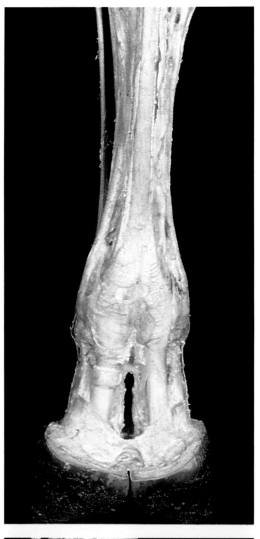

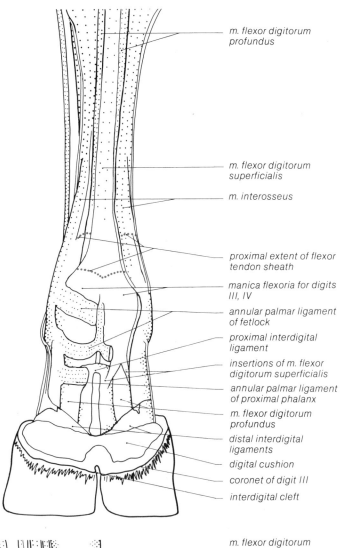

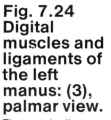

m. flexor digitorum profundus

m. flexor digitorum superficialis

m. interosseus

proximal extent of flexor tendon sheath

manica flexoria for digits III, IV

annular palmar ligament of fetlock

proximal interdigital ligament

insertions of m. flexor digitorum superficialis

annular palmar ligament of proximal phalanx

m. flexor digitorum profundus

distal interdigital ligaments

digital cushion

coronet of digit III

interdigital cleft

Fig. 7.24 Digital muscles and ligaments of the left manus: (3), palmar view.

The annular ligaments have been dissected on the lateral digit (IV) and removed on the medial digit (III). The voluminous flexor tendon sheaths have not been completely removed proximally (blue lines). Distally the shiny surfaces of the flexor tendons have been exposed; the sheaths end just distal to the distal interdigital ligaments. The synovial structures of the digit are also shown in fig. 7.27.

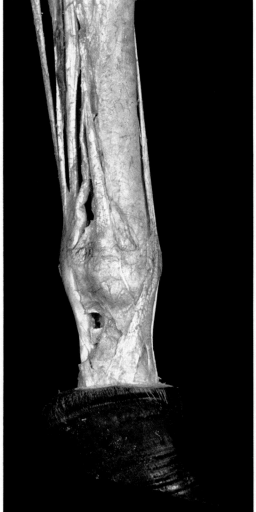

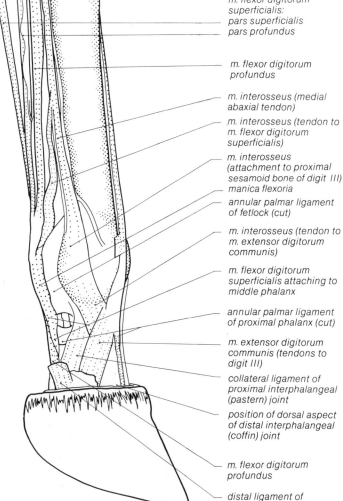

m. flexor digitorum superficialis:
pars superficialis
pars profundus

m. flexor digitorum profundus

m. interosseus (medial abaxial tendon)

m. interosseus (tendon to m. flexor digitorum superficialis)

m. interosseus (attachment to proximal sesamoid bone of digit III)

manica flexoria

annular palmar ligament of fetlock (cut)

m. interosseus (tendon to m. extensor digitorum communis)

m. flexor digitorum superficialis attaching to middle phalanx

annular palmar ligament of proximal phalanx (cut)

m. extensor digitorum communis (tendons to digit III)

collateral ligament of proximal interphalangeal (pastern) joint

position of dorsal aspect of distal interphalangeal (coffin) joint

m. flexor digitorum profundus

distal ligament of accessory digit II

Fig. 7.25 Digital muscles and ligaments of the left manus: (4), medial view.

Removal of the palmar annular ligaments exposes the manica flexoria of the superficial flexor which ensheaths the deep flexor muscle at the region of the fetlock joint.

The specimen is at the stage of dissection shown in fig. 3.22. A glass rod has been inserted to display the interosseous tendons more clearly. The axial tendon of the interosseous muscle divides in the interdigital space and joins the extensor tendons as shown in fig. 7.22.

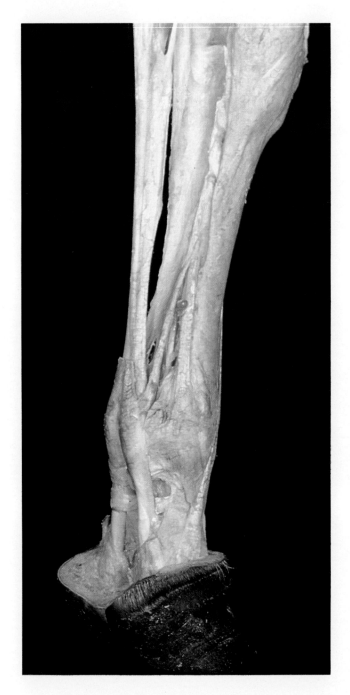

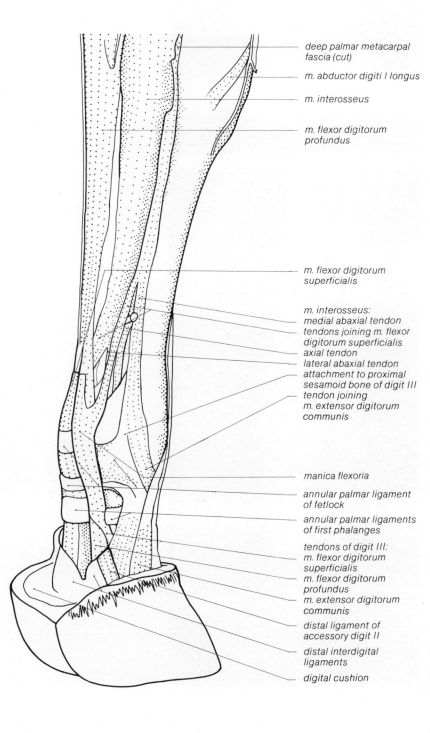

deep palmar metacarpal fascia (cut)

m. abductor digiti I longus

m. interosseus

m. flexor digitorum profundus

m. flexor digitorum superficialis

m. interosseus:
medial abaxial tendon
tendons joining m. flexor digitorum superficialis
axial tendon
lateral abaxial tendon
attachment to proximal sesamoid bone of digit III
tendon joining m. extensor digitorum communis

manica flexoria

annular palmar ligament of fetlock

annular palmar ligaments of first phalanges

tendons of digit III:
m. flexor digitorum superficialis
m. flexor digitorum profundus
m. extensor digitorum communis

distal ligament of accessory digit II

distal interdigital ligaments

digital cushion

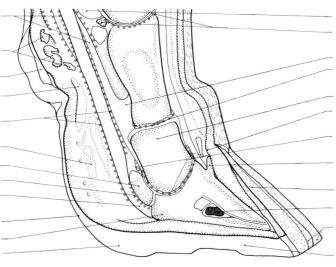

m. flexor digitorum superficialis (manica flexoria)

phalanges of digit V

hoof of digit V

annular ligament of proximal phalanx

synovial sheath of flexor tendons

distal interdigital ligament

distal sesamoid bone

bursa podotrochlearis

m. flexor digitorum profundus

"heel" of digit IV

flexor tuberosity

bulb of hoof

proximal sesamoid bone

metacarpophalangeal joint

palmar ligament

proximal interphalangeal joint

middle phalanx

m. extensor digitorum communis

distal interphalangeal joint

extensor process of distal phalanx

wall of hoof

vessels in solar canal

"toes" of hooves, digits III, IV

sole of hoof

Fig. 7.27 The fourth digit of the right manus, in sagittal section.

This figure is a lateral view of the fourth digit of the manus and is a close-up of fig. 3.24. The integumentary structures are dealt with in fig. 7.17. The plane of sectioning is shown in fig. 3.23. Synovial structures are indicated by blue dotted lines.

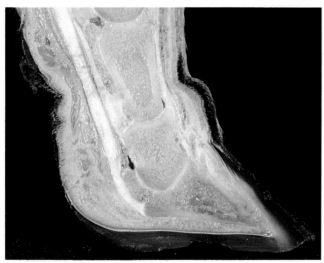

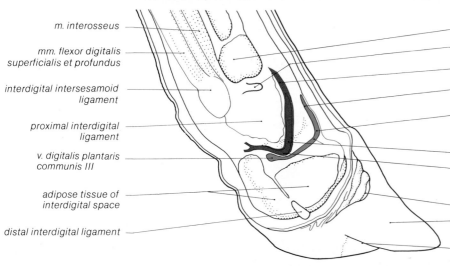

m. interosseus

mm. flexor digitalis superficialis et profundus

interdigital intersesamoid ligament

proximal interdigital ligament

v. digitalis plantaris communis III

adipose tissue of interdigital space

distal interdigital ligament

metatarsal bone IV

m. interosseus, axial tendon

a. metatarsea dorsalis III

v. digitalis dorsalis communis III

origins of vv. digitales dorsales propriae III, IV axiales

a.v. interdigitalis III

origins of aa. digitales plantares propriae III, IV axiales

coronet

axial part of hoof wall, digit III

axial groove

Fig. 7.28 The interdigital region of the right pes, in median section.

The plane of sectioning is shown in fig. 7.14. In this figure, the medial half of the sectioned limb is viewed from the lateral aspect. The integumentary structures are fully labelled in fig. 7.15. In the pes, the main arterial supply to the interdigital region is from the dorsal side. In the manus, however, most of the supply is from the palmar side; compare with figs. 7.18 and 7.20.

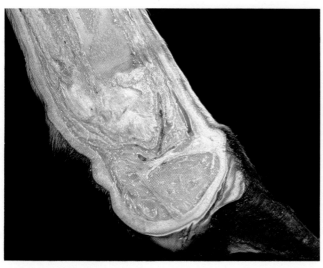

Fig. 7.29 Superficial veins and nerves in the right forelimb of a one-week old calf: (1), dorsal view.

Figs. 7.29 – 7.32 provide a general view of the vessels and nerves to show how those of the manus are related to those in the more proximal regions of the limb.

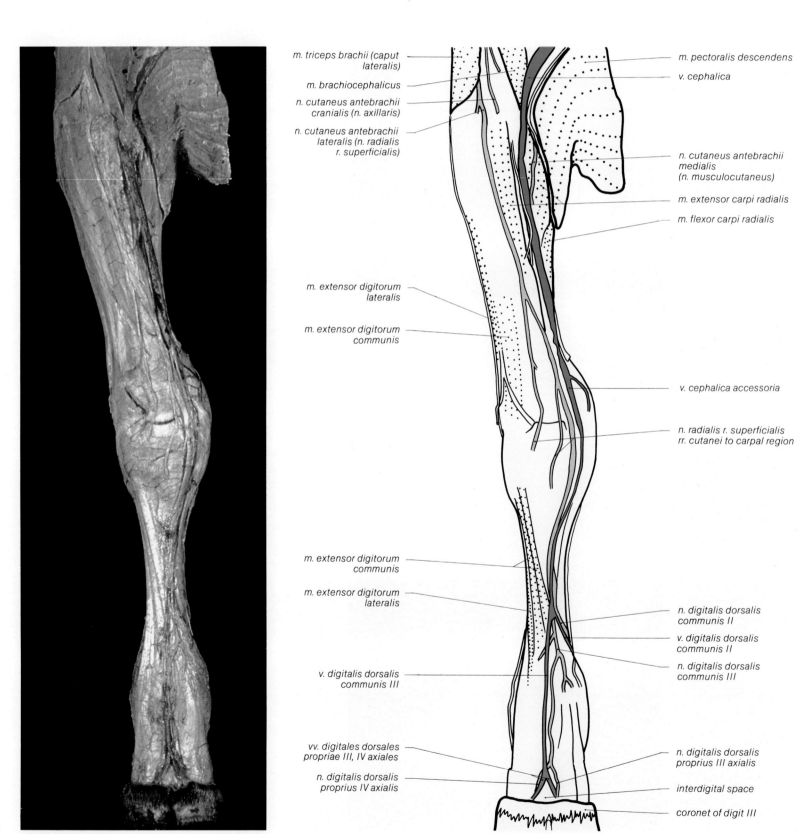

m. triceps brachii (caput lateralis)

m. brachiocephalicus

n. cutaneus antebrachii cranialis (n. axillaris)

n. cutaneus antebrachii lateralis (n. radialis r. superficialis)

m. extensor digitorum lateralis

m. extensor digitorum communis

m. extensor digitorum communis

m. extensor digitorum lateralis

v. digitalis dorsalis communis III

vv. digitales dorsales propriae III, IV axiales

n. digitalis dorsalis proprius IV axialis

m. pectoralis descendens

v. cephalica

n. cutaneus antebrachii medialis (n. musculocutaneus)

m. extensor carpi radialis

m. flexor carpi radialis

v. cephalica accessoria

n. radialis r. superficialis rr. cutanei to carpal region

n. digitalis dorsalis communis II

v. digitalis dorsalis communis II

n. digitalis dorsalis communis III

n. digitalis dorsalis proprius III axialis

interdigital space

coronet of digit III

Fig. 7.30 Superficial veins and nerves in the right forelimb of the calf: (2), lateral view.

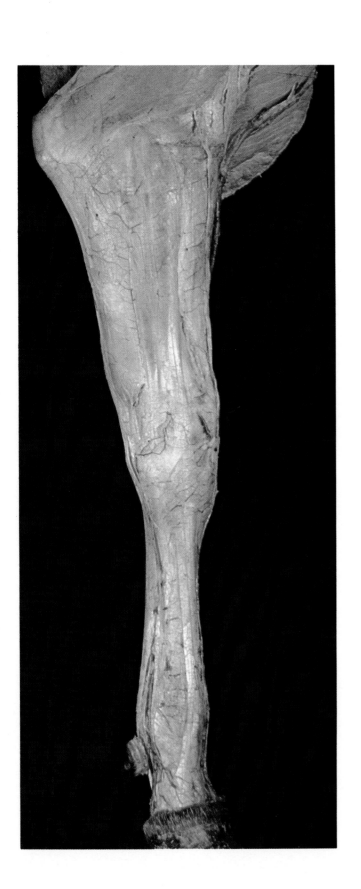

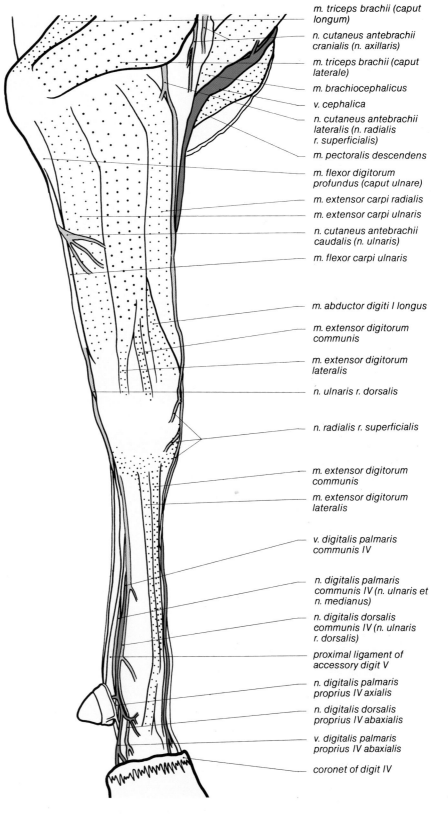

m. triceps brachii (caput longum)

n. cutaneus antebrachii cranialis (n. axillaris)

m. triceps brachii (caput laterale)

m. brachiocephalicus

v. cephalica

n. cutaneus antebrachii lateralis (n. radialis r. superficialis)

m. pectoralis descendens

m. flexor digitorum profundus (caput ulnare)

m. extensor carpi radialis

m. extensor carpi ulnaris

n. cutaneus antebrachii caudalis (n. ulnaris)

m. flexor carpi ulnaris

m. abductor digiti I longus

m. extensor digitorum communis

m. extensor digitorum lateralis

n. ulnaris r. dorsalis

n. radialis r. superficialis

m. extensor digitorum communis

m. extensor digitorum lateralis

v. digitalis palmaris communis IV

n. digitalis palmaris communis IV (n. ulnaris et n. medianus)

n. digitalis dorsalis communis IV (n. ulnaris r. dorsalis)

proximal ligament of accessory digit V

n. digitalis palmaris proprius IV axialis

n. digitalis dorsalis proprius IV abaxialis

v. digitalis palmaris proprius IV abaxialis

coronet of digit IV

Fig. 7.31 Superficial vessels and nerves in the right forelimb of the calf: (3), palmar view.

In the distal metacarpus, the deep fascia has been partially removed to display the vessels and nerves, but the ligaments of the accessory digits have been preserved to demonstrate the fascial levels of the vessels and nerves.

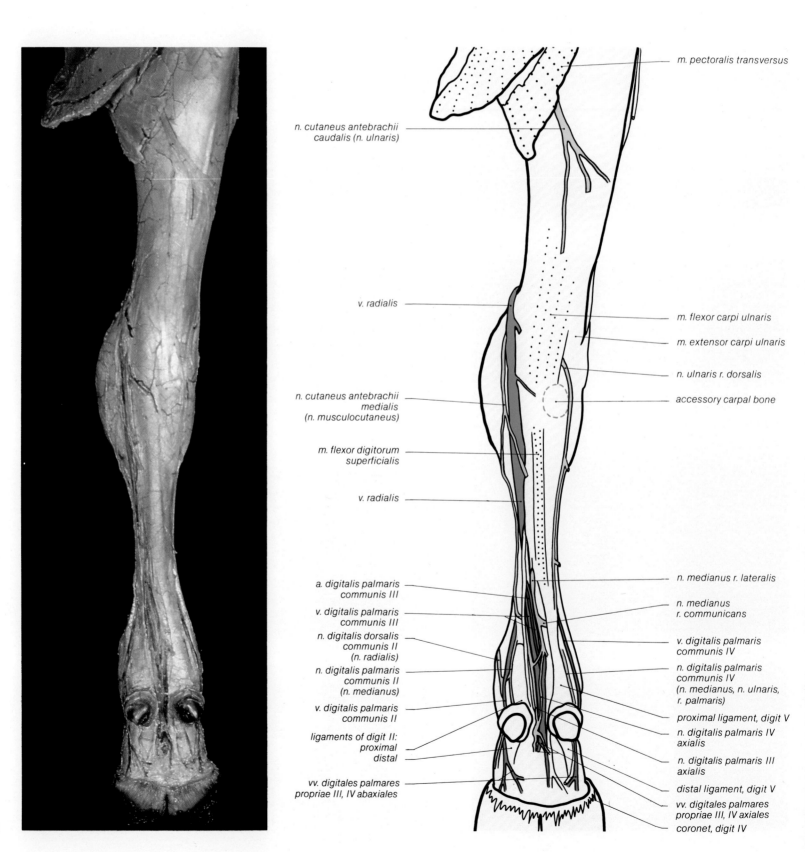

m. pectoralis transversus

n. cutaneus antebrachii caudalis (n. ulnaris)

v. radialis

m. flexor carpi ulnaris

m. extensor carpi ulnaris

n. ulnaris r. dorsalis

n. cutaneus antebrachii medialis (n. musculocutaneus)

accessory carpal bone

m. flexor digitorum superficialis

v. radialis

n. medianus r. lateralis

a. digitalis palmaris communis III

v. digitalis palmaris communis III

n. medianus r. communicans

n. digitalis dorsalis communis II (n. radialis)

v. digitalis palmaris communis IV

n. digitalis palmaris communis II (n. medianus)

n. digitalis palmaris communis IV (n. medianus, n. ulnaris, r. palmaris)

v. digitalis palmaris communis II

proximal ligament, digit V

n. digitalis palmaris IV axialis

ligaments of digit II: proximal distal

n. digitalis palmaris III axialis

distal ligament, digit V

vv. digitales palmares propriae III, IV abaxiales

vv. digitales palmares propriae III, IV axiales

coronet, digit IV

Fig. 7.32 Superficial veins and nerves in the right forelimb of the calf: (4), medial view.

In this specimen, the musculocutaneous nerve extends, as a distinct nerve, into the distal parts of the limb but appeared to play no major part in forming the second dorsal common digital nerve.

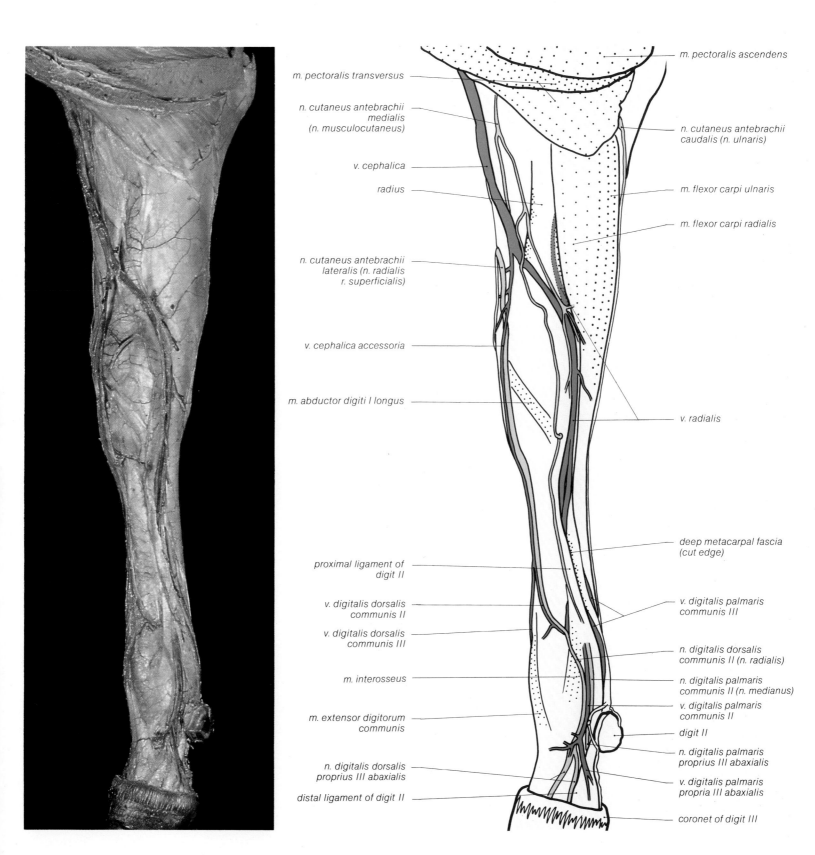

m. pectoralis transversus

n. cutaneus antebrachii medialis (n. musculocutaneus)

v. cephalica

radius

n. cutaneus antebrachii lateralis (n. radialis r. superficialis)

v. cephalica accessoria

m. abductor digiti I longus

proximal ligament of digit II

v. digitalis dorsalis communis II

v. digitalis dorsalis communis III

m. interosseus

m. extensor digitorum communis

n. digitalis dorsalis proprius III abaxialis

distal ligament of digit II

m. pectoralis ascendens

n. cutaneus antebrachii caudalis (n. ulnaris)

m. flexor carpi ulnaris

m. flexor carpi radialis

v. radialis

deep metacarpal fascia (cut edge)

v. digitalis palmaris communis III

n. digitalis dorsalis communis II (n. radialis)

n. digitalis palmaris communis II (n. medianus)

v. digitalis palmaris communis II

digit II

n. digitalis palmaris proprius III abaxialis

v. digitalis palmaris propria III abaxialis

coronet of digit III

7.17

Fig. 7.33 Superficial veins and nerves of the right hindlimb of the calf: (1), dorsal view.

Figs. 7.33 – 7.36 provide a general view of the vessels and nerves to show how those of the pes are related to those in the more proximal regions of the limb. Only the pes is included in this figure because the contour of the more proximal regions of the limb produces excessive foreshortening.

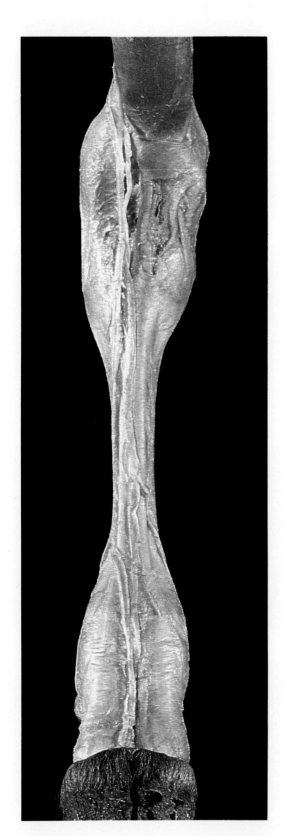

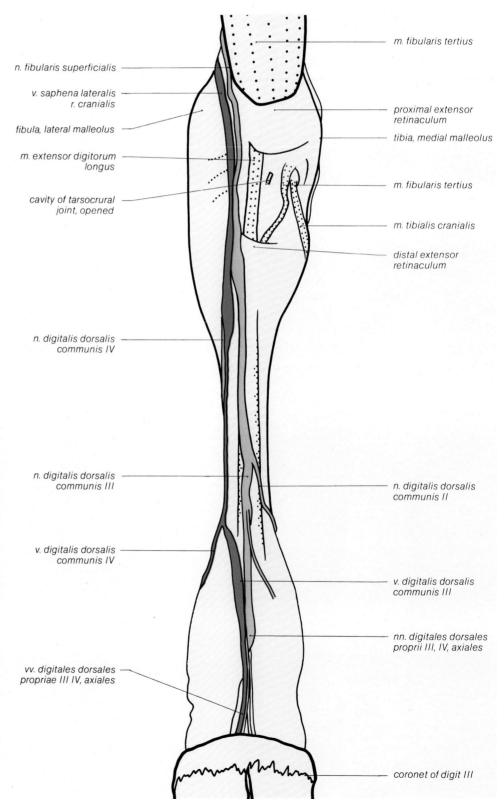

n. fibularis superficialis

v. saphena lateralis
r. cranialis

fibula, lateral malleolus

m. extensor digitorum
longus

cavity of tarsocrural
joint, opened

n. digitalis dorsalis
communis IV

n. digitalis dorsalis
communis III

v. digitalis dorsalis
communis IV

vv. digitales dorsales
propriae III IV, axiales

m. fibularis tertius

proximal extensor
retinaculum

tibia, medial malleolus

m. fibularis tertius

m. tibialis cranialis

distal extensor
retinaculum

n. digitalis dorsalis
communis II

v. digitalis dorsalis
communis III

nn. digitales dorsales
proprii III, IV, axiales

coronet of digit III

Fig. 7.34 Superficial veins and nerves of the right hindlimb of the calf: (2), lateral view.

The crural fascia has been incised and pinned back to reveal the course of the lateral cutaneous sural nerve. The nerve is large in this specimen; when it is small, its territory is partly supplied by the caudal cutaneous sural nerve.

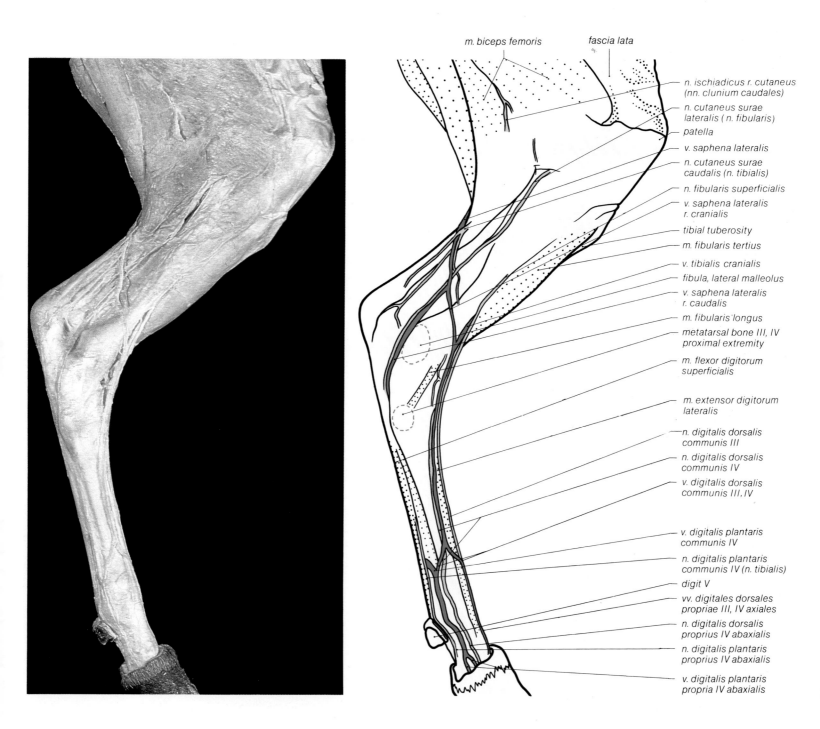

m. biceps femoris

fascia lata

n. ischiadicus r. cutaneus (nn. clunium caudales)

n. cutaneus surae lateralis (n. fibularis)

patella

v. saphena lateralis

n. cutaneus surae caudalis (n. tibialis)

n. fibularis superficialis

v. saphena lateralis r. cranialis

tibial tuberosity

m. fibularis tertius

v. tibialis cranialis

fibula, lateral malleolus

v. saphena lateralis r. caudalis

m. fibularis longus

metatarsal bone III, IV proximal extremity

m. flexor digitorum superficialis

m. extensor digitorum lateralis

n. digitalis dorsalis communis III

n. digitalis dorsalis communis IV

v. digitalis dorsalis communis III, IV

v. digitalis plantaris communis IV

n. digitalis plantaris communis IV (n. tibialis)

digit V

vv. digitales dorsales propriae III, IV axiales

n. digitalis dorsalis proprius IV abaxialis

n. digitalis plantaris proprius IV abaxialis

v. digitalis plantaris propria IV abaxialis

7.19

Fig. 7.35 Superficial vessels and nerves of the right hindlimb of the calf: (3), plantar view.

The contour of the more proximal regions of the limb produces considerable foreshortening. The deep fascia has not been removed from the distal metatarsal region and only the superficial structures are visible (compare with fig. 7.31).

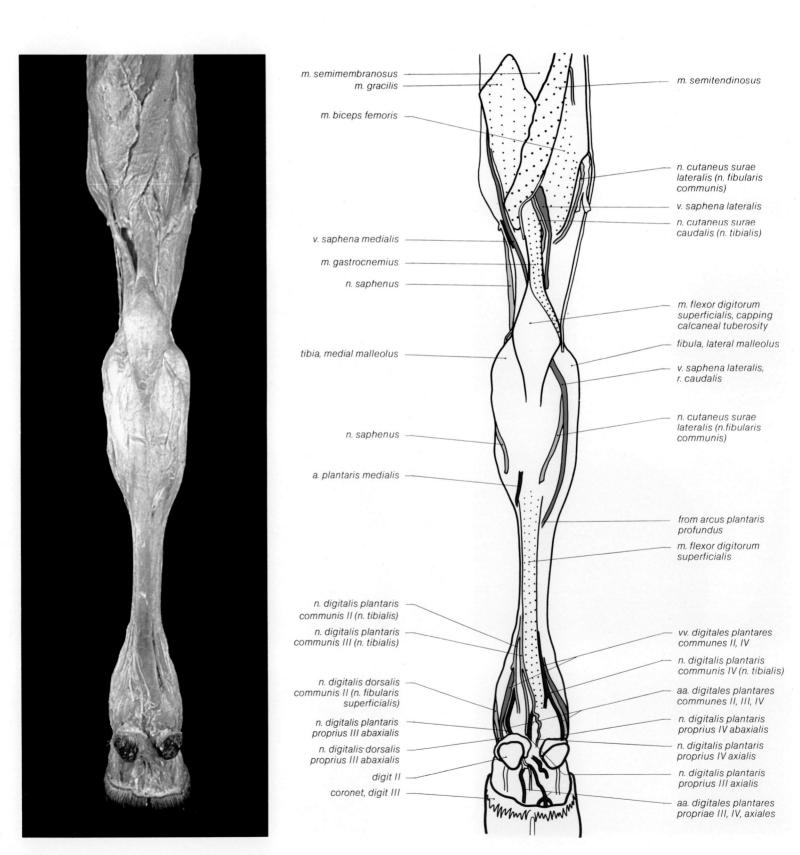

m. semimembranosus
m. gracilis

m. biceps femoris

v. saphena medialis

m. gastrocnemius

n. saphenus

tibia, medial malleolus

n. saphenus

a. plantaris medialis

n. digitalis plantaris communis II (n. tibialis)

n. digitalis plantaris communis III (n. tibialis)

n. digitalis dorsalis communis II (n. fibularis superficialis)

n. digitalis plantaris proprius III abaxialis

n. digitalis·dorsalis proprius III abaxialis

digit II

coronet, digit III

m. semitendinosus

n. cutaneus surae lateralis (n. fibularis communis)

v. saphena lateralis

n. cutaneus surae caudalis (n. tibialis)

m. flexor digitorum superficialis, capping calcaneal tuberosity

fibula, lateral malleolus

v. saphena lateralis, r. caudalis

n. cutaneus surae lateralis (n.fibularis communis)

from arcus plantaris profundus

m. flexor digitorum superficialis

vv. digitales plantares communes II, IV

n. digitalis plantaris communis IV (n. tibialis)

aa. digitales plantares communes II, III, IV

n. digitalis plantaris proprius IV abaxialis

n. digitalis plantaris proprius IV axialis

n. digitalis plantaris proprius III axialis

aa. digitales plantares propriae III, IV, axiales

Fig. 7.36 Superficial vessels and nerves of the right hindlimb of the calf: (4), medial view.

The course of the medial plantar nerve, artery and vein beneath the deep fascia, alongside the deep flexor tendon, is indicated by broken lines.

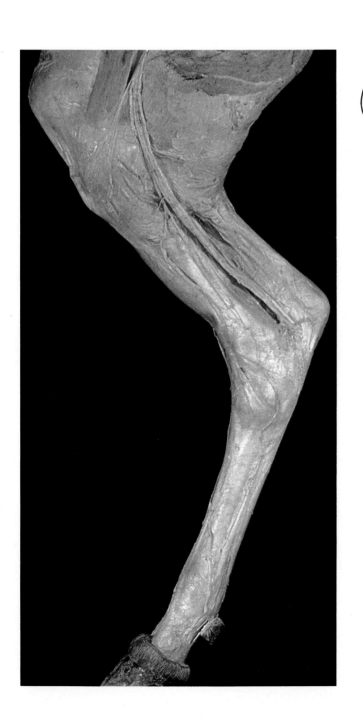

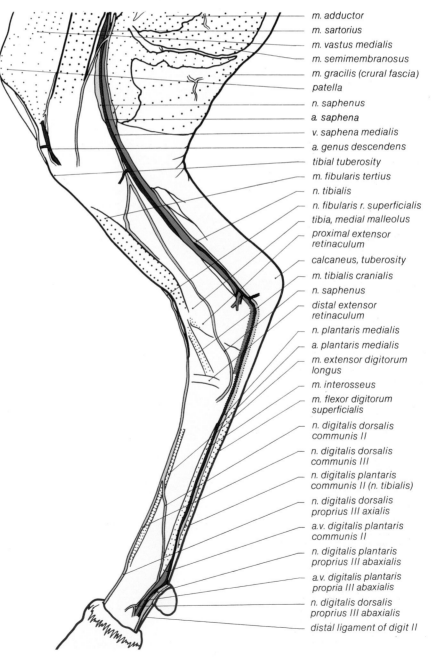

m. adductor
m. sartorius
m. vastus medialis
m. semimembranosus
m. gracilis (crural fascia)
patella
n. saphenus
a. saphena
v. saphena medialis
a. genus descendens
tibial tuberosity
m. fibularis tertius
n. tibialis
n. fibularis r. superficialis
tibia, medial malleolus
proximal extensor retinaculum
calcaneus, tuberosity
m. tibialis cranialis
n. saphenus
distal extensor retinaculum
n. plantaris medialis
a. plantaris medialis
m. extensor digitorum longus
m. interosseus
m. flexor digitorum superficialis
n. digitalis dorsalis communis II
n. digitalis dorsalis communis III
n. digitalis plantaris communis II (n. tibialis)
n. digitalis dorsalis proprius III axialis
a.v. digitalis plantaris communis II
n. digitalis plantaris proprius III abaxialis
a.v. digitalis plantaris propria III abaxialis
n. digitalis dorsalis proprius III abaxialis
distal ligament of digit II

Fig. 7.37 Solar surfaces of the hooves of the right pes of a sheep.

The limb was fixed in the standing position. The foot has been divided into lateral and medial halves by a median sagittal incision, and the lateral part (digits IV and V) has been clipped. Figs. 7.38 and 7.39 show further views of the lateral half of this specimen. This figure should be compared with that of the ox in fig. 7.16.

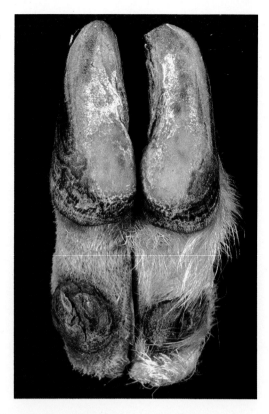

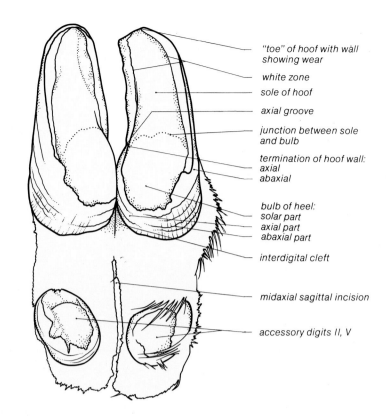

- "toe" of hoof with wall showing wear
- white zone
- sole of hoof
- axial groove
- junction between sole and bulb
- termination of hoof wall: axial abaxial
- bulb of heel: solar part axial part abaxial part
- interdigital cleft
- midaxial sagittal incision
- accessory digits II, V

Fig. 7.38 Digital region of the right pes of a sheep, in lateral view.

This is a lateral view of half of the foot shown in fig. 7.37 showing the fourth digit. The hair has been clipped to show the coronet region. This figure should be compared with that of the ox in fig. 7.13. The axial line of the coronet is shown by blue dots.

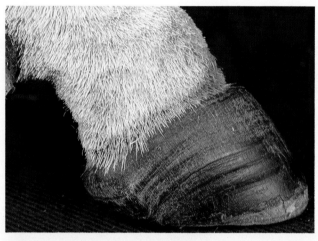

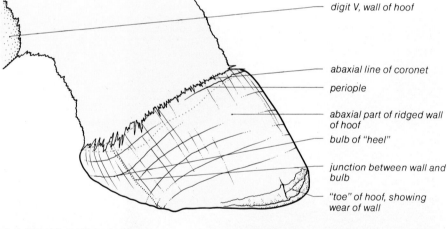

- digit V, wall of hoof
- abaxial line of coronet
- periople
- abaxial part of ridged wall of hoof
- bulb of "heel"
- junction between wall and bulb
- "toe" of hoof, showing wear of wall

Fig. 7.39 The interdigital region of the right pes of the sheep, in median section.

The interdigital cleft and interdigital region are revealed by the median sagittal incision (see fig. 7.37). This is a medial view of the clipped lateral half of the specimen showing the fourth digit. The interdigital sinus is not found in the ox (fig. 7.28) or in the goat.

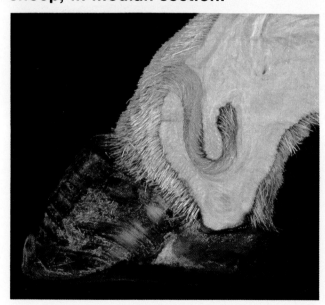

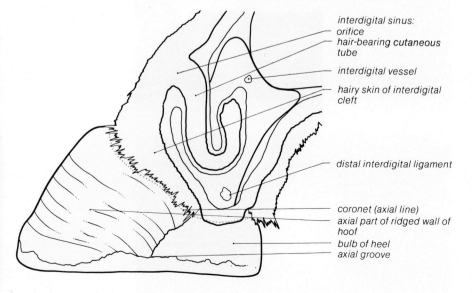

- interdigital sinus: orifice hair-bearing cutaneous tube
- interdigital vessel
- hairy skin of interdigital cleft
- distal interdigital ligament
- coronet (axial line) axial part of ridged wall of hoof
- bulb of heel axial groove

8 The Pelvis

Fig. 8.1 Surface features of the pelvic regions, in left lateral view.

In older cattle, the first caudal vertebra may fuse with the sacrum. The first moveable joint caudal to the sacrum is then the first intervertebral joint of the tail.

Fig. 8.2 Pelvis, vertebrae and proximal femur, in left lateral view.

The palpable bony features shown in fig. 8.1 are coloured red. Note also that in this skeleton the tail is not sufficiently elevated. The caudal border of the sacrotuberous ligament is attached to the dorsal and transverse processes of the sacrocaudal junction, and the dorsal tuberosity of the tuber ischiadicum.

ilium, tuber coxae   *ilium, tuber sacrale*   *sacrocaudal articulation*

Cau 1, 2, dorsal spinous processes
Cau 1, 2, 3, transverse processes
ischiorectal fossa
sacrotuberous ligament
tuber ischiadicum:
dorsal tuberosity
ventral tuberosity
lateral tuberosity
vulva, ventral commissure
femur, great trochanter

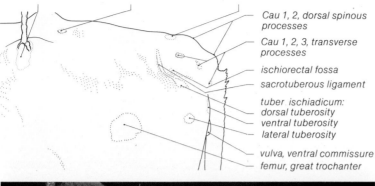

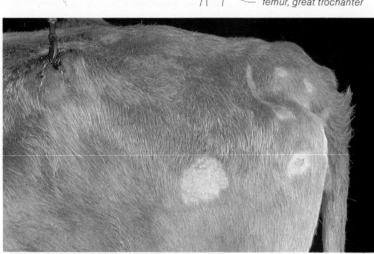

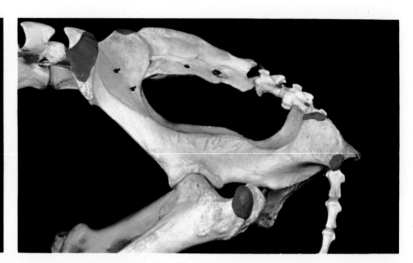

Fig. 8.3 Surface features of the pelvic regions, in caudolateral view.

Strictly, the escutcheon is the region in which the hairs lie in a dorsal direction. The skin of the perineum is said to lie between the anus and the scrotum. However, it is difficult to define in female ruminants because the scrotal swellings of the foetus are not incorporated into the perivulvar region but gradually disappear in the inguinal region. Therefore, the udder forms the ventral boundary of the perineum in the female.

Fig. 8.4 Pelvis and vertebrae, in caudolateral view.

The palpable bony features shown in fig. 8.3 are coloured red. The caudal border of the sacrotuberous ligament is attached to the dorsal and transverse processes of the sacrocaudal junction and the dorsal tuberosity of the tuber ischiadicum.

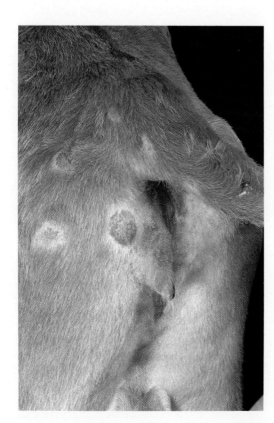

moveable sacrocaudal junction

Cau 1, dorsal spinous process
palpable caudal border of sacrotuberous ligament
Cau 1, 2, 3, transverse processes
abrasion on tail
anus
ischiorectal fossa
vulva
left vulval labium
ventral vulval commissure
tuber ischiadicum:
ventral tuberosity
dorsal tuberosity
lateral tuberosity
escutcheon
base of udder

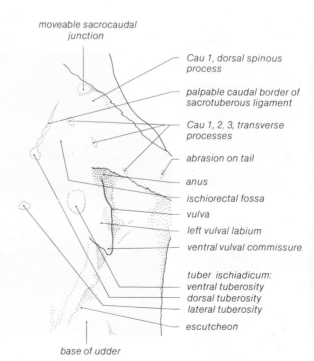

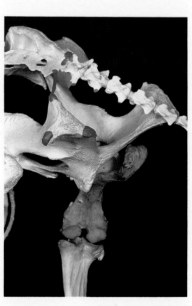

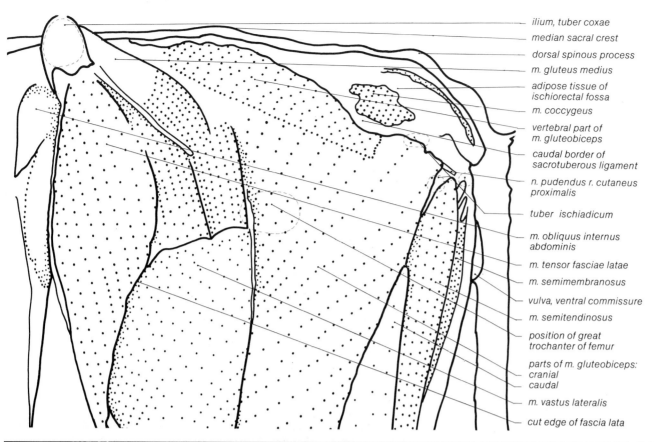

ilium, tuber coxae
median sacral crest
dorsal spinous process
m. gluteus medius
adipose tissue of ischiorectal fossa
m. coccygeus
vertebral part of m. gluteobiceps
caudal border of sacrotuberous ligament
n. pudendus r. cutaneus proximalis
tuber ischiadicum
m. obliquus internus abdominis
m. tensor fasciae latae
m. semimembranosus
vulva, ventral commissure
m. semitendinosus
position of great trochanter of femur
parts of m. gluteobiceps:
cranial
caudal
m. vastus lateralis
cut edge of fascia lata

**Fig. 8.5
Superficial
muscles of
the left lateral
pelvic wall.**
The cutaneous nerves
and superficial lymph
nodes of the region
are shown in fig. 8.29.

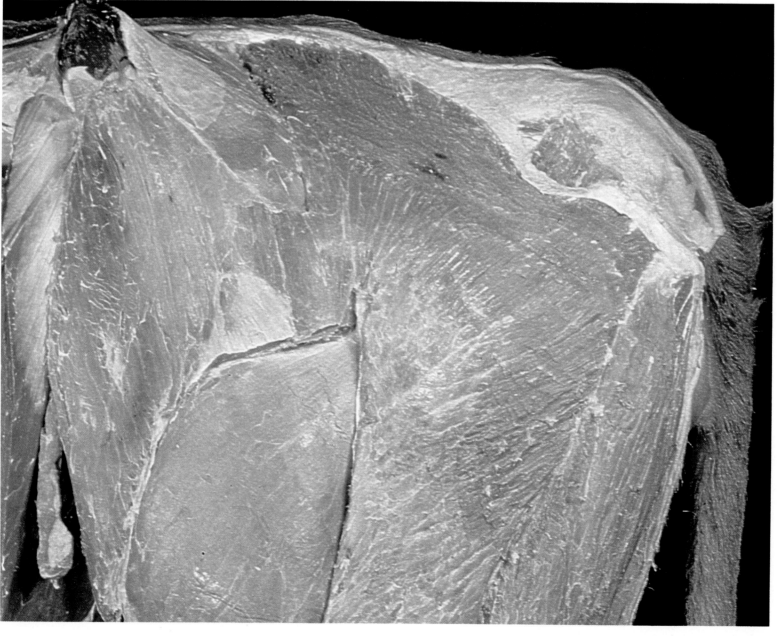

Fig. 8.6 Deeper muscles of the left lateral pelvic wall.

Removal of the large gluteobiceps muscle reveals part of the sacrotuberous ligament caudal to the medial gluteal muscle.

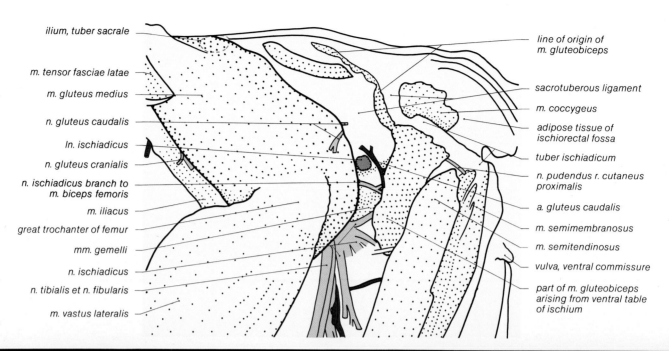

ilium, tuber sacrale

m. tensor fasciae latae

m. gluteus medius

n. gluteus caudalis

ln. ischiadicus

n. gluteus cranialis

n. ischiadicus branch to m. biceps femoris

m. iliacus

great trochanter of femur

mm. gemelli

n. ischiadicus

n. tibialis et n. fibularis

m. vastus lateralis

line of origin of m. gluteobiceps

sacrotuberous ligament

m. coccygeus

adipose tissue of ischiorectal fossa

tuber ischiadicum

n. pudendus r. cutaneus proximalis

a. gluteus caudalis

m. semimembranosus

m. semitendinosus

vulva, ventral commissure

part of m. gluteobiceps arising from ventral table of ischium

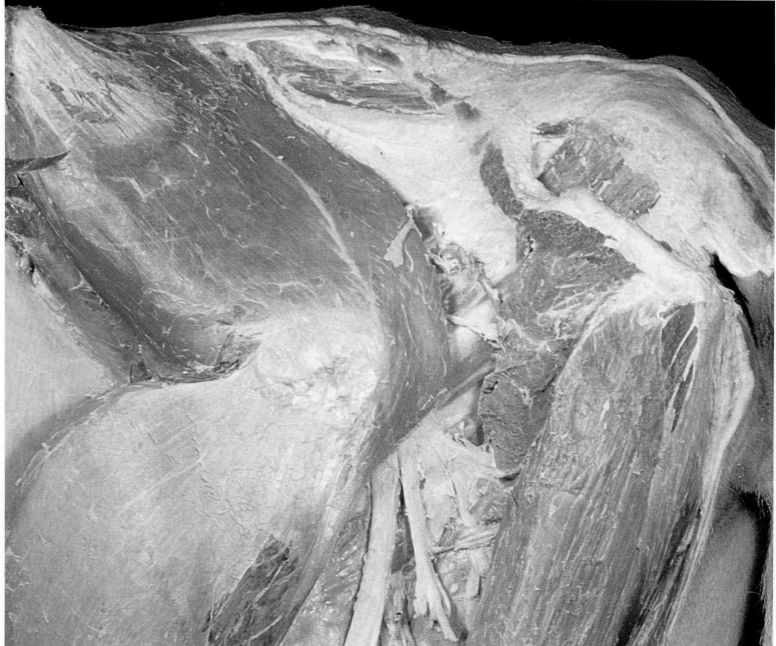

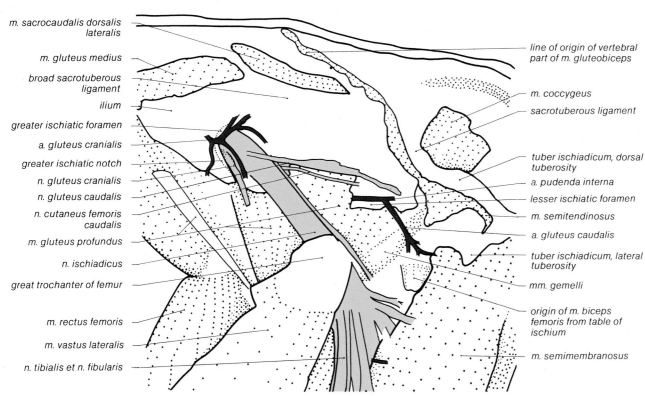

m. sacrocaudalis dorsalis lateralis

m. gluteus medius

broad sacrotuberous ligament

ilium

greater ischiatic foramen

a. gluteus cranialis

greater ischiatic notch

n. gluteus cranialis

n. gluteus caudalis

n. cutaneus femoris caudalis

m. gluteus profundus

n. ischiadicus

great trochanter of femur

m. rectus femoris

m. vastus lateralis

n. tibialis et n. fibularis

line of origin of vertebral part of m. gluteobiceps

m. coccygeus

sacrotuberous ligament

tuber ischiadicum, dorsal tuberosity

a. pudenda interna

lesser ischiatic foramen

m. semitendinosus

a. gluteus caudalis

tuber ischiadicum, lateral tuberosity

mm. gemelli

origin of m. biceps femoris from table of ischium

m. semimembranosus

**Fig. 8.7
The broad sacrotuberous ligament and its foramina, in left lateral view.**
Removal of the middle gluteal muscle reveals the full extent of the sacrotuberous ligament, the two foramina and the vessels and nerves that traverse them.

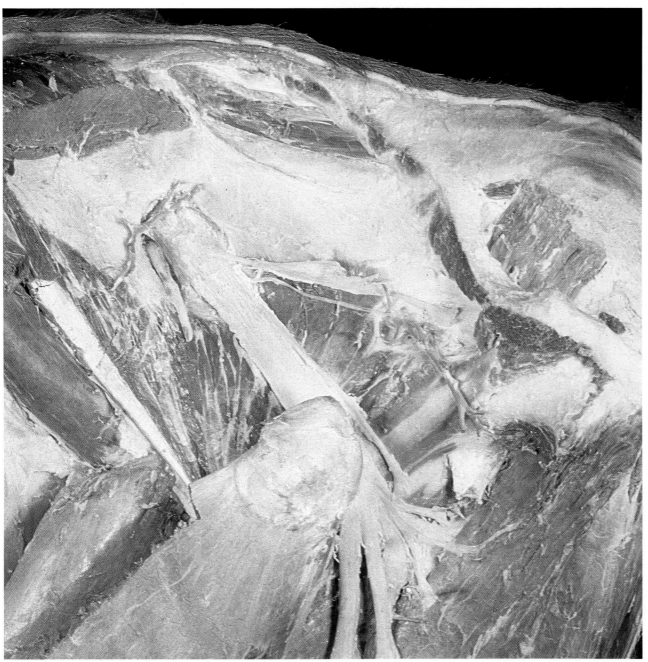

Fig. 8.8 The pelvis after partial removal of the left lateral pelvic wall.

The wing of the ilium and most of the broad sacrotuberous ligament have been removed. This figure shows the nerves and arteries of the pelvic cavity surrounded by massive adipose deposits as in life. A further dissection is shown in fig. 8.11.

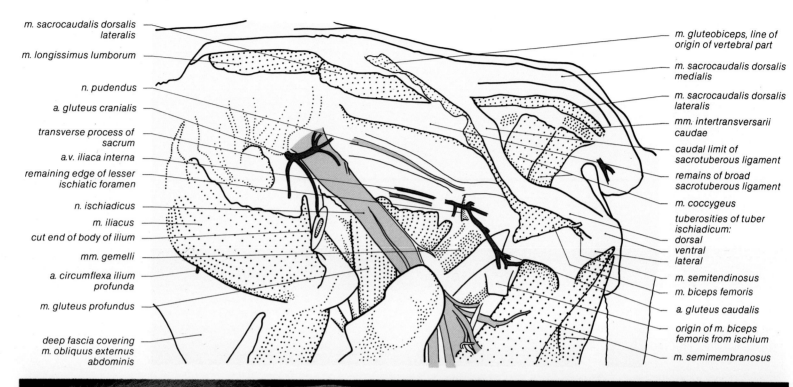

m. sacrocaudalis dorsalis lateralis

m. longissimus lumborum

n. pudendus

a. gluteus cranialis

transverse process of sacrum

a.v. iliaca interna

remaining edge of lesser ischiatic foramen

n. ischiadicus

m. iliacus

cut end of body of ilium

mm. gemelli

a. circumflexa ilium profunda

m. gluteus profundus

deep fascia covering m. obliquus externus abdominis

m. gluteobiceps, line of origin of vertebral part

m. sacrocaudalis dorsalis medialis

m. sacrocaudalis dorsalis lateralis

mm. intertransversarii caudae

caudal limit of sacrotuberous ligament

remains of broad sacrotuberous ligament

m. coccygeus

tuberosities of tuber ischiadicum:
dorsal
ventral
lateral

m. semitendinosus

m. biceps femoris

a. gluteus caudalis

origin of m. biceps femoris from ischium

m. semimembranosus

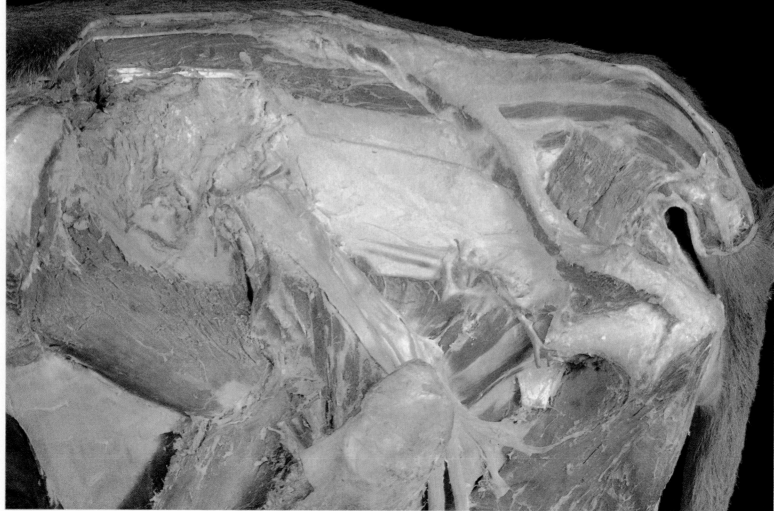

Fig. 8.9 The median caudal artery and ischiorectal fossa: left lateral view.

In fat animals the ischiorectal fossa is occupied by a large adipose mass and externally this forms a bulge rather than a concavity.

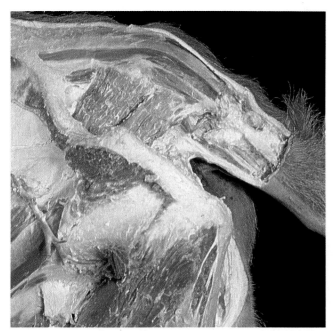

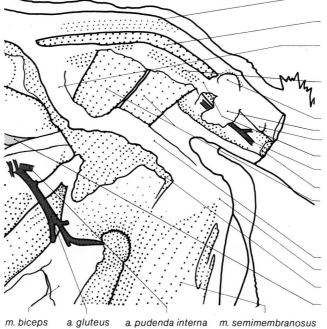

m. sacrocaudalis dorsalis medialis

m. sacrocaudalis dorsalis lateralis

sacrotuberous ligament, forming laterodorsal wall of ischiorectal fossa

mm. intertransversarii caudae

Cau 3:
cranial articular process
haemal arch
transverse process

Cau 2, transverse process

a. caudalis mediana

m. sacrocaudalis ventralis

m. coccygeus, forming medial wall of ischiorectal fossa

tuber ischiadicum:
dorsal tuberosity
ventral tuberosity

m. semitendinosus

n. pudendus

m. biceps femoris   a. gluteus caudalis   a. pudenda interna   m. semimembranosus

Fig. 8.10 Superficial muscles of the perineal region and the ischiorectal fossa: left caudolateral view.

The fascia of the urogenital diaphragm, which forms the medial wall of the ischiorectal fossa, has been dissected away to reveal the retractor muscle of the clitoris.

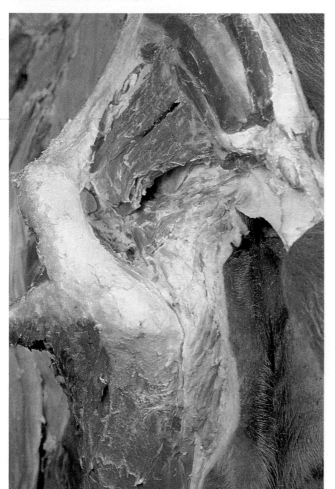

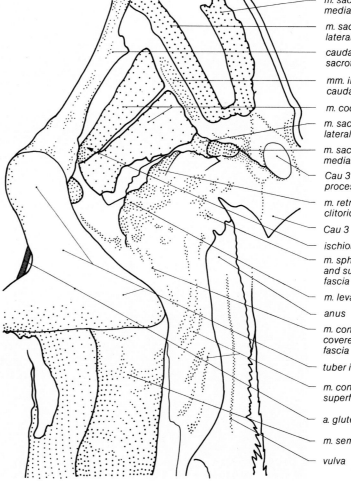

m. sacrocaudalis dorsalis medialis

m. sacrocaudalis dorsalis lateralis

caudal border of sacrotuberous ligament

mm. intertransversarii caudae

m. coccygeus

m. sacrocaudalis ventralis lateralis

m. sacrocaudalis ventralis medialis

Cau 3 cranial articular process

m. retractor clitoridis (pars clitoridea)

Cau 3 transverse process

ischiorectal fossa

m. sphincter ani externus and superficial perineal fascia

m. levator ani

anus

m. constrictor vestibuli covered by deep perineal fascia

tuber ischiadicum

m. constrictor vulvae and superficial perineal fascia

a. gluteus caudalis

m. semimembranosus

vulva

Fig. 8.11
Nerves and blood vessels of the pelvis, in left lateral view.

The caudal cutaneous femoral nerve enters the pelvis through the lesser sciatic foramen and joins a branch of the pudendal nerve; this union is not shown here but can be seen in figs. 8.31 – 8.33. The origin of the pelvic nerve can be seen in figs. 8.13 and 8.33.

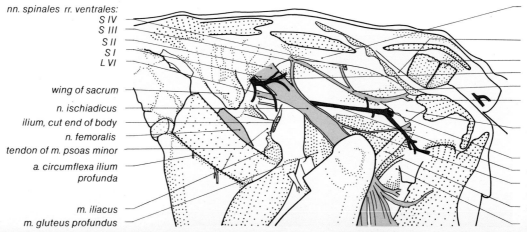

nn. spinales rr. ventrales:
S IV
S III
S II
S I
L VI
wing of sacrum
n. ischiadicus
ilium, cut end of body
n. femoralis
tendon of m. psoas minor
a. circumflexa ilium profunda
m. iliacus
m. gluteus profundus

broad sacrotuberous ligament
caudal edge of sacrotuberous ligament
m. coccygeus
a. glutea cranialis
n. pudendus
n. pudendus, r. cutaneus proximalis
pelvic fascia at lesser ischiatic foramen
a. pudenda interna
a. iliaca interna
n. cutaneus femoris caudalis (displaced)
mm. gemelli
m. quadratus femoris

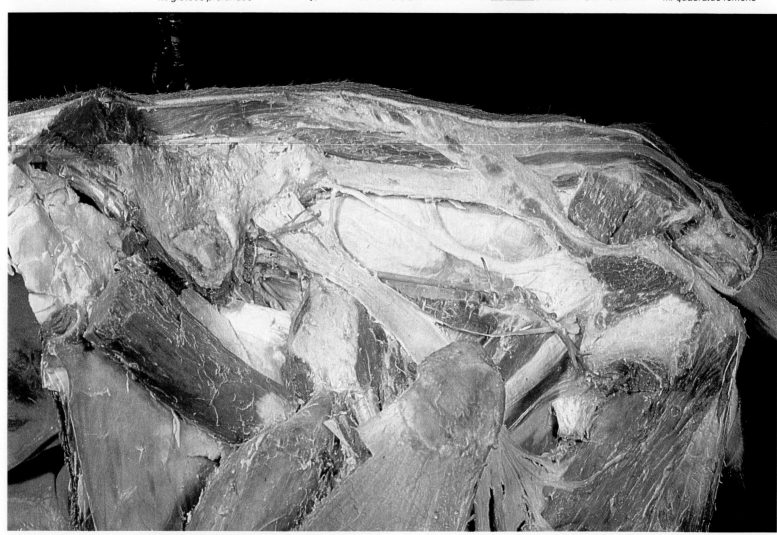

Fig. 8.12
Nerves and blood vessels at the pelvic inlet, in left lateral view.

This is a close up of part of fig. 8.11 after removal of the abdominal wall and the iliacus and rectus femoris muscles

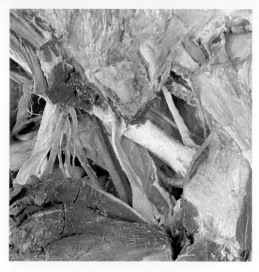

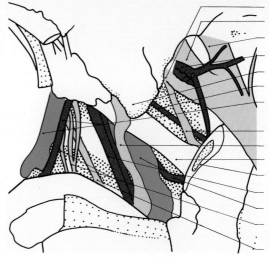

LVI
SI
SII
a. glutea cranialis
sacrum
a. umbilicalis
a. v. circumflexa ilium profunda
n. obturatorius
n. femoralis
tendon of m. psoas minor
ilium, cut end of body
a.v. iliaca externa
a. uterina
n. cutaneus femoris lateralis
n. genitofemoralis

Fig. 8.13 Nerves and arteries of the pelvis, after removal of the limb: left lateral view.

The origin of the pudendal nerve from SIV has been cut and reflected to reveal the pelvic nerve.

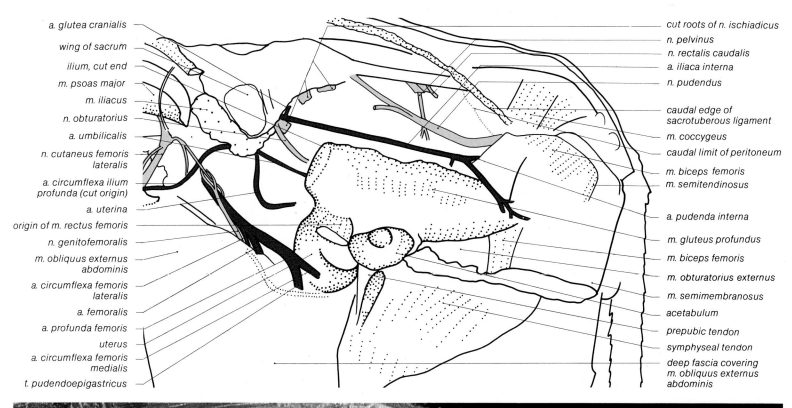

a. glutea cranialis
wing of sacrum
ilium, cut end
m. psoas major
m. iliacus
n. obturatorius
a. umbilicalis
n. cutaneus femoris lateralis
a. circumflexa ilium profunda (cut origin)
a. uterina
origin of m. rectus femoris
n. genitofemoralis
m. obliquus externus abdominis
a. circumflexa femoris lateralis
a. femoralis
a. profunda femoris
uterus
a. circumflexa femoris medialis
t. pudendoepigastricus

cut roots of n. ischiadicus
n. pelvinus
n. rectalis caudalis
a. iliaca interna
n. pudendus
caudal edge of sacrotuberous ligament
m. coccygeus
caudal limit of peritoneum
m. biceps femoris
m. semitendinosus
a. pudenda interna
m. gluteus profundus
m. biceps femoris
m. obturatorius externus
m. semimembranosus
acetabulum
prepubic tendon
symphyseal tendon
deep fascia covering m. obliquus externus abdominis

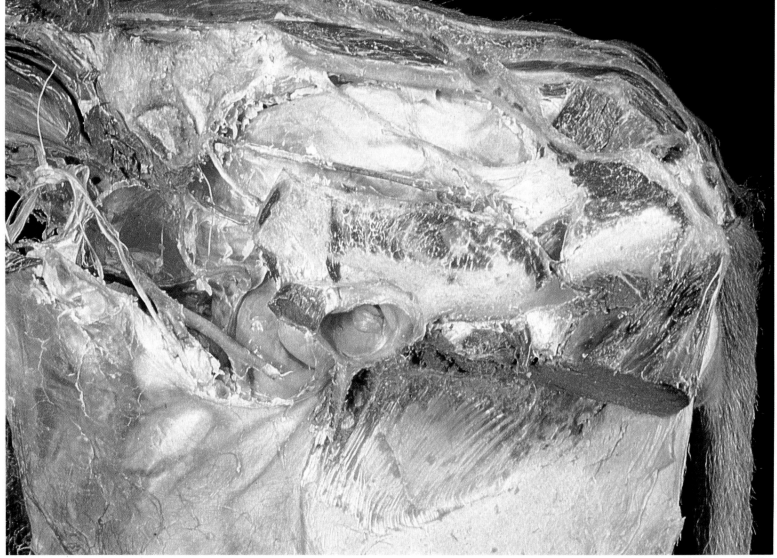

8.9

Fig. 8.14 Pelvic viscera before removal of the left side of the bony pelvis.

The adipose tissue of the pelvic wall has been removed together with the coccygeus muscle to show the positions of the viscera. A more complete topographical display is seen in fig. 8.15.

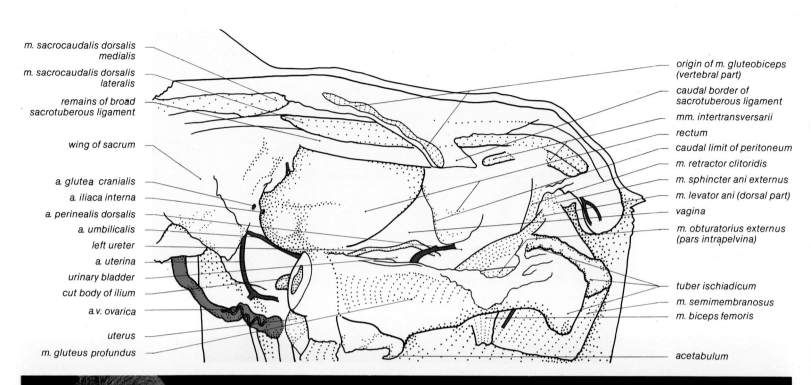

m. sacrocaudalis dorsalis medialis

m. sacrocaudalis dorsalis lateralis

remains of broad sacrotuberous ligament

wing of sacrum

a. glutea cranialis

a. iliaca interna

a. perinealis dorsalis

a. umbilicalis

left ureter

a. uterina

urinary bladder

cut body of ilium

a.v. ovarica

uterus

m. gluteus profundus

origin of m. gluteobiceps (vertebral part)

caudal border of sacrotuberous ligament

mm. intertransversarii

rectum

caudal limit of peritoneum

m. retractor clitoridis

m. sphincter ani externus

m. levator ani (dorsal part)

vagina

m. obturatorius externus (pars intrapelvina)

tuber ischiadicum

m. semimembranosus

m. biceps femoris

acetabulum

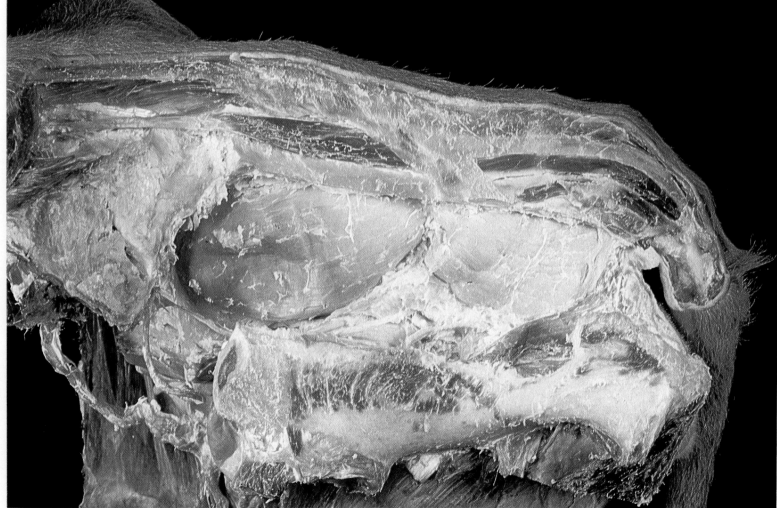

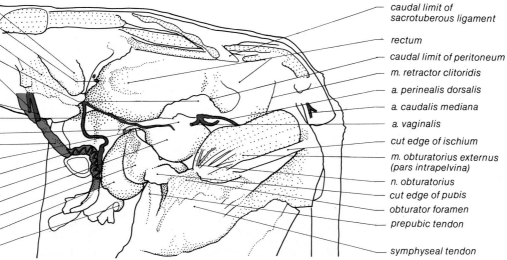

wing of sacrum
a. iliaca interna
m. iliopsoas
vagina
a. circumflexa ilium profunda
a. iliaca externa
a. uterina
left ureter
v. ovarica
lateral ligament of bladder
a. ovarica
colon, descending part
urinary bladder
left uterine horn
right uterine horn
left ovary with corpus luteum

caudal limit of sacrotuberous ligament
rectum
caudal limit of peritoneum
m. retractor clitoridis
a. perinealis dorsalis
a. caudalis mediana
a. vaginalis
cut edge of ischium
m. obturatorius externus (pars intrapelvina)
n. obturatorius
cut edge of pubis
obturator foramen
prepubic tendon
symphyseal tendon

**Fig. 8.15
Pelvic viscera after removal of the left bony pelvis.**
The paramedian saw cut passes through the obturator foramen; the intrapelvic part of the obturator muscle remains *in situ*. Figs. 8.17 and 8.18 show the uterus and ovary at this stage of the dissection from a more cranial view.

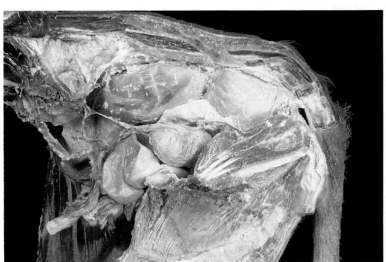

broad sacrotuberous ligament
rectum
vagina
a. vesicalis cranialis
a. umbilicalis
urinary bladder
a. vaginalis:
a. vaginalis r. uterinus
a. vaginalis r. urethralis
left uterine horn
pubis
obturator foramen
ovary

caudal limit of sacrotuberous ligament
Cau 2
m. retractor clitoridis
caudal limit of peritoneum
n. pudendus
external fascia of pelvic diaphragm
m. levator ani
m. constrictor vulvae and superficial perineal fascia
ischium
vulva, ventral commissure
a. perinealis dorsalis

**Fig. 8.16
Pelvic viscera after removal of the left bony pelvis and the obturator muscle.**
Comparison with the usual text book accounts shows the contracted urinary bladder in this cow to be rotated dorsally and to the left, while the uterus is displaced ventrally towards the right.

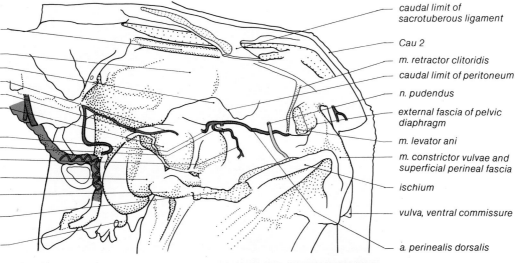

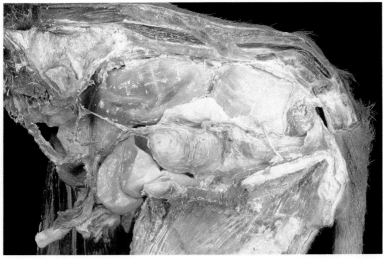

8.11

Fig. 8.17 Structures at the pelvic inlet, in left lateral view.

This is a slightly more cranial part of the dissection shown in fig. 8.16. Further details of the ovary and the ovarian bursa are shown by another series of dissections in figs. 8.24-8.28.

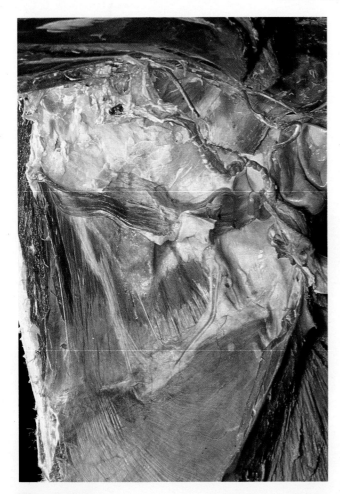

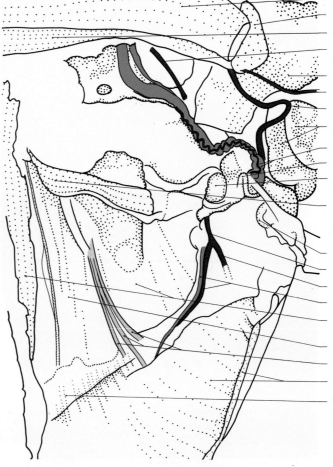

- m. psoas major
- m. iliacus
- m. psoas minor
- a. circumflexa ilium profunda
- rectum
- a. umbilicalis
- a. uterina
- uterus
- a.v. ovarica (sinistra)
- right uterine horn
- right ovary in ovarian bursa
- suspensory ligament of right ovary (cranial edge of broad ligament)
- left ovary
- t. pudendoepigastricus
- a. pudenda externa
- a.v. epigastrica caudalis
- m. obliquus internus abdominis
- m. transversus abdominis
- n. lumbalis II r. ventralis
- m. rectus abdominis
- vagina m. recti abdominis, lamina interna (covered by peritoneum)

Fig. 8.18 Structures at the pelvic inlet, in left craniolateral view.

The tissues covering the right inguinal region in fig. 8.17 have been partially removed to expose the positions of the vessels and lymph node.

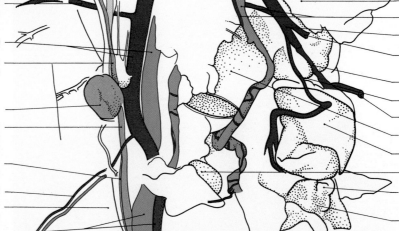

- a. circumflexa ilium profunda (dextra)
- a.v. iliaca externa (dextra)
- vasa efferentia lymphatica
- ln. iliofemoralis
- vasa afferentia from lnn. inguinales superficiales
- n. genitofemoralis (L III, IV)
- muscular branch
- m. obliquus internus abdominis (caudal border)
- t.v. pudendoepigastricus

- m. psoas major
- a.v. ovarica sinistra
- a. iliaca externa (sinistra)
- a. circumflexa ilium profunda
- a. umbilicalis (sinistra)
- a. uterina (sinistra)
- cut end of a. iliaca interna
- descending colon
- uterus
- right ovary
- corpus luteum in left ovary
- wall of ovarian bursa

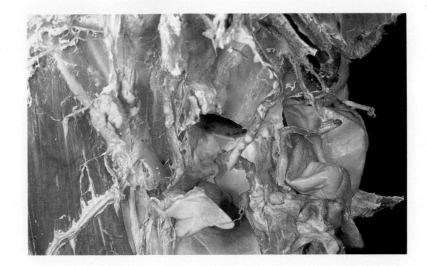

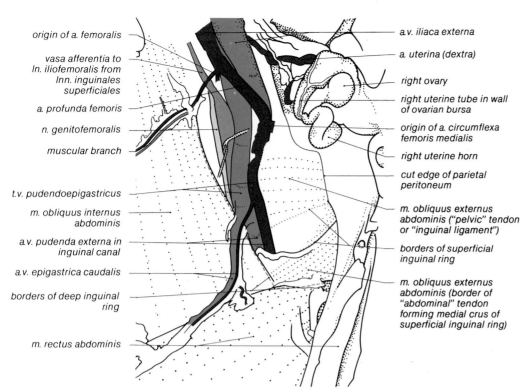

origin of a. femoralis

vasa afferentia to
ln. iliofemoralis from
lnn. inguinales
superficiales

a. profunda femoris

n. genitofemoralis

muscular branch

t.v. pudendoepigastricus

m. obliquus internus
abdominis

a.v. pudenda externa in
inguinal canal

a.v. epigastrica caudalis

borders of deep inguinal
ring

m. rectus abdominis

a.v. iliaca externa

a. uterina (dextra)

right ovary

right uterine tube in wall
of ovarian bursa

origin of a. circumflexa
femoris medialis

right uterine horn

cut edge of parietal
peritoneum

m. obliquus externus
abdominis ("pelvic" tendon
or "inguinal ligament")

borders of superficial
inguinal ring

m. obliquus externus
abdominis (border of
"abdominal" tendon
forming medial crus of
superficial inguinal ring)

Fig. 8.19 The right inguinal canal and structures traversing it: left craniolateral view.

This is a further dissection of part of the specimen shown in fig.8.17, partly overlapping with that shown in fig. 8.18. The cranial and ventral borders of the deep inguinal ring are shown with a broken blue line. The medial and lateral borders of the superficial inguinal ring are shown with a line of blue dots; the lateral border is not very distinct.

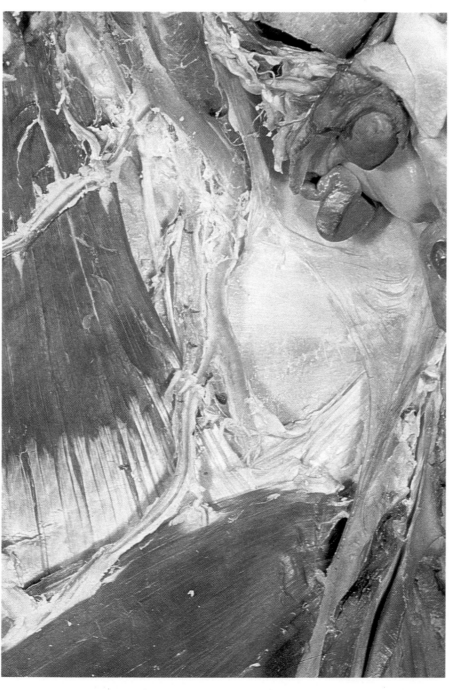

Fig. 8.20 Structures of the right inguinal canal, in cranial view (1).

In figs. 8.20-8.23 the anatomy of the superficial and deep inguinal rings and the disposition of the structures traversing the inguinal canal are shown by progressively reflecting the layers of the abdominal wall. The female reproductive tract has been displaced caudally into the pelvis.

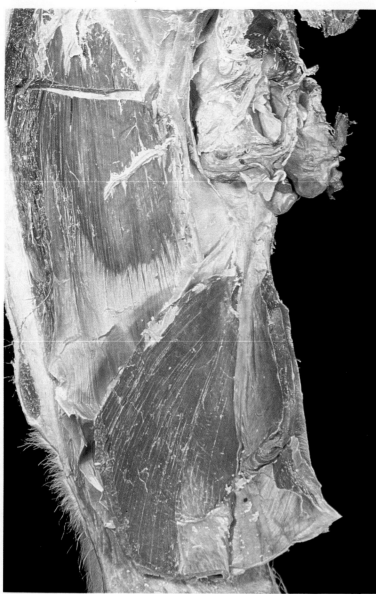

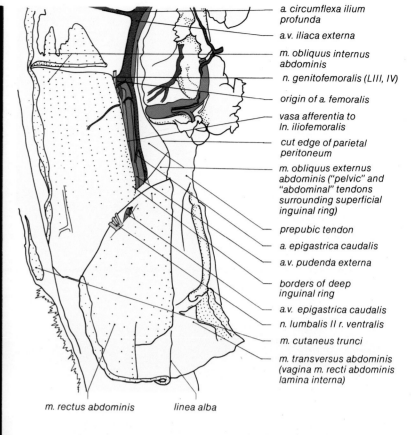

a. circumflexa ilium profunda

a.v. iliaca externa

m. obliquus internus abdominis

n. genitofemoralis (LIII, IV)

origin of a. femoralis

vasa afferentia to ln. iliofemoralis

cut edge of parietal peritoneum

m. obliquus externus abdominis ("pelvic" and "abdominal" tendons surrounding superficial inguinal ring)

prepubic tendon

a. epigastrica caudalis

a.v. pudenda externa

borders of deep inguinal ring

a.v. epigastrica caudalis

n. lumbalis II r. ventralis

m. cutaneus trunci

m. transversus abdominis (vagina m. recti abdominis lamina interna)

m. rectus abdominis   linea alba

Fig. 8.21 Structures of the right inguinal canal, in cranial view (2).

Medial reflection of the right rectus abdominal muscle opens the deep inguinal ring.

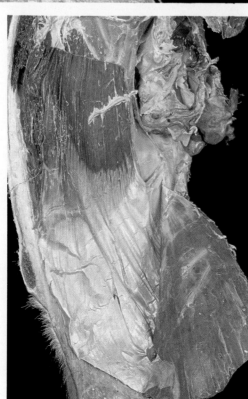

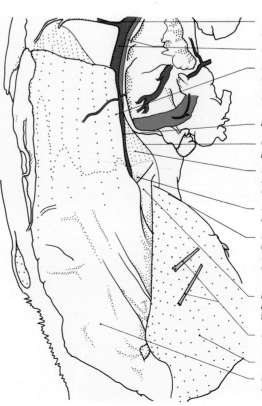

a. circumflexa ilium profunda

a.v. iliaca externa

m. obliquus internus abdominis (caudal border forming cranial rim of deep inguinal ring)

a. pudenda externa

cut edge of parietal peritoneum

m. obliquus externus abdominis ("pelvic" tendon or "inguinal ligament")

superficial inguinal ring

m. rectus abdominis (dorsal border which formed ventral border of deep inguinal ring)

m. obliquus externus abdominis ("abdominal" tendon)

n. lumbalis II r. cutaneus ventralis medialis

m. rectus abdominis

m. obliquus internus abdominis

Fig. 8.22 Structures of the right inguinal canal, in cranial view (3).

Reflection of the ventral part of the internal oblique abdominal muscle removes the cranial border of the deep inguinal ring and exposes the cranial part of the superficial ring.

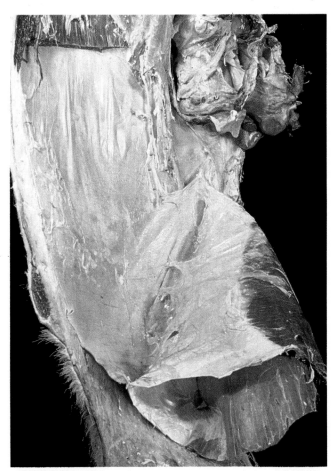

- a.v. iliaca externa
- n. genitofemoralis (LIII, IV)
- a. femoralis
- pelvic viscera and vessels
- vasa afferentia to ln. iliofemoralis
- m. obliquus externus abdominis, "pelvic" tendon (or "inguinal ligament")
- prepubic tendon
- a. pudenda externa
- superficial inguinal ring
- "abdominal" tendon of m. obliquus externus abdominis
- m. obliquus internus abdominis (reflected medially)
- fusion between m. obliquus internus and m. obliquus externus abdominis
- m. rectus abdominis (reflected medially)
- vagina m. recti abdominis, lamina externa

Fig. 8.23 Structures of the right inguinal canal, in cranial view (4).

The "pelvic" tendon of the external oblique abdominal muscle has been incised and the rest of the muscle has been reflected medially, leaving the pelvic tendon *in situ*. In this way the superficial inguinal ring is opened up.

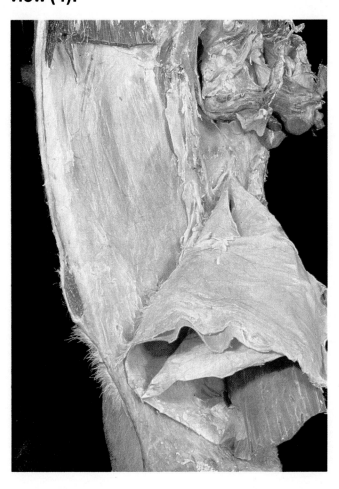

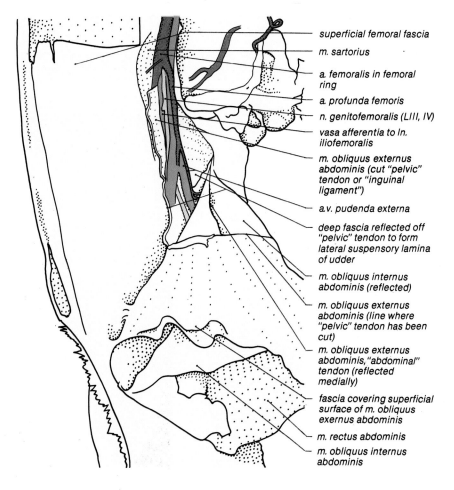

- superficial femoral fascia
- m. sartorius
- a. femoralis in femoral ring
- a. profunda femoris
- n. genitofemoralis (LIII, IV)
- vasa afferentia to ln. iliofemoralis
- m. obliquus externus abdominis (cut "pelvic" tendon or "inguinal ligament")
- a.v. pudenda externa
- deep fascia reflected off "pelvic" tendon to form lateral suspensory lamina of udder
- m. obliquus internus abdominis (reflected)
- m. obliquus externus abdominis (line where "pelvic" tendon has been cut)
- m. obliquus externus abdominis, "abdominal" tendon (reflected medially)
- fascia covering superficial surface of m. obliquus exernus abdominis
- m. rectus abdominis
- m. obliquus internus abdominis

Fig. 8.24 The pelvic inlet of a cow aged six years: cranial view.

The trunk has been transected at fifth lumbar level and the incision continued ventrally, removing all but the floor of the abdominal wall. The figure shows the structures as they were when embalmed in the standing position. No part of the female tract (non-pregnant, but adult) lay in the abdomen and the empty bladder was entirely pelvic in position. Figs. 8.25 – 8.28 show further details.

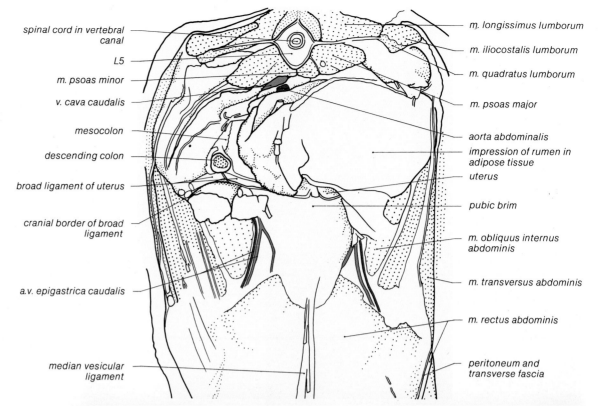

spinal cord in vertebral canal
L5
m. psoas minor
v. cava caudalis
mesocolon
descending colon
broad ligament of uterus
cranial border of broad ligament
a.v. epigastrica caudalis
median vesicular ligament

m. longissimus lumborum
m. iliocostalis lumborum
m. quadratus lumborum
m. psoas major
aorta abdominalis
impression of rumen in adipose tissue
uterus
pubic brim
m. obliquus internus abdominis
m. transversus abdominis
m. rectus abdominis
peritoneum and transverse fascia

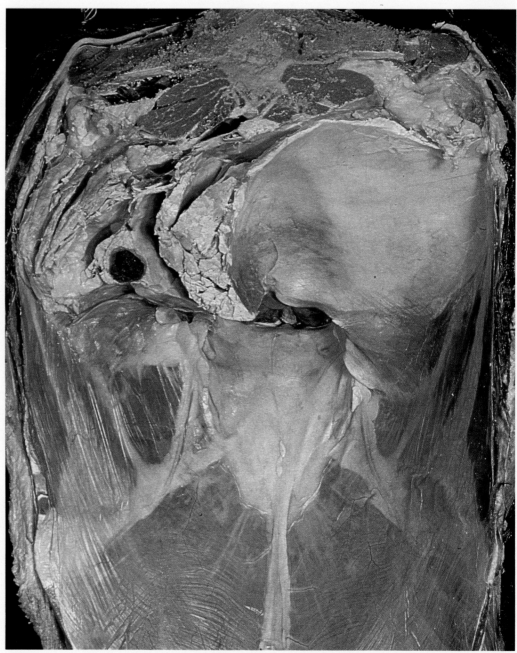

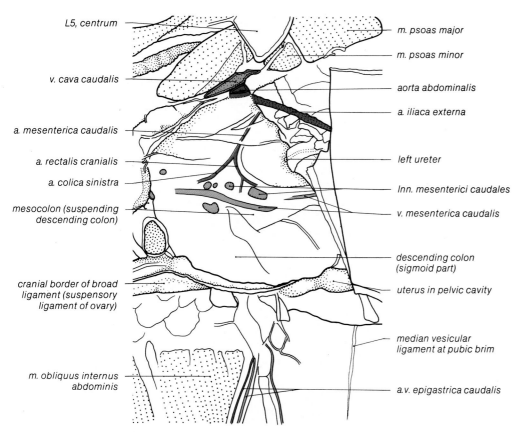

L5, centrum

v. cava caudalis

a. mesenterica caudalis

a. rectalis cranialis

a. colica sinistra

mesocolon (suspending descending colon)

cranial border of broad ligament (suspensory ligament of ovary)

m. obliquus internus abdominis

m. psoas major

m. psoas minor

aorta abdominalis

a. iliaca externa

left ureter

lnn. mesenterici caudales

v. mesenterica caudalis

descending colon (sigmoid part)

uterus in pelvic cavity

median vesicular ligament at pubic brim

a.v. epigastrica caudalis

Fig. 8.25 The descending colon at the pelvic inlet, in cranial view.
Removal of a part of the large mass of adipose tissue, shown in fig. 8.24, reveals further details of the descending colon just cranial to the pelvic inlet. This view is taken from a slightly lateral angle to show the right side of the inlet.

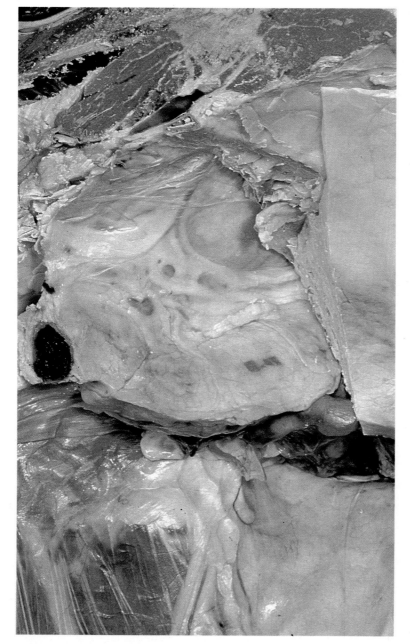

Fig. 8.26 The ovary and associated structures at the pelvic inlet, in cranial view (1).
Removal of the sigmoid descending colon at its junction with the rectum now reveals the position of the right ovary and its associated structures in relation to the pubic brim.

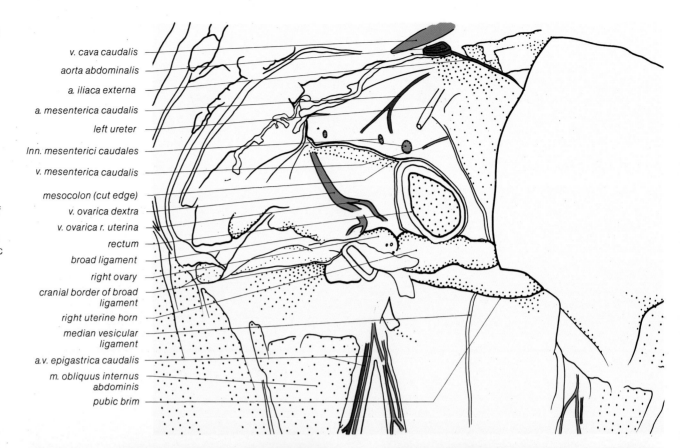

v. cava caudalis
aorta abdominalis
a. iliaca externa
a. mesenterica caudalis
left ureter
lnn. mesenterici caudales
v. mesenterica caudalis
mesocolon (cut edge)
v. ovarica dextra
v. ovarica r. uterina
rectum
broad ligament
right ovary
cranial border of broad ligament
right uterine horn
median vesicular ligament
a.v. epigastrica caudalis
m. obliquus internus abdominis
pubic brim

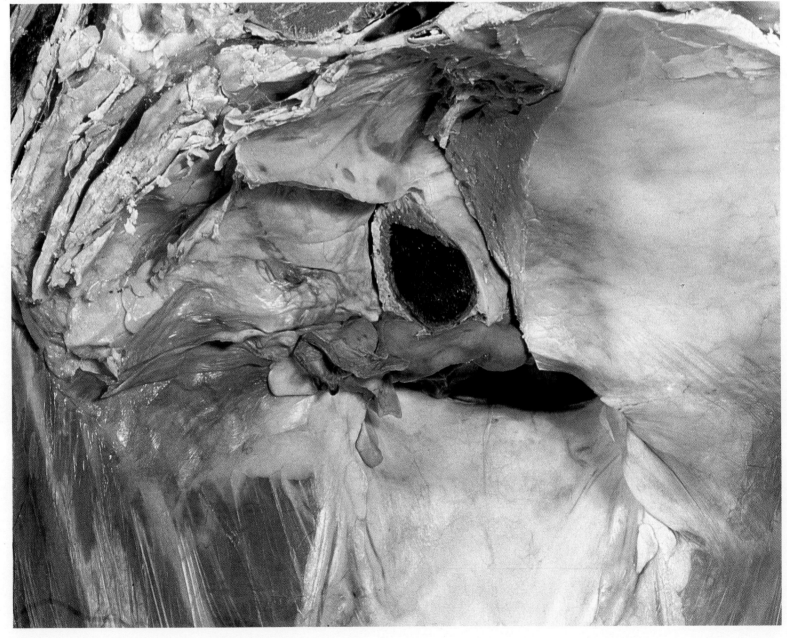

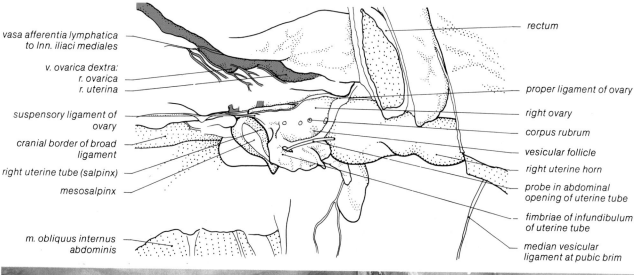

vasa afferentia lymphatica to lnn. iliaci mediales

v. ovarica dextra:
r. ovarica
r. uterina

suspensory ligament of ovary

cranial border of broad ligament

right uterine tube (salpinx)

mesosalpinx

m. obliquus internus abdominis

rectum

proper ligament of ovary

right ovary

corpus rubrum

vesicular follicle

right uterine horn

probe in abdominal opening of uterine tube

fimbriae of infundibulum of uterine tube

median vesicular ligament at pubic brim

Fig. 8.27 The ovary and associated structures at the pelvic inlet, in cranial view (2).
The fimbriae of the infundibulum have been turned ventrally to expose the abdominal opening of the uterine tube and the surface of the ovary.

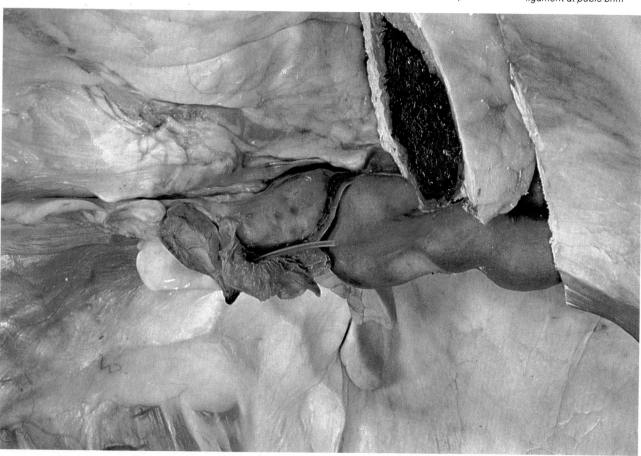

Fig. 8.28 The ovary and associated structures at the pelvic inlet, in cranial view (3).

The fimbriae of the infundibulum have been replaced after filling the ovarian bursa with cotton wool. This cotton wool is clearly visible through the thin mesosalpinx which forms the wall of the bursa.

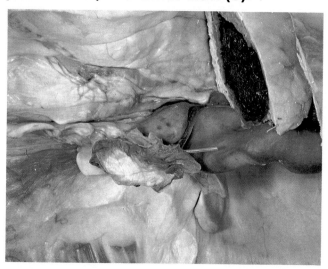

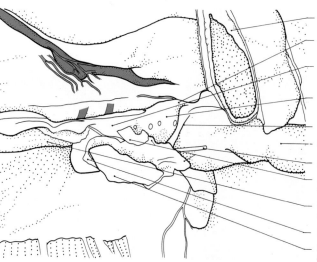

rectum

proper ligament of ovary

suspensory ligament of ovary

right ovary, lying partly in ovarian bursa

free edge of mesosalpinx

right uterine horn

probe in uterine tube

fimbriae of infundibulum of uterine tube

cranial border of broad ligament

right uterine tube (salpinx)

mesosalpinx, forming wall of ovarian bursa

Fig. 8.29 Superficial muscles, nerves and lymph nodes of the pelvic regions in a bull calf aged one week: lateral view.

The lymph nodes shown here are not always present in the ox.

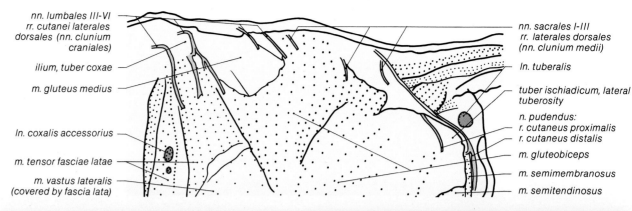

nn. lumbales III-VI
rr. cutanei laterales dorsales (nn. clunium craniales)

ilium, tuber coxae

m. gluteus medius

ln. coxalis accessorius

m. tensor fasciae latae

m. vastus lateralis (covered by fascia lata)

nn. sacrales I-III
rr. laterales dorsales (nn. clunium medii)

ln. tuberalis

tuber ischiadicum, lateral tuberosity

n. pudendus:
r. cutaneus proximalis
r. cutaneus distalis

m. gluteobiceps

m. semimembranosus

m. semitendinosus

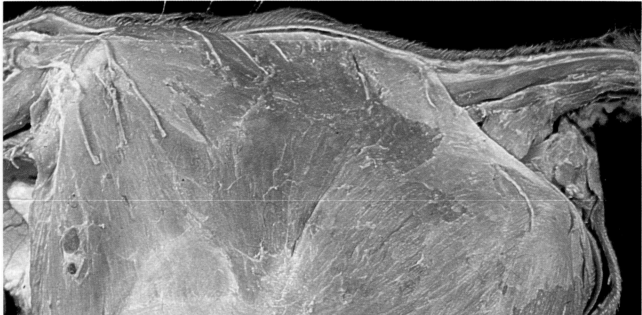

Fig. 8.30 The perineal region and the root of the tail in the calf: left caudolateral view.

The dissection is at the stage shown in the previous figure but the tail has been raised to show the median caudal artery and the related muscles more clearly.

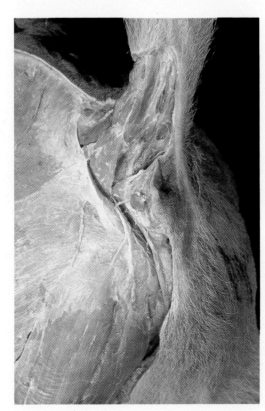

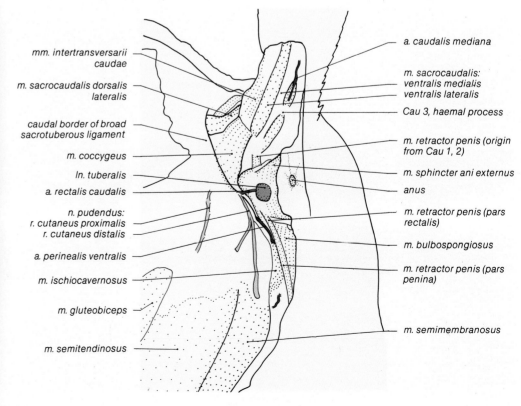

mm. intertransversarii caudae

m. sacrocaudalis dorsalis lateralis

caudal border of broad sacrotuberous ligament

m. coccygeus

ln. tuberalis

a. rectalis caudalis

n. pudendus:
r. cutaneus proximalis
r. cutaneus distalis

a. perinealis ventralis

m. ischiocavernosus

m. gluteobiceps

m. semitendinosus

a. caudalis mediana

m. sacrocaudalis:
ventralis medialis
ventralis lateralis

Cau 3, haemal process

m. retractor penis (origin from Cau 1, 2)

m. sphincter ani externus

anus

m. retractor penis (pars rectalis)

m. bulbospongiosus

m. retractor penis (pars penina)

m. semimembranosus

Fig. 8.31 The lateral wall of the pelvis and associated structures in the calf: lateral view.

Removal of the gluteobiceps and middle gluteal muscles exposes the structures that lie superficial to the broad sacrotuberous ligament.

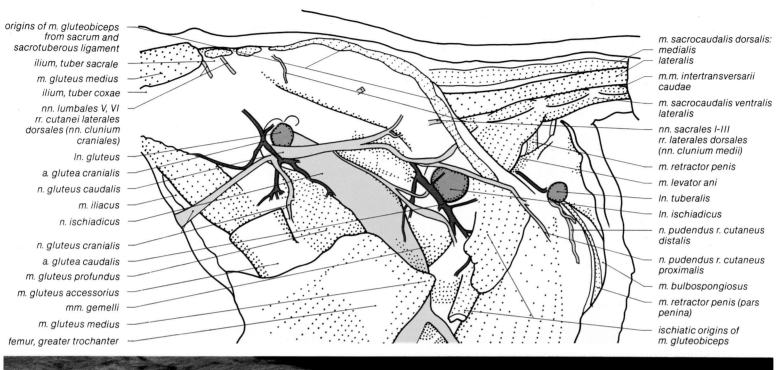

origins of m. gluteobiceps from sacrum and sacrotuberous ligament
ilium, tuber sacrale
m. gluteus medius
ilium, tuber coxae
nn. lumbales V, VI rr. cutanei laterales dorsales (nn. clunium craniales)
ln. gluteus
a. glutea cranialis
n. gluteus caudalis
m. iliacus
n. ischiadicus
n. gluteus cranialis
a. glutea caudalis
m. gluteus profundus
m. gluteus accessorius
mm. gemelli
m. gluteus medius
femur, greater trochanter

m. sacrocaudalis dorsalis:
medialis
lateralis
m.m. intertransversarii caudae
m. sacrocaudalis ventralis lateralis
nn. sacrales I-III rr. laterales dorsales (nn. clunium medii)
m. retractor penis
m. levator ani
ln. tuberalis
ln. ischiadicus
n. pudendus r. cutaneus distalis
n. pudendus r. cutaneus proximalis
m. bulbospongiosus
m. retractor penis (pars penina)
ischiatic origins of m. gluteobiceps

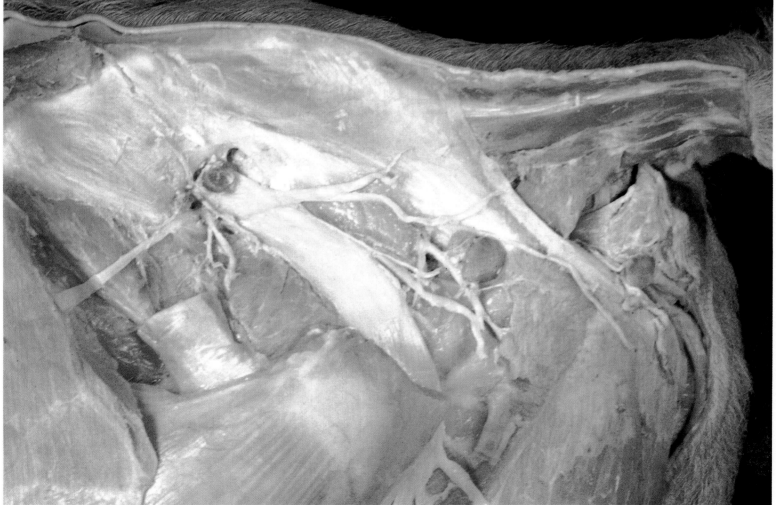

Fig. 8.32 The greater and lesser ischiatic foramina of the calf, in lateral view.

The broad sacrotuberous ligament has been incised (broken blue line) in preparation for partial removal to display the structures lying medial to it (see fig. 8.33). The incision passes round the borders of the ischiatic foramina without damaging them or the structures traversing them.

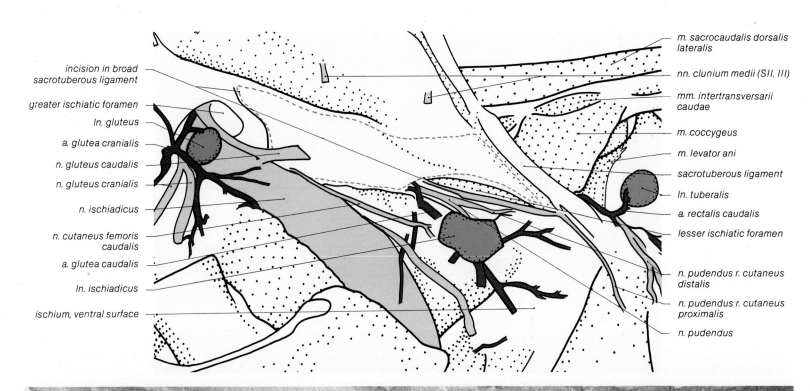

incision in broad sacrotuberous ligament
greater ischiatic foramen
ln. gluteus
a. glutea cranialis
n. gluteus caudalis
n. gluteus cranialis
n. ischiadicus
n. cutaneus femoris caudalis
a. glutea caudalis
ln. ischiadicus
ischium, ventral surface

m. sacrocaudalis dorsalis lateralis
nn. clunium medii (SII, III)
mm. intertransversarii caudae
m. coccygeus
m. levator ani
sacrotuberous ligament
ln. tuberalis
a. rectalis caudalis
lesser ischiatic foramen
n. pudendus r. cutaneus distalis
n. pudendus r. cutaneus proximalis
n. pudendus

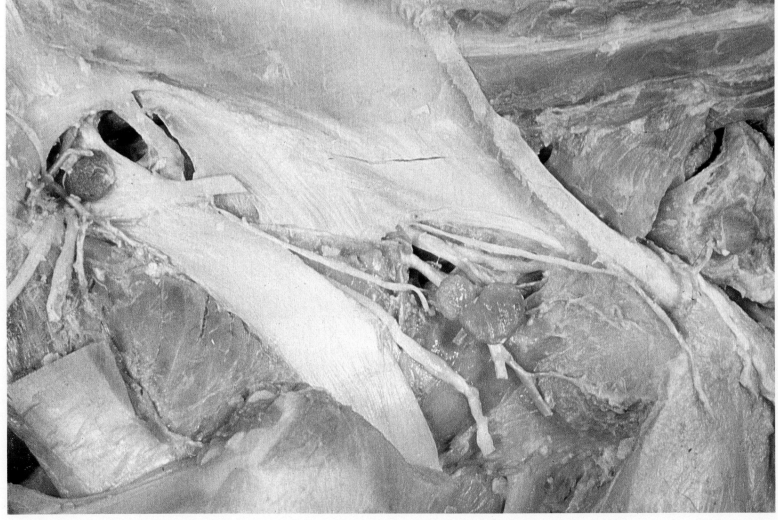

Fig. 8.33 Vessels and nerves related to the broad sacrotuberous ligament in the calf: left lateral view.

Excision of a part of the ligament (as indicated in figs. 8.32 and 8.33 by a broken blue line) and removal of the ischiatic lymph node, reveals the course of the branches of the third and fourth sacral nerves and the internal pudendal artery. Their relationships at the lesser ischiatic foramen are also displayed.

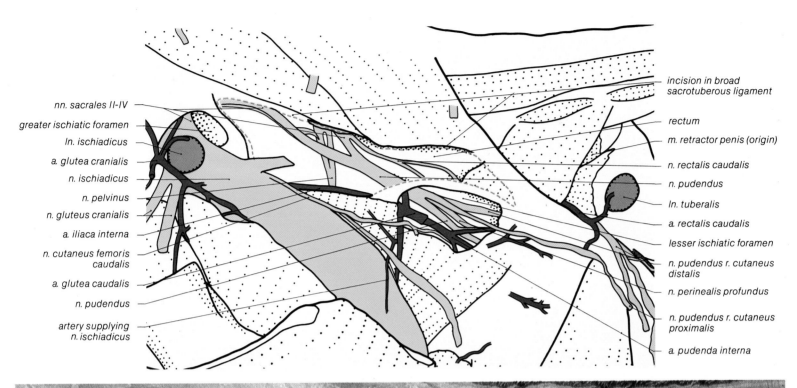

- nn. sacrales II-IV
- greater ischiatic foramen
- ln. ischiadicus
- a. glutea cranialis
- n. ischiadicus
- n. pelvinus
- n. gluteus cranialis
- a. iliaca interna
- n. cutaneus femoris caudalis
- a. glutea caudalis
- n. pudendus
- artery supplying n. ischiadicus

- incision in broad sacrotuberous ligament
- rectum
- m. retractor penis (origin)
- n. rectalis caudalis
- n. pudendus
- ln. tuberalis
- a. rectalis caudalis
- lesser ischiatic foramen
- n. pudendus r. cutaneus distalis
- n. perinealis profundus
- n. pudendus r. cutaneus proximalis
- a. pudenda interna

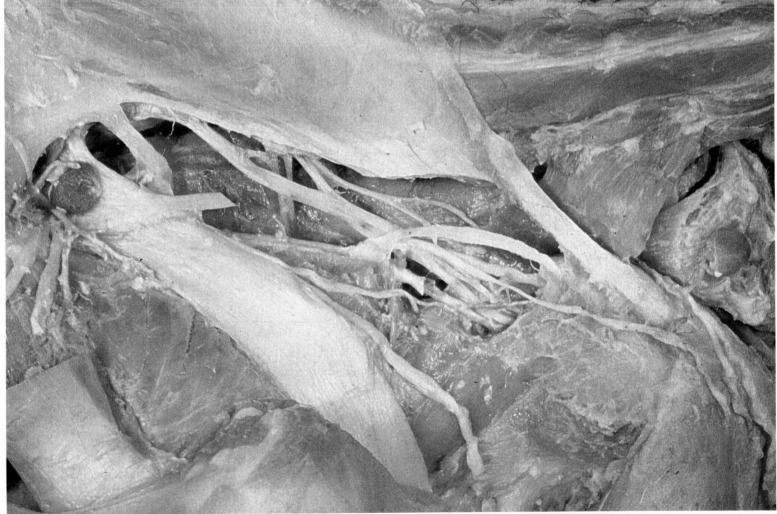

Fig. 8.34 Surface features of the anal, perineal and scrotal regions in a bull calf aged five months: caudal view.

In this preserved specimen the contour of the scrotum differs from that in life. The escutcheon (in which the hairs lie pointing dorsally) is variable in size and includes the caudal scrotal wall. In this calf it was not extensive.

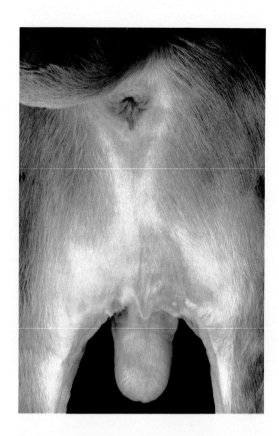

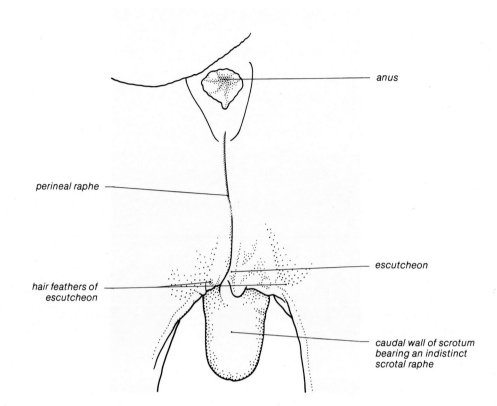

anus

perineal raphe

escutcheon

hair feathers of escutcheon

caudal wall of scrotum bearing an indistinct scrotal raphe

Fig. 8.35 Superficial structures of the perineal and scrotal regions in the calf: right caudolateral view.

The skin has been removed from left and right sides but on the left side the superficial and deep fasciae have also been taken away. This calf was in prime condition at slaughter, and the adipose deposits in the superficial fascia, especially around the neck of the scrotum, were very large.

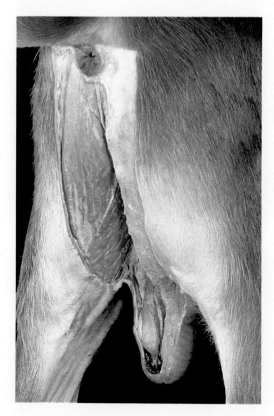

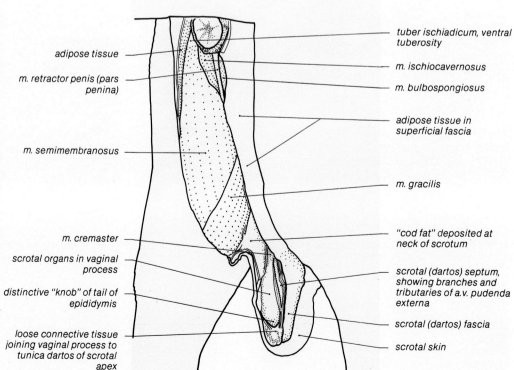

adipose tissue

m. retractor penis (pars penina)

m. semimembranosus

m. cremaster

scrotal organs in vaginal process

distinctive "knob" of tail of epididymis

loose connective tissue joining vaginal process to tunica dartos of scrotal apex

tuber ischiadicum, ventral tuberosity

m. ischiocavernosus

m. bulbospongiosus

adipose tissue in superficial fascia

m. gracilis

"cod fat" deposited at neck of scrotum

scrotal (dartos) septum, showing branches and tributaries of a.v. pudenda externa

scrotal (dartos) fascia

scrotal skin

Fig. 8.36 Topography of the penis in the perineal region of the calf: left caudolateral view.

The superficial and deep fasciae of the perineum and scrotum remain intact on the right side, showing the depth within the perineum of the retractor penis muscle and the penile body (including the sigmoid flexure).

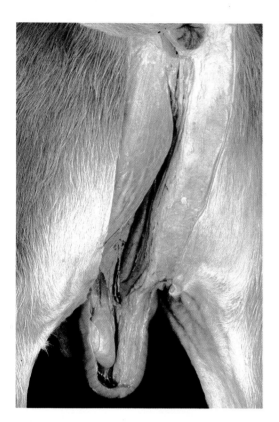

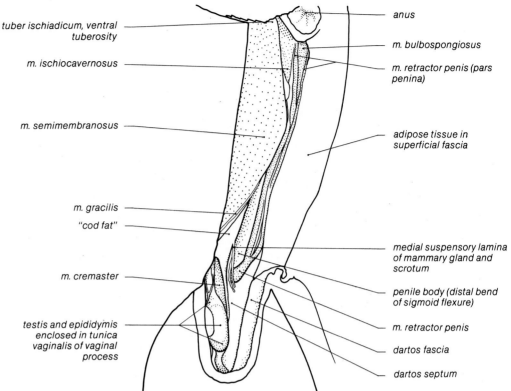

- anus
- m. bulbospongiosus
- m. retractor penis (pars penina)
- adipose tissue in superficial fascia
- medial suspensory lamina of mammary gland and scrotum
- penile body (distal bend of sigmoid flexure)
- m. retractor penis
- dartos fascia
- dartos septum

- tuber ischiadicum, ventral tuberosity
- m. ischiocavernosus
- m. semimembranosus
- m. gracilis
- "cod fat"
- m. cremaster
- testis and epididymis enclosed in tunica vaginalis of vaginal process

Fig. 8.37 Structures situated in the scrotum and at the scrotal neck in the calf: left caudolateral view.

This figure is a closer view of a part of fig. 8.36.

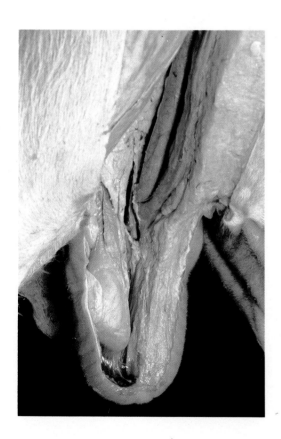

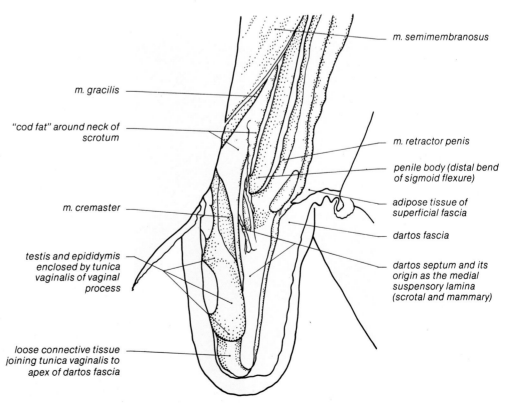

- m. semimembranosus
- m. retractor penis
- penile body (distal bend of sigmoid flexure)
- adipose tissue of superficial fascia
- dartos fascia
- dartos septum and its origin as the medial suspensory lamina (scrotal and mammary)

- m. gracilis
- "cod fat" around neck of scrotum
- m. cremaster
- testis and epididymis enclosed by tunica vaginalis of vaginal process
- loose connective tissue joining tunica vaginalis to apex of dartos fascia

8.25

Fig. 8.38 Contents of the left vaginal process within the left side of the scrotum of the calf: caudal view.

The parietal tunica vaginalis has been incised to display the testis and epididymis suspended within the cavity of the vaginal process. Note the medial location of the body of the epididymis (compare with fig. 9.27).

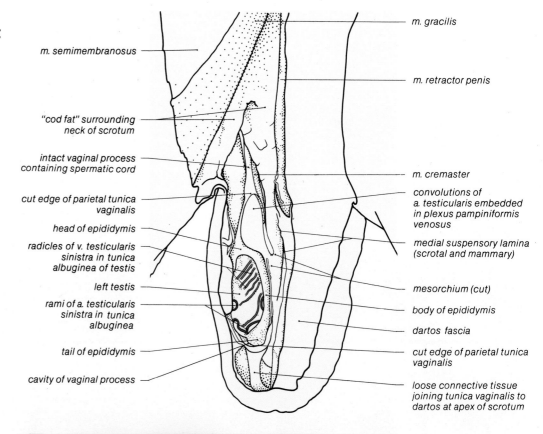

m. semimembranosus

"cod fat" surrounding neck of scrotum

intact vaginal process containing spermatic cord

cut edge of parietal tunica vaginalis

head of epididymis

radicles of v. testicularis sinistra in tunica albuginea of testis

left testis

rami of a. testicularis sinistra in tunica albuginea

tail of epididymis

cavity of vaginal process

m. gracilis

m. retractor penis

m. cremaster

convolutions of a. testicularis embedded in plexus pampiniformis venosus

medial suspensory lamina (scrotal and mammary)

mesorchium (cut)

body of epididymis

dartos fascia

cut edge of parietal tunica vaginalis

loose connective tissue joining tunica vaginalis to dartos at apex of scrotum

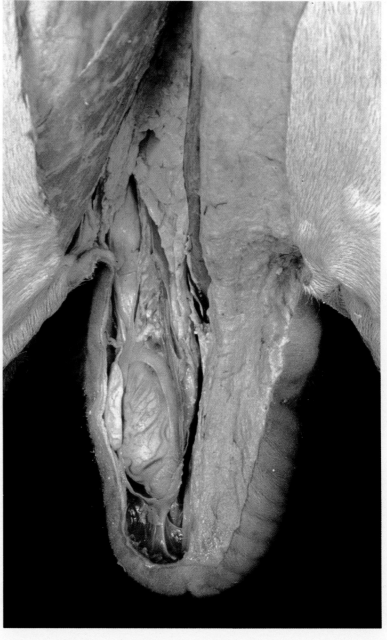

Fig. 8.39 Muscles of the penile root in the perineal region: caudal view (1).

The small flap of fascia left attached, but reflected from the surface of the bulbospongiosus muscle, emphasises the thickness and density of the deep fascia in the perineal region of the bull.

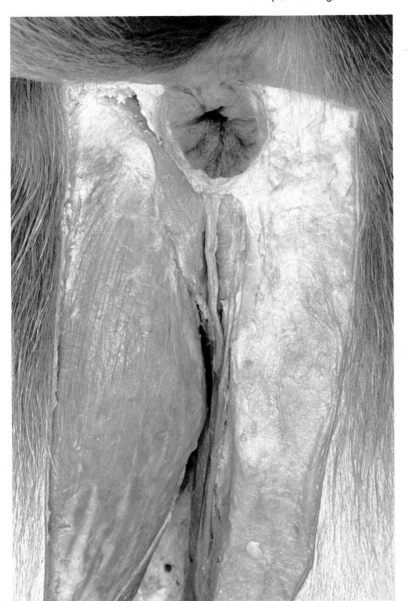

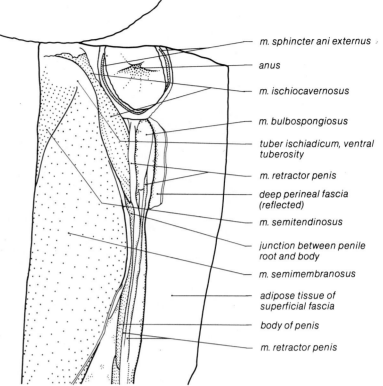

- m. sphincter ani externus
- anus
- m. ischiocavernosus
- m. bulbospongiosus
- tuber ischiadicum, ventral tuberosity
- m. retractor penis
- deep perineal fascia (reflected)
- m. semitendinosus
- junction between penile root and body
- m. semimembranosus
- adipose tissue of superficial fascia
- body of penis
- m. retractor penis

Fig. 8.40 Muscles of the penile root in the perineal region: caudal view (2).

The origin of the retractor penis muscle from the coccygeal vertebrae is shown in fig. 8.49.

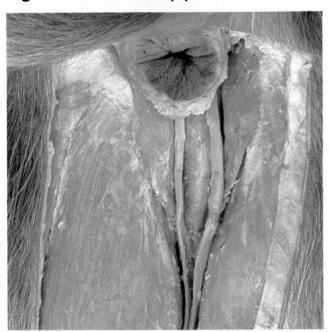

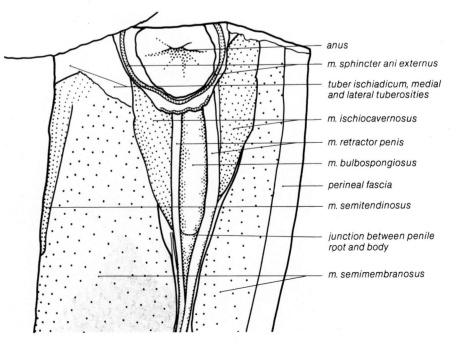

- anus
- m. sphincter ani externus
- tuber ischiadicum, medial and lateral tuberosities
- m. ischiocavernosus
- m. retractor penis
- m. bulbospongiosus
- perineal fascia
- m. semitendinosus
- junction between penile root and body
- m. semimembranosus

Fig. 8.41 The superficial inguinal ring of a male goat aged five months, in left lateral view.

The left hind limb has been removed, and the superficial inguinal ring exposed by removal of the lateral lamina along the line indicated in blue. Further dissections of the pelvic regions and reproductive organs of this male goat are shown in figs. 8.42-8.50.

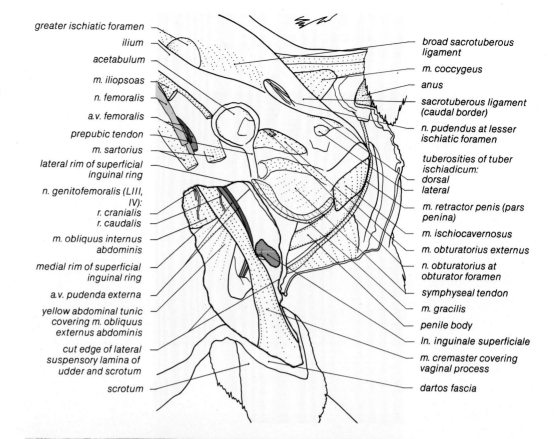

greater ischiatic foramen
ilium
acetabulum
m. iliopsoas
n. femoralis
a.v. femoralis
prepubic tendon
m. sartorius
lateral rim of superficial inguinal ring
n. genitofemoralis (LIII, IV):
r. cranialis
r. caudalis
m. obliquus internus abdominis
medial rim of superficial inguinal ring
a.v. pudenda externa
yellow abdominal tunic covering m. obliquus externus abdominis
cut edge of lateral suspensory lamina of udder and scrotum
scrotum

broad sacrotuberous ligament
m. coccygeus
anus
sacrotuberous ligament (caudal border)
n. pudendus at lesser ischiatic foramen
tuberosities of tuber ischiadicum:
dorsal
lateral
m. retractor penis (pars penina)
m. ischiocavernosus
m. obturatorius externus
n. obturatorius at obturator foramen
symphyseal tendon
m. gracilis
penile body
ln. inguinale superficiale
m. cremaster covering vaginal process
dartos fascia

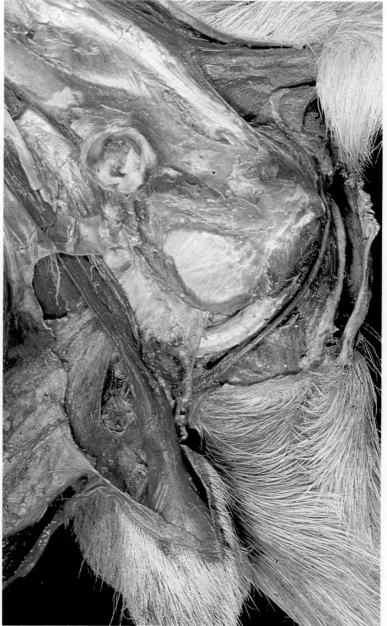

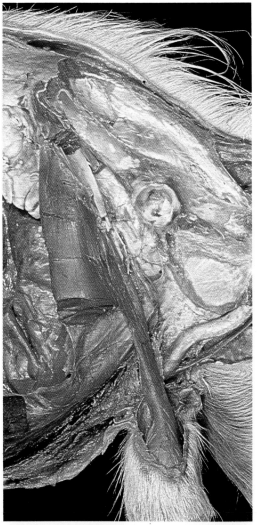

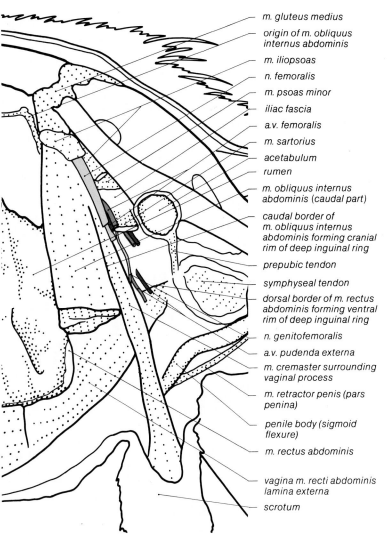

m. gluteus medius
origin of m. obliquus internus abdominis
m. iliopsoas
n. femoralis
m. psoas minor
iliac fascia
a.v. femoralis
m. sartorius
acetabulum
rumen
m. obliquus internus abdominis (caudal part)
caudal border of m. obliquus internus abdominis forming cranial rim of deep inguinal ring
prepubic tendon
symphyseal tendon
dorsal border of m. rectus abdominis forming ventral rim of deep inguinal ring
n. genitofemoralis
a.v. pudenda externa
m. cremaster surrounding vaginal process
m. retractor penis (pars penina)
penile body (sigmoid flexure)
m. rectus abdominis
vagina m. recti abdominis lamina externa
scrotum

Fig. 8.42 The deep inguinal ring of the goat, in left lateral view.

The external oblique abdominal muscle has been removed, with its superficial inguinal ring (see fig. 8.41). The caudal part of the internal oblique abdominal muscle was preserved when the abdominal viscera were displayed (see fig. 5.61). The deep inguinal ring lies caudal to the caudal border of the internal oblique muscle.

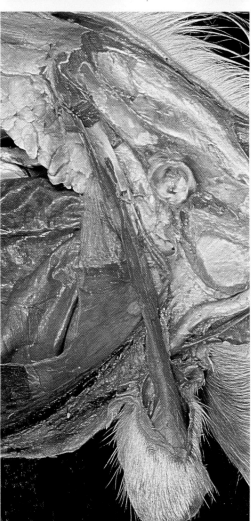

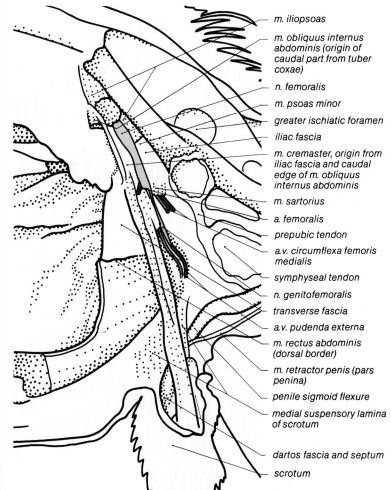

m. iliopsoas
m. obliquus internus abdominis (origin of caudal part from tuber coxae)
n. femoralis
m. psoas minor
greater ischiatic foramen
iliac fascia
m. cremaster, origin from iliac fascia and caudal edge of m. obliquus internus abdominis
m. sartorius
a. femoralis
prepubic tendon
a.v. circumflexa femoris medialis
symphyseal tendon
n. genitofemoralis
transverse fascia
a.v. pudenda externa
m. rectus abdominis (dorsal border)
m. retractor penis (pars penina)
penile sigmoid flexure
medial suspensory lamina of scrotum
dartos fascia and septum
scrotum

Fig. 8.43 Inguinal structures of the goat, in left lateral view.

Removal of the caudal border of the internal oblique abdominal muscle displays the origin of the cremaster muscle and the transverse fascia of the inguinal region. The orifice of the vaginal process is shown in fig. 8.45.

Fig. 8.44 The broad sacrotuberous ligament and the structures related to the iliac fascia in the male goat: left lateral view.

This is a closer view of a part of the dissection shown in fig.8.43.

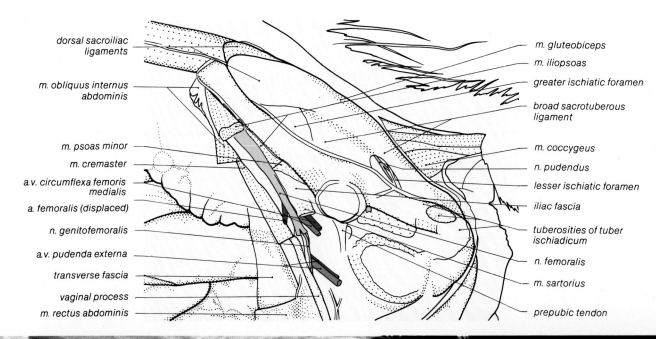

dorsal sacroiliac ligaments

m. obliquus internus abdominis

m. psoas minor

m. cremaster

a.v. circumflexa femoris medialis

a. femoralis (displaced)

n. genitofemoralis

a.v. pudenda externa

transverse fascia

vaginal process

m. rectus abdominis

m. gluteobiceps

m. iliopsoas

greater ischiatic foramen

broad sacrotuberous ligament

m. coccygeus

n. pudendus

lesser ischiatic foramen

iliac fascia

tuberosities of tuber ischiadicum

n. femoralis

m. sartorius

prepubic tendon

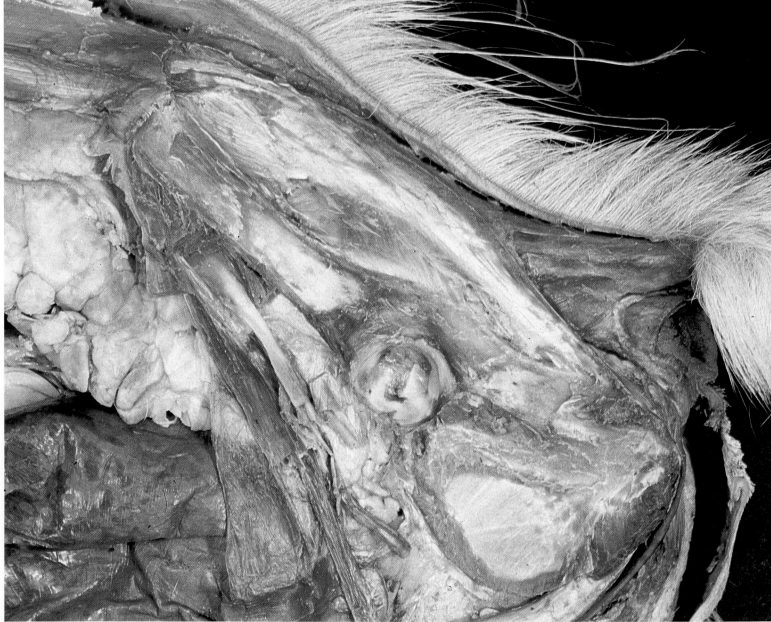

Fig. 8.45 Nerves and blood vessels of the pelvis of the goat: left lateral view.

The left pelvic bone has been removed, as shown in fig. 8.46. The damaged internal pudendal and caudal gluteal arteries are shown by broken lines.

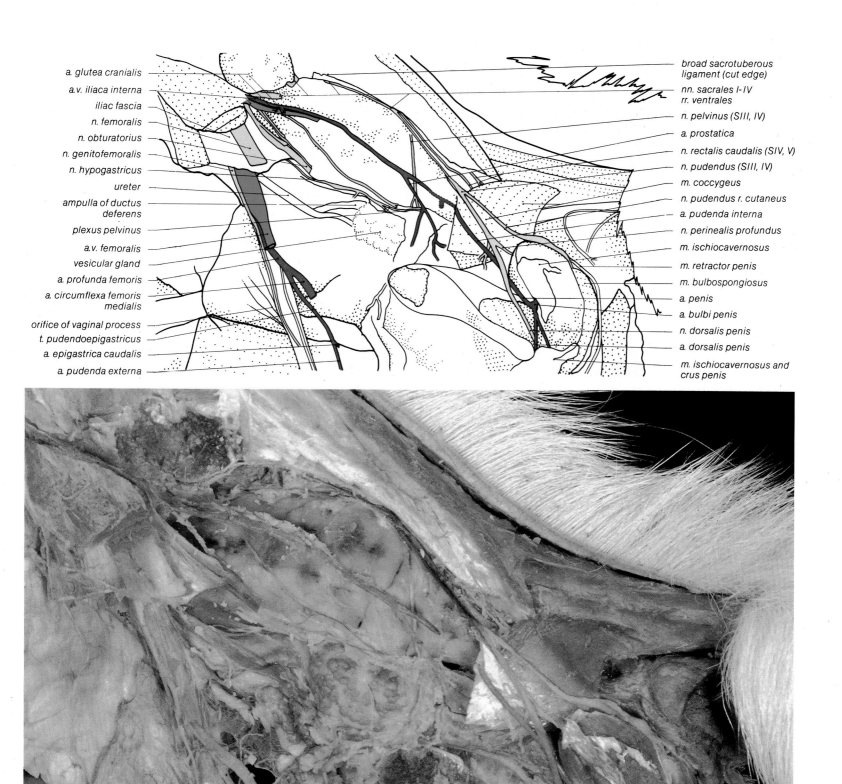

a. glutea cranialis
a.v. iliaca interna
iliac fascia
n. femoralis
n. obturatorius
n. genitofemoralis
n. hypogastricus
ureter
ampulla of ductus deferens
plexus pelvinus
a.v. femoralis
vesicular gland
a. profunda femoris
a. circumflexa femoris medialis
orifice of vaginal process
t. pudendoepigastricus
a. epigastrica caudalis
a. pudenda externa

broad sacrotuberous ligament (cut edge)
nn. sacrales I-IV rr. ventrales
n. pelvinus (SIII, IV)
a. prostatica
n. rectalis caudalis (SIV, V)
n. pudendus (SIII, IV)
m. coccygeus
n. pudendus r. cutaneus
a. pudenda interna
n. perinealis profundus
m. ischiocavernosus
m. retractor penis
m. bulbospongiosus
a. penis
a. bulbi penis
n. dorsalis penis
a. dorsalis penis
m. ischiocavernosus and crus penis

8.31

Fig. 8.46 Relationships of the pelvic bone of the goat, in left lateral view.

The left pelvic bone has been replaced, after the dissection shown in fig. 8.45, to show its relationships to the dissected structures.

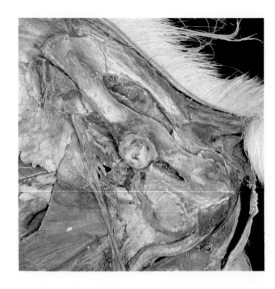

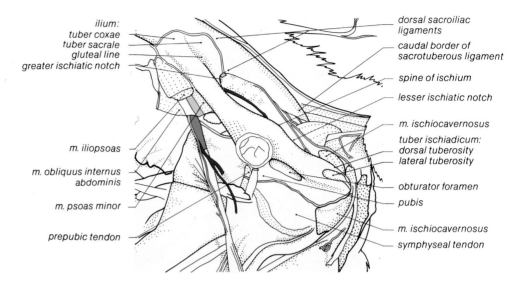

ilium:
tuber coxae
tuber sacrale
gluteal line
greater ischiatic notch

m. iliopsoas

m. obliquus internus abdominis

m. psoas minor

prepubic tendon

dorsal sacroiliac ligaments

caudal border of sacrotuberous ligament

spine of ischium

lesser ischiatic notch

m. ischiocavernosus

tuber ischiadicum:
dorsal tuberosity
lateral tuberosity

obturator foramen

pubis

m. ischiocavernosus

symphyseal tendon

Fig. 8.47 The right vaginal ring of the goat, in left lateral view.

The specimen is at the same stage of dissection as that shown in fig. 8.48, but the abdominal contents have been pushed cranially to reveal the orifice of the vaginal process in the peritoneum of the right abdominal wall.

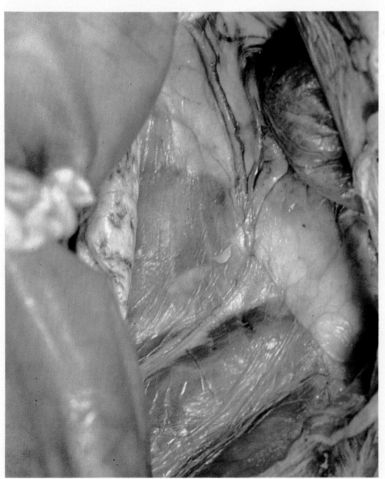

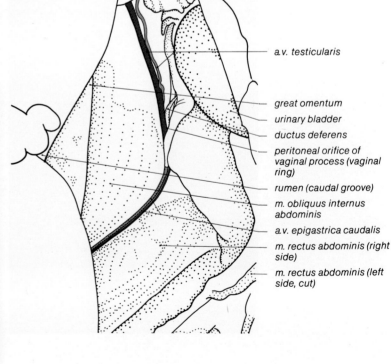

a.v. testicularis

great omentum

urinary bladder

ductus deferens

peritoneal orifice of vaginal process (vaginal ring)

rumen (caudal groove)

m. obliquus internus abdominis

a.v. epigastrica caudalis

m. rectus abdominis (right side)

m. rectus abdominis (left side, cut)

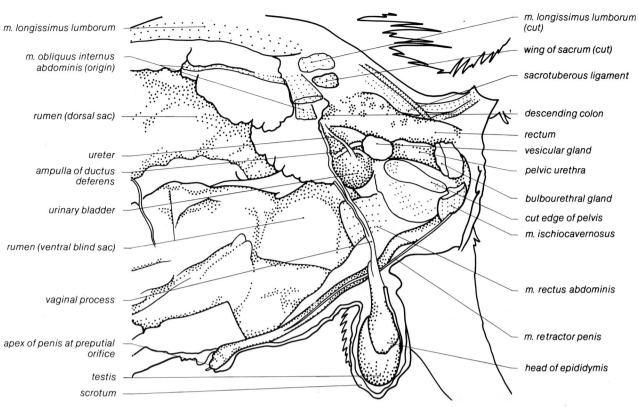

m. longissimus lumborum

m. obliquus internus abdominis (origin)

rumen (dorsal sac)

ureter

ampulla of ductus deferens

urinary bladder

rumen (ventral blind sac)

vaginal process

apex of penis at preputial orifice

testis

scrotum

m. longissimus lumborum (cut)

wing of sacrum (cut)

sacrotuberous ligament

descending colon

rectum

vesicular gland

pelvic urethra

bulbourethral gland

cut edge of pelvis

m. ischiocavernosus

m. rectus abdominis

m. retractor penis

head of epididymis

Fig. 8.48 The reproductive organs of the male goat, in left lateral view.
Removal of the bony pelvis and the parietal structures now displays the major organs. Further details of the reproductive organs in this dissection are shown in figs. 8.49 and 8.50.

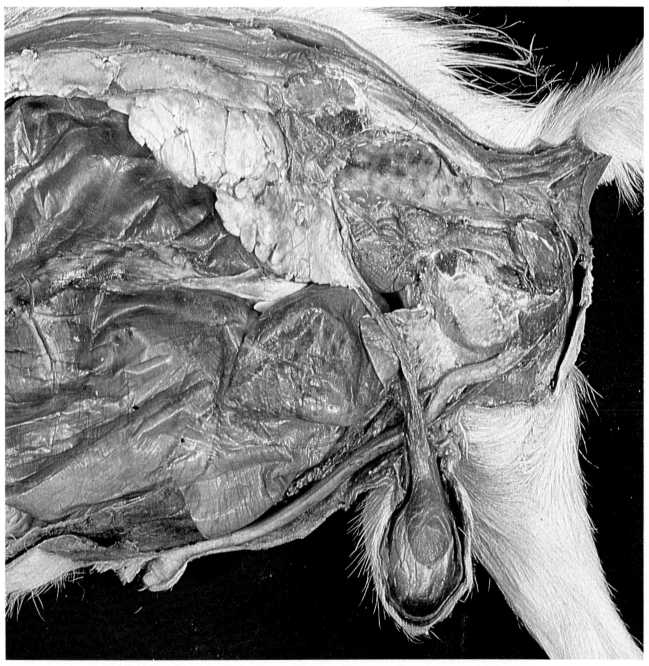

Fig. 8.49 Pelvic viscera of the goat, in left lateral view.

The left side of the bony pelvis has been removed, as shown in fig. 8.46, and the vessels and nerves of the pelvis removed. Note also that the dorsal and medial part of the ischiocavernosus muscle has been removed to display the bulbourethral gland more completely. Three black pins in the wall of the rectum mark the caudal limit of the peritoneal cavity.

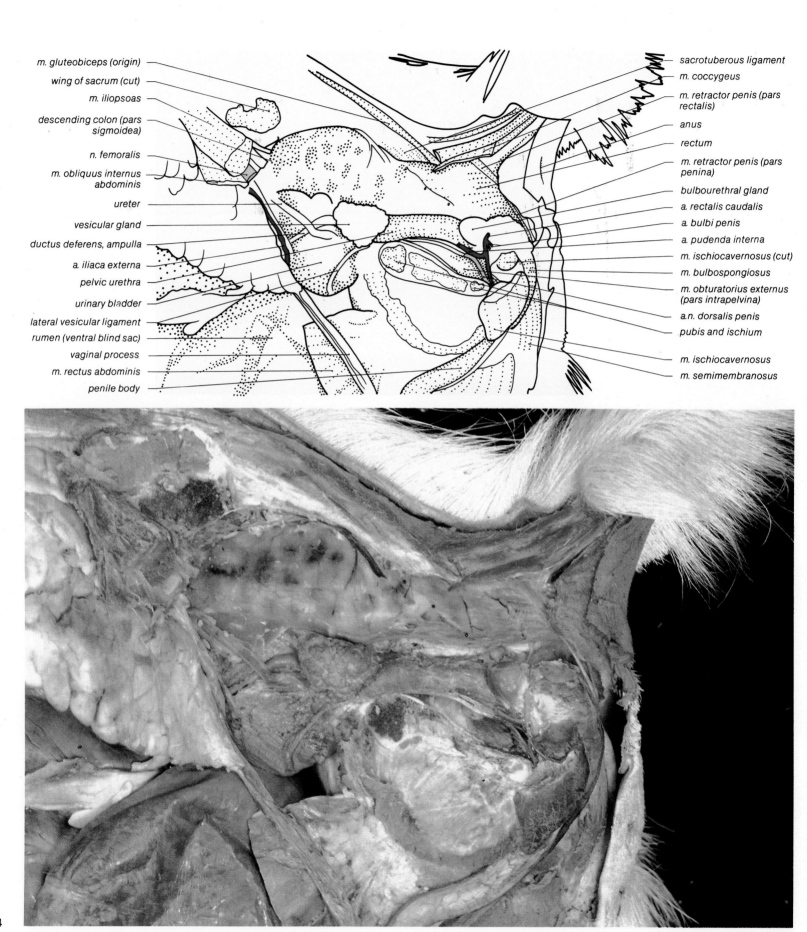

m. gluteobiceps (origin)

wing of sacrum (cut)

m. iliopsoas

descending colon (pars sigmoidea)

n. femoralis

m. obliquus internus abdominis

ureter

vesicular gland

ductus deferens, ampulla

a. iliaca externa

pelvic urethra

urinary bladder

lateral vesicular ligament

rumen (ventral blind sac)

vaginal process

m. rectus abdominis

penile body

sacrotuberous ligament

m. coccygeus

m. retractor penis (pars rectalis)

anus

rectum

m. retractor penis (pars penina)

bulbourethral gland

a. rectalis caudalis

a. bulbi penis

a. pudenda interna

m. ischiocavernosus (cut)

m. bulbospongiosus

m. obturatorius externus (pars intrapelvina)

a.n. dorsalis penis

pubis and ischium

m. ischiocavernosus

m. semimembranosus

Fig. 8.50 The penis and scrotum of the goat, in left lateral view.

The sigmoid flexure is effaced to a considerable extent and therefore the apex of the penis lies at the preputial orifice. When the tonus of the retractor penis muscle is raised the apex of the penis can be retracted to scrotal level; this draws out the prepuce into an integumentary sheath of considerable length.

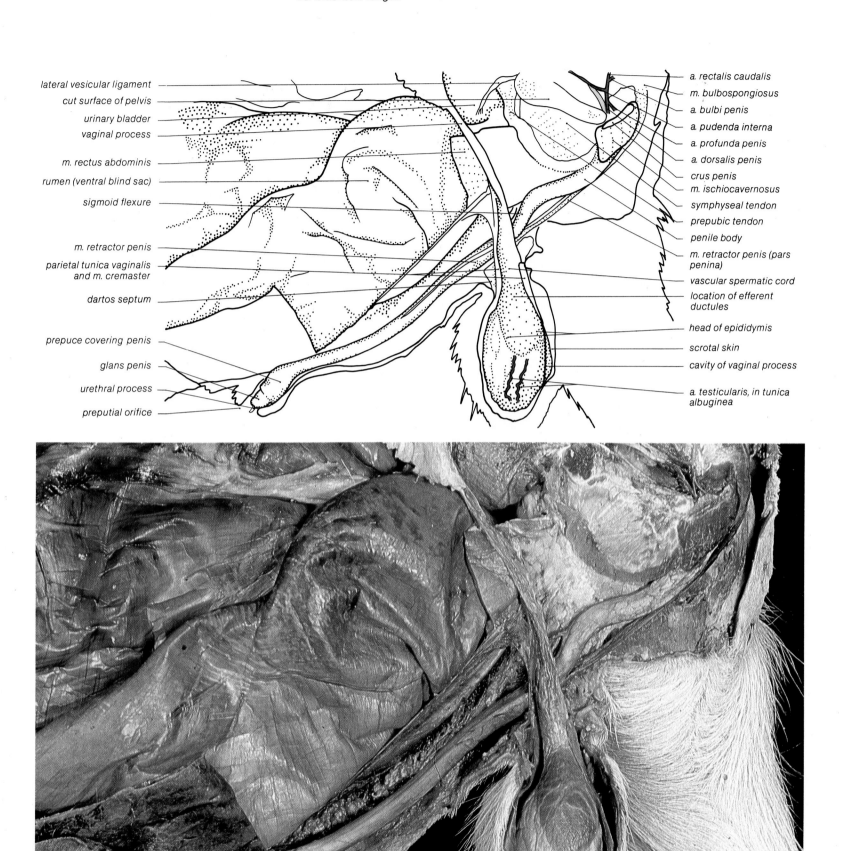

lateral vesicular ligament
cut surface of pelvis
urinary bladder
vaginal process
m. rectus abdominis
rumen (ventral blind sac)
sigmoid flexure
m. retractor penis
parietal tunica vaginalis and m. cremaster
dartos septum
prepuce covering penis
glans penis
urethral process
preputial orifice

a. rectalis caudalis
m. bulbospongiosus
a. bulbi penis
a. pudenda interna
a. profunda penis
a. dorsalis penis
crus penis
m. ischiocavernosus
symphyseal tendon
prepubic tendon
penile body
m. retractor penis (pars penina)
vascular spermatic cord
location of efferent ductules
head of epididymis
scrotal skin
cavity of vaginal process
a. testicularis, in tunica albuginea

8.35

9 The Udder and Scrotum

Fig. 9.1 Surface features of the udder and hindlimb, in left lateral view.

The dissection of the udder is covered in figs. 9.1 – 9.18; the rest of the chapter deals with the dissection of the scrotum. The lateral fold of the flank is also called the 'knee' fold because of its proximity to the stifle joint. This Jersey cow was almost at the end of her lactation, but the 'milk vein' was clearly visible in life. The hind legs are positioned in normal level standing, and the udder shows good dairy conformation.

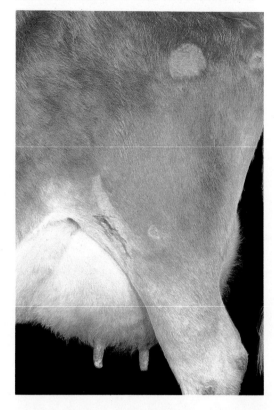

Fig. 9.2 Bones of the pelvis and hindlimb related to the udder: left lateral view.

The palpable bony prominences which are shaved in fig. 9.1 are coloured red. Note, however, that the tuberculum of the trochlea of the femur, lying dorsomedial to the patella, has not been coloured.

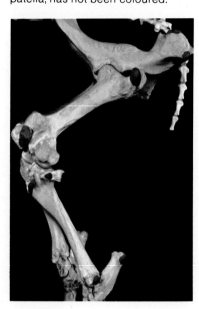

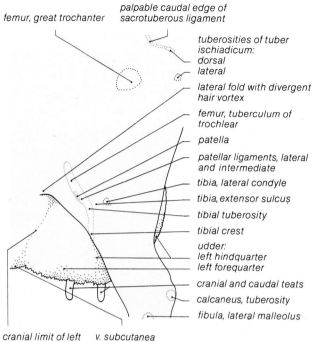

femur, great trochanter

palpable caudal edge of sacrotuberous ligament

tuberosities of tuber ischiadicum:
dorsal
lateral

lateral fold with divergent hair vortex

femur, tuberculum of trochlear

patella

patellar ligaments, lateral and intermediate

tibia, lateral condyle

tibia, extensor sulcus

tibial tuberosity

tibial crest

udder:
left hindquarter
left forequarter

cranial and caudal teats

calcaneus, tuberosity

fibula, lateral malleolus

cranial limit of left forequarter

v. subcutanea abdominis location of "milk vein"

Fig. 9.3 Surface features of the udder and hindlimb, in caudolateral view.

The shape of the escutcheon and the extent of the hair feathers (penna pilorum) vary greatly between individuals and attempts have been made to relate this to variations in milk production. Supernumerary teats may be seen on the caudal surface of the udder, but these are generally removed from calves destined for use as dairy cows.

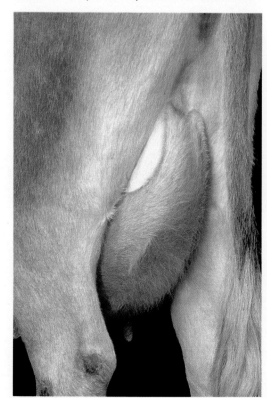

Fig. 9.4 Bones of the hindlimb related to the udder: caudolateral view.

The palpable prominences which are shaved in fig. 9.3 are coloured red.

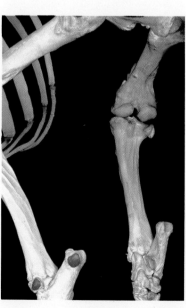

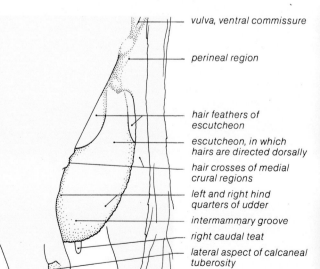

vulva, ventral commissure

perineal region

hair feathers of escutcheon

escutcheon, in which hairs are directed dorsally

hair crosses of medial crural regions

left and right hind quarters of udder

intermammary groove

right caudal teat

lateral aspect of calcaneal tuberosity

fibula, lateral malleolus

a. iliaca externa

n. genitofemoralis (LIII, IV)

a. profunda femoris

t. pudendoepigastricus

a. femoralis

a. circumflexa femoris medialis

m. obliquus internus abdominis

aponeurosis of m. obliquus externus abdominis (cut edge)

deep fascia of abdominal wall (yellow abdominal tunic)

nn. lumbales I, II rr. cutanei mediales ventrales

left cranial teat

m. iliacus

m. rectus femoris

acetabulum

m. biceps femoris

m. semimembranosus

m. obturatorius externus

n. obturatorius

m. adductor

m. gracilis

m. pectineus

position of lnn. inguinales superficiales

deep fascia of udder (lateral suspensory lamina)

superficial fascia of udder (reflected)

tuberosity of right calcaneus

Fig. 9.5 The superficial and deep fasciae of the udder after removal of the left hind-limb: lateral view.

This stage of the dissection is slightly earlier than that shown in fig. 8.13. The superficial inguinal (mammary) lymph nodes lie deep to the deep fascia, in the transverse plane of the acetabulum and the caudal teat

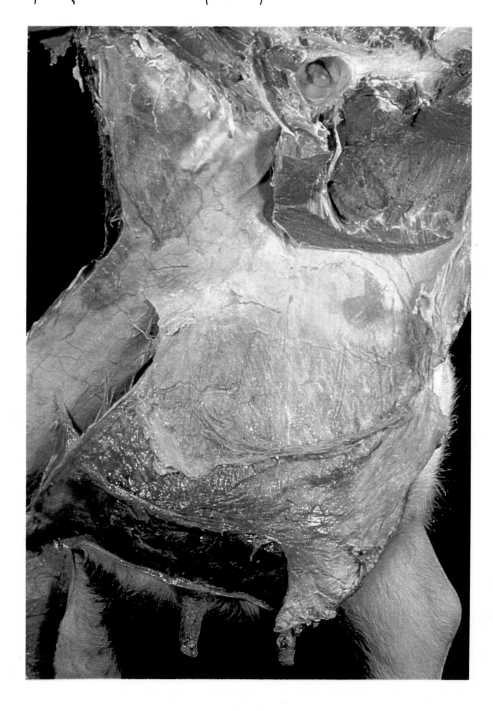

Fig. 9.6 The left lateral suspensory lamina of the udder, in lateral view.

This ligament is continuous with the yellow abdominal tunic. Its attachment to the prepubic and symphyseal tendons is shown, but the details of the origins of the adductor muscles (pectineus, gracilis, adductor) from these tendons are not shown.

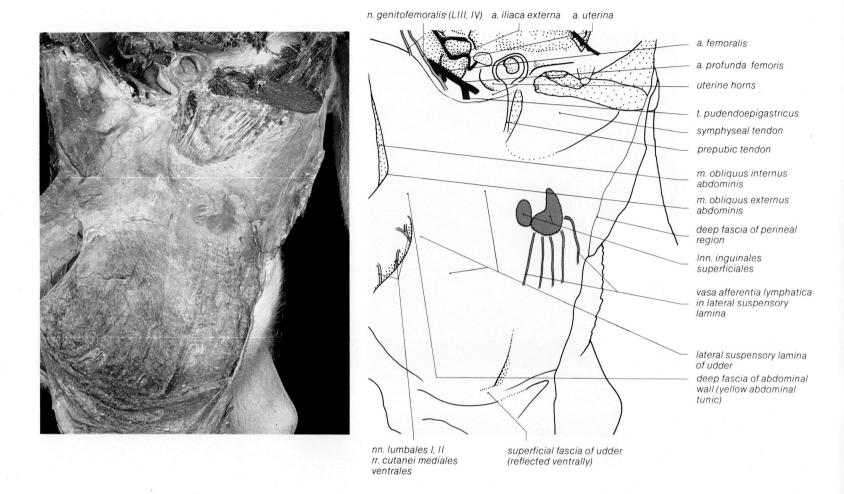

n. genitofemoralis (LIII, IV) a. iliaca externa a. uterina

a. femoralis

a. profunda femoris

uterine horns

t. pudendoepigastricus

symphyseal tendon

prepubic tendon

m. obliquus internus abdominis

m. obliquus externus abdominis

deep fascia of perineal region

lnn. inguinales superficiales

vasa afferentia lymphatica in lateral suspensory lamina

lateral suspensory lamina of udder

deep fascia of abdominal wall (yellow abdominal tunic)

nn. lumbales I, II
rr. cutanei mediales ventrales

superficial fascia of udder (reflected ventrally)

Fig. 9.7 The 'milk vein' and nerves of the ventral abdominal wall, in left lateral view.

The abdominal wall is traversed by the ventral cutaneous branches of the thoracic nerves. Where the 'milk vein' also uses a nerve canal, the palpable superficial foramen becomes greatly enlarged and is called a 'milk well'. In this cow, only that of ThX is utilised. Further details of the internal course of the milk vein are shown in figs. 9.8 and 9.9.

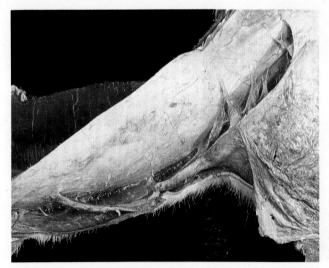

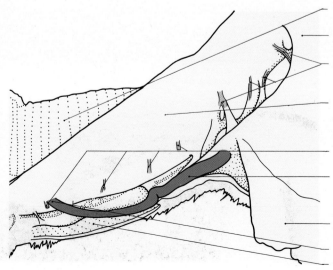

m. transversus abdominis dexter

lateral suspensory lamina of udder

nn. lumbales I, II
rr. cutanei mediales ventrales

m. obliquus externus abdominis, sinister (covered by yellow abdominal tunic)

nn. thoracici X- XIII
rr. cutanei ventrales

v. subcutanea abdominis ("milk vein" or v. epigastrica cranialis superficialis)

superficial fascia of udder (reflected)

"milk well"

m. cutaneus trunci

Fig. 9.8 The left 'milk well' and the structures traversing it: left dorsolateral view.

The subcutaneous abdominal, or 'milk', vein pierces the oblique and straight abdominal muscles. The xiphoid cartilage, transverse fascia and transverse abdominal muscle have been removed from a paramedian sagittal incision on the left side; this reveals the course of the vein and its accompanying artery as it runs in a cranial direction within the abdominal and thoracic wall. Further details of the course of these vessels are shown in fig. 9.9.

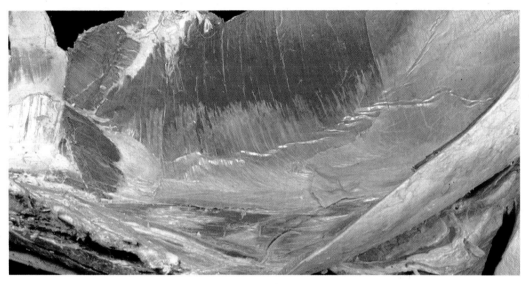

costal arch   m. transversus thoracis

a.v. thoracica interna   diaphragm   sternum, xiphoid cartilage

m. transversus abdominis dexter

peritoneum of right side

m. transversus abdominis, sinister (cut edge)

a.v. epigastrica cranialis

midline linea alba

m. rectus abdominis sinister

m. obliquus externus abdominis sinister

v. subcutanea abdominis at "milk well"

n. thoracicus X r. cutaneus ventralis

Fig. 9.9 The abdominal and thoracic course of the left cranial epigastric vessels: right dorsolateral view.

The epigastric vessels do not pierce the transverse muscles of the trunk. Their caudal connections, as seen from the left side, are shown in fig. 9.8; fig. 4.16 shows the cranial connections.

m. rectus abdominis sinister   a.v. epigastrica cranialis   a.v. intercostalis ventralis   rib 6   midline   a.v. thoracica interna

ln. sternalis cranialis

lnn. sternales caudales

m. transversus thoracis

parts of diaphragm: sternal costal

aponeurosis of m. transversus abdominis sinister   linea alba   costal arch   xiphoid cartilage

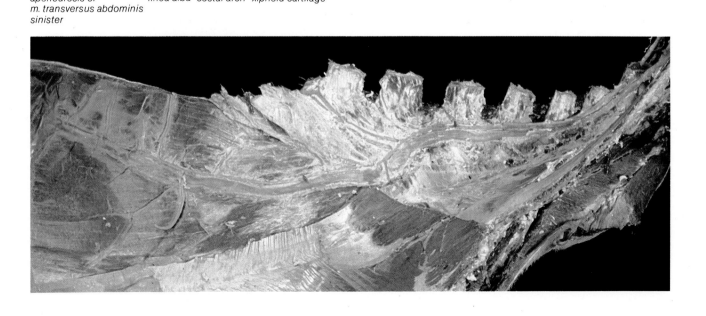

Fig. 9.10 The lateral suspensory lamina of the udder and the superficial inguinal ring, in left lateral view.

The attachments of the suspensory lamina to the abdominal wall, prepubic tendon and symphyseal tendon have been incised to reveal the position of the superficial inguinal ring (the outer limit of the inguinal canal).

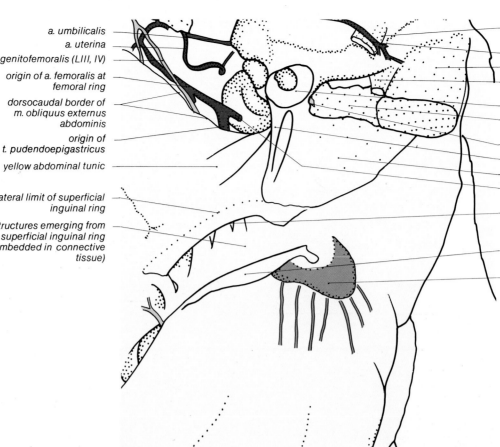

a. umbilicalis
a. uterina
n. genitofemoralis (LIII, IV)
origin of a. femoralis at femoral ring
dorsocaudal border of m. obliquus externus abdominis
origin of t. pudendoepigastricus
yellow abdominal tunic

lateral limit of superficial inguinal ring
structures emerging from superficial inguinal ring (embedded in connective tissue)

mm. gemelli (pars caudalis)
a. gluteus caudalis
m. semimembranosus
m. biceps femoris (ischiatic tendon)
acetabulum
m. obturatorius externus in obturator foramen
n. obturatorius
prepubic tendon
symphyseal tendon
a. circumflexa femoris medialis
cut edge of deep fascia (lateral suspensory lamina of udder)
lateral suspensory lamina of udder (reflected)
position of lnn. inguinales superficiales

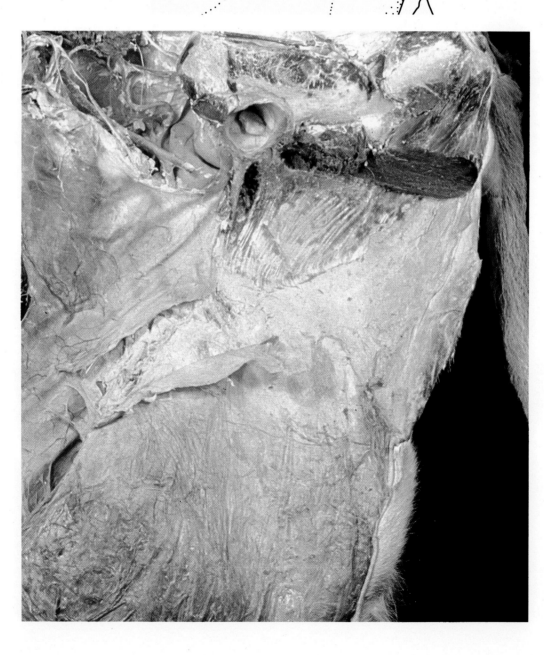

Fig. 9.11 The superficial inguinal (mammary) lymph nodes, in left lateral view.

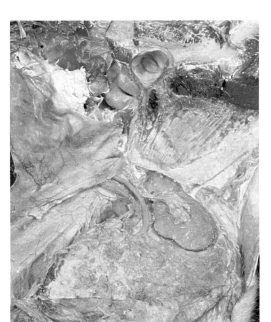

The 'pelvic' tendon of the external oblique abdominal muscle has been incised. The lateral suspensory lamina of the udder has been reflected ventrally. In this way the structures which traverse the inguinal canal are exposed; their pathway through the canal is shown better in fig. 9.13.

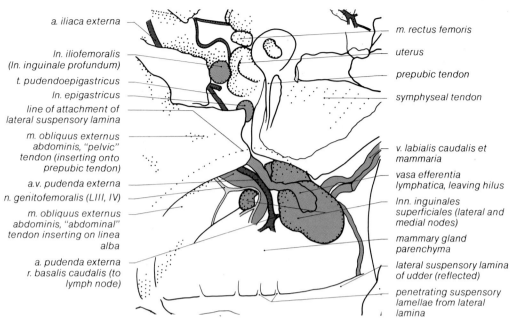

a. iliaca externa

In. iliofemoralis
(In. inguinale profundum)

t. pudendoepigastricus

In. epigastricus

line of attachment of
lateral suspensory lamina

m. obliquus externus
abdominis, "pelvic"
tendon (inserting onto
prepubic tendon)

a.v. pudenda externa

n. genitofemoralis (LIII, IV)

m. obliquus externus
abdominis, "abdominal"
tendon inserting on linea
alba

a. pudenda externa
r. basalis caudalis (to
lymph node)

m. rectus femoris

uterus

prepubic tendon

symphyseal tendon

v. labialis caudalis et
mammaria

vasa efferentia
lymphatica, leaving hilus

Inn. inguinales
superficiales (lateral and
medial nodes)

mammary gland
parenchyma

lateral suspensory lamina
of udder (reflected)

penetrating suspensory
lamellae from lateral
lamina

Fig. 9.12 The dorsal surface of the udder, in craniolateral view.

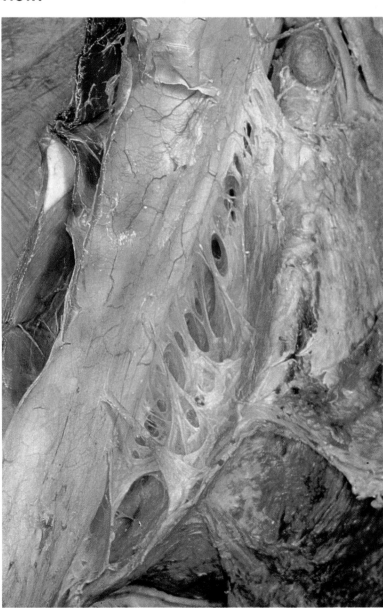

This figure shows a closer view of a part of the dissection seen in fig. 9.11. The dorsal surface of the udder is supported from the deep fascia of the abdominal wall by numerous connective tissue lamellae in which run small blood vessels and nerves.

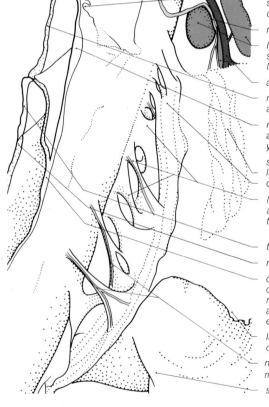

origin of lateral
suspensory lamina of
udder (reflected)

n. genitofemoralis (LIII, IV)

Inn. inguinales
superficiales (medial and
lateral nodes)

a.v. pudenda externa

m. obliquus internus
abdominis

m. obliquus externus
abdominis (covered by
yellow abdominal tunic)

surfaces of udder:
lateral
dorsal

lamellae from yellow
abdominal tunic passing
to dorsal surface of udder

transverse fascia

m. rectus abdominis

conjoint aponeurosis of
oblique abdominal
muscles (vagina m. recti
abdominis, lamina
externa)

lateral suspensory lamina
of udder

nn. lumbales I, II rr. cutanei
mediales ventrales

superficial fascia of udder

Fig. 9.13 The inguinal canal and associated structures, in left lateral view.

Reflection of the 'pelvic' tendon of the external abdominal muscle opens up the inguinal canal. The dorsal border of the 'abdominal' tendon is now visible; this forms the medial rim of the superficial inguinal ring. The cranial rim of the deep ring, formed by the dorsocaudal border of the internal oblique muscle, can also be seen. The genitofemoral nerve (the most caudal of the ventromedial cutaneous branches of the lumbar spinal nerves) and associated vessels traverse the abdominal wall by way of the inguinal canal. In males, the vaginal process persists and also traverses the canal (see fig. 9.27).

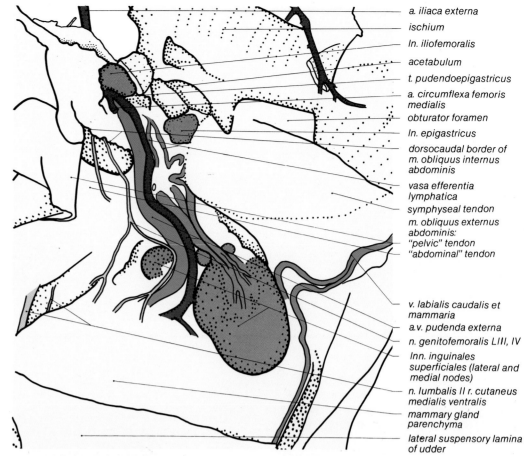

a. iliaca externa

ischium

ln. iliofemoralis

acetabulum

t. pudendoepigastricus

a. circumflexa femoris medialis

obturator foramen

ln. epigastricus

dorsocaudal border of m. obliquus internus abdominis

vasa efferentia lymphatica

symphyseal tendon

m. obliquus externus abdominis:
"pelvic" tendon
"abdominal" tendon

v. labialis caudalis et mammaria

a.v. pudenda externa

n. genitofemoralis LIII, IV

lnn. inguinales superficiales (lateral and medial nodes)

n. lumbalis II r. cutaneus medialis ventralis

mammary gland parenchyma

lateral suspensory lamina of udder

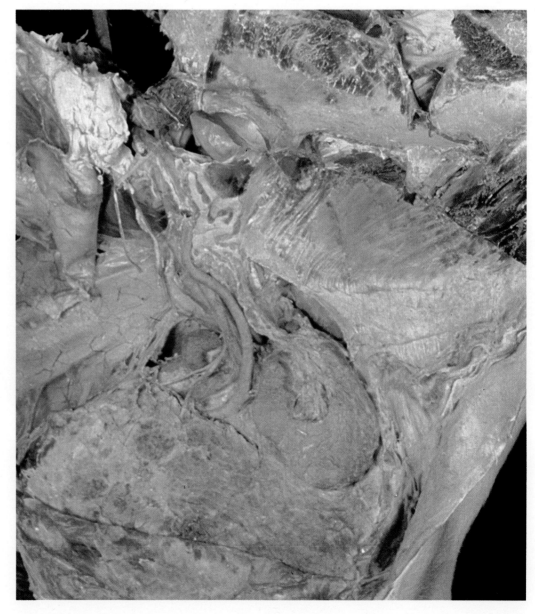

Fig. 9.14 The yellow abdominal tunic and ventromedial cutaneous nerves, in left lateral view.

The ventromedial cutaneous branches of LI, LII, traverse the abdominal wall in the same way that the ventromedial cutaneous branches of LIII, LIV (the genitofemoral nerve) traverse the inguinal canal. This dissection is a closer view of fig. 9.15, but at a slightly earlier stage of dissection.

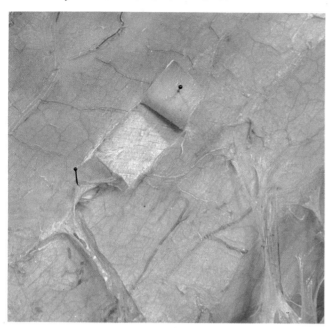

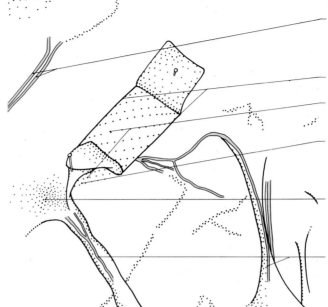

twigs of a ventromedial cutaneous nerve (LI, LII) supplying skin of ventral abdominal wall in region of udder

window in yellow abdominal tunic

aponeurosis of m. obliquus externus abdominis

dorsal rim of foramen in aponeurosis, by which cutaneous nerve passes through muscle of abdominal wall

"canal" between aponeurosis and deep fascia, traversed by rr. cutanei mediales ventrales, LI, LII

twigs of a ventromedial cutaneous nerve (LI, II) running in fascial lamellae of udder

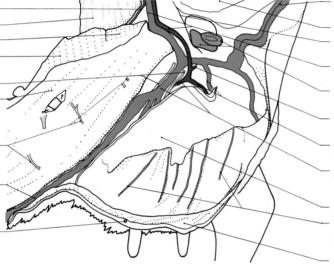

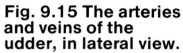

a. epigastrica caudalis

right abdominal wall

m. rectus abdominis

m. obliquus internus abdominis

n. genitofemoralis

m. obliquus externus abdominis ("abdominal" tendon) covered by yellow abdominal tunic

nn. spinales ThXIII-LII rr. cutanei mediales ventrales

v. subcutanea abdominis ("milk vein" or v. epigastrica cranialis superficialis)

superficial vein draining venous plexus of left cranial teat

v. labialis caudalis et mammaria

symphyseal tendon

caudal edge of medial suspensory lamina

a.v. pudenda externa, in inguinal canal

lnn. inguinales superficiales (dexter)

a. pudenda externa r. basalis caudalis

a.v. mammaria caudalis (v. labialis cranialis)

a.v. mammaria cranialis (v. epigastrica caudalis superficialis)

parenchyma of udder

vasa afferentia lymphatica in lateral suspensory lamina

superficial fascia of udder

Fig. 9.15 The arteries and veins of the udder, in lateral view.

The superficial inguinal lymph node of the left side has been cut away from its union with that on the right side. The paths of dorsal venous trunks in the substance of the udder have been dissected to show the three venous drainage routes.

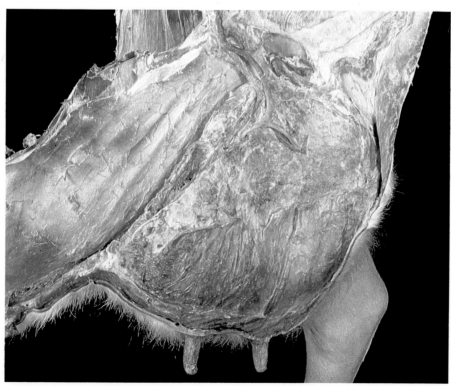

Fig. 9.16 Internal structure of the left forequarter of the udder: lateral view.

An incision has been made through the axis of the teat, slanting obliquely and laterally through the lateral part of the forequarter. The cut also passes through the parenchyma of the hindquarter. There is no visible demarcation in the udder parenchyma between fore and hindquarters, but the two glands do not intercommunicate.

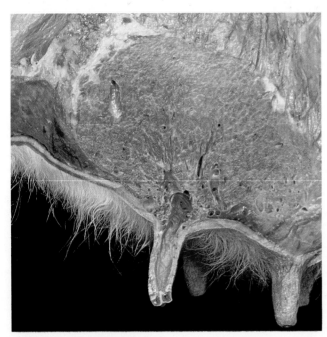

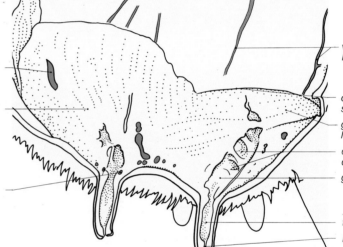

vasa afferentia lymphatica in lateral suspensory lamina of udder

large tributary of v. mammaria cranialis

collecting ducts

one terminal collecting duct, showing entry into gland sinus

gland sinus

veins draining from venous circles of teats

components of venous circle which drains erectile venous plexus in teat wall

teat sinus

position of teat sphincter

left caudal teat

slight concavity at apex of teat

teat rosette

teat duct

teat orifice

Fig. 9.17 Internal structure of the left half of the udder: lateral view.

A second cut passes through the lateral part of the left hindquarter. The two cuts do not define the extent of each gland system; there is no clear demarcation between fore and hindquarters. Left and right halves of the udder are distinctly separated by the medial suspensory laminae (see fig. 9.18).

large tributary of v. mammaria cranialis

glandular parenchyma of left cranial quarter

components of venous circle at base of teat

vasa afferentia lymphatica

cut edge of lateral suspensory lamina

glandular parenchyma of left caudal quarter

orifices of terminal collecting ducts

gland sinus

teat sinus

keratinised teat duct

teat orifice

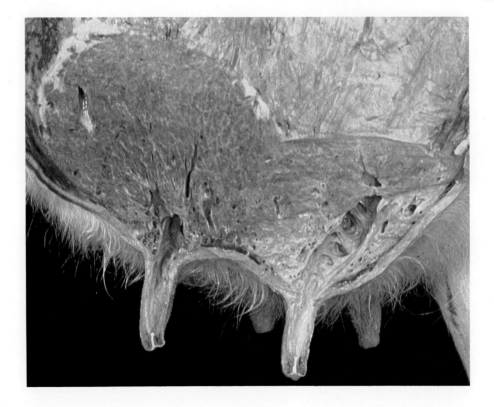

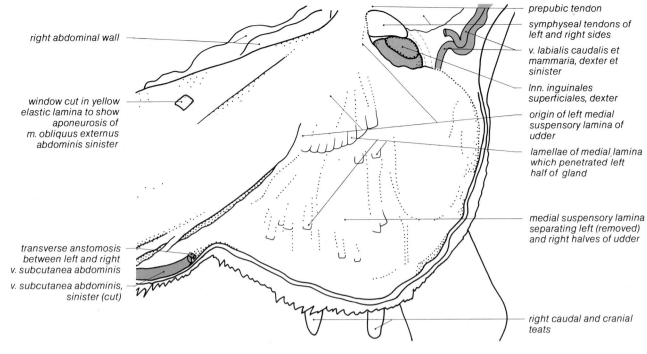

right abdominal wall

window cut in yellow
elastic lamina to show
aponeurosis of
m. obliquus externus
abdominis sinister

transverse anstomosis
between left and right
v. subcutanea abdominis

v. subcutanea abdominis,
sinister (cut)

prepubic tendon

symphyseal tendons of
left and right sides

v. labialis caudalis et
mammaria, dexter et
sinister

lnn. inguinales
superficiales, dexter

origin of left medial
suspensory lamina of
udder

lamellae of medial lamina
which penetrated left
half of gland

medial suspensory lamina
separating left (removed)
and right halves of udder

right caudal and cranial
teats

Fig. 9.18 The left medial suspensory lamina after removal of the left half of the udder: lateral view.
Left and right laminae arise from the yellow abdominal tunic near the midline of the abdominal wall. A small caudal elastic lamina often arises from the symphyseal tendon as indicated by the broken blue lines, but it was not recognisable on this specimen.

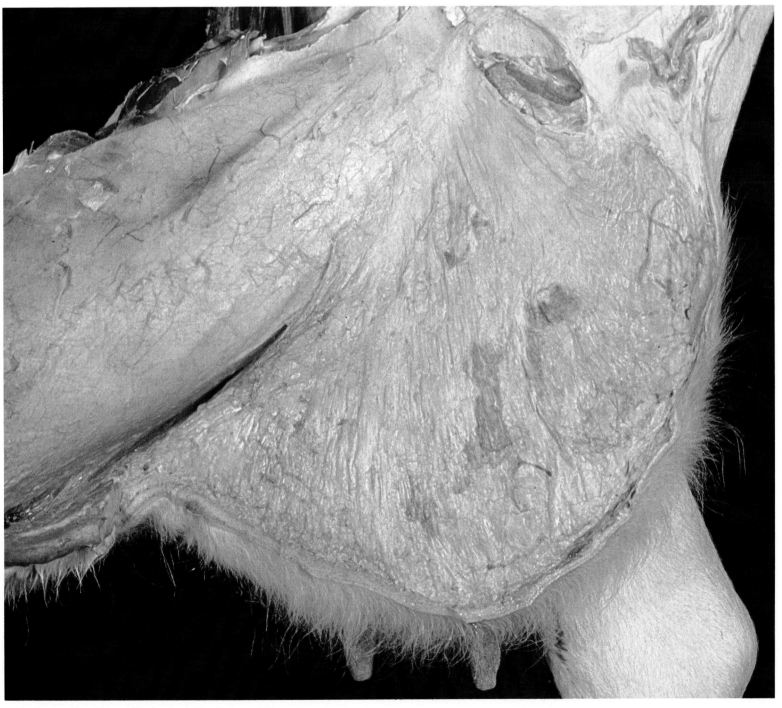

Fig. 9.19 Caudal abdominal and pelvic regions of a week-old bull calf, in right lateral view.

The male structures occupying the same regions as the udder are displayed in figures 9.19 to 9.27. This facilitates comparisons between the two sexes. In female ruminants the foetal scrotum regresses in the inguinal region, just caudal to the udder. In male ruminants the mammary gland persists, just cranial to the scrotum. Scrotum and udder are both components of the escutcheon and the two regions are strictly comparable.

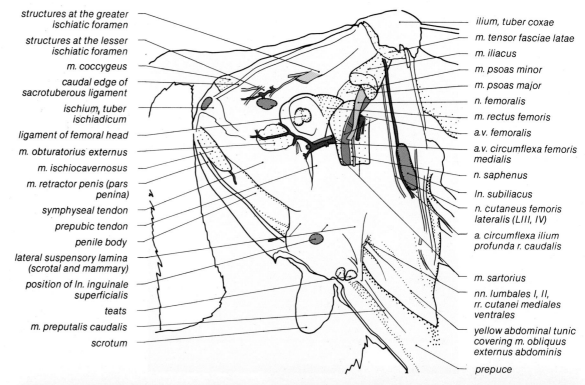

structures at the greater ischiatic foramen
structures at the lesser ischiatic foramen
m. coccygeus
caudal edge of sacrotuberous ligament
ischium, tuber ischiadicum
ligament of femoral head
m. obturatorius externus
m. ischiocavernosus
m. retractor penis (pars penina)
symphyseal tendon
prepubic tendon
penile body
lateral suspensory lamina (scrotal and mammary)
position of ln. inguinale superficialis
teats
m. preputalis caudalis
scrotum

ilium, tuber coxae
m. tensor fasciae latae
m. iliacus
m. psoas minor
m. psoas major
n. femoralis
m. rectus femoris
a.v. femoralis
a.v. circumflexa femoris medialis
n. saphenus
ln. subiliacus
n. cutaneus femoris lateralis (LIII, IV)
a. circumflexa ilium profunda r. caudalis
m. sartorius
nn. lumbales I, II, rr. cutanei mediales ventrales
yellow abdominal tunic covering m. obliquus externus abdominis
prepuce

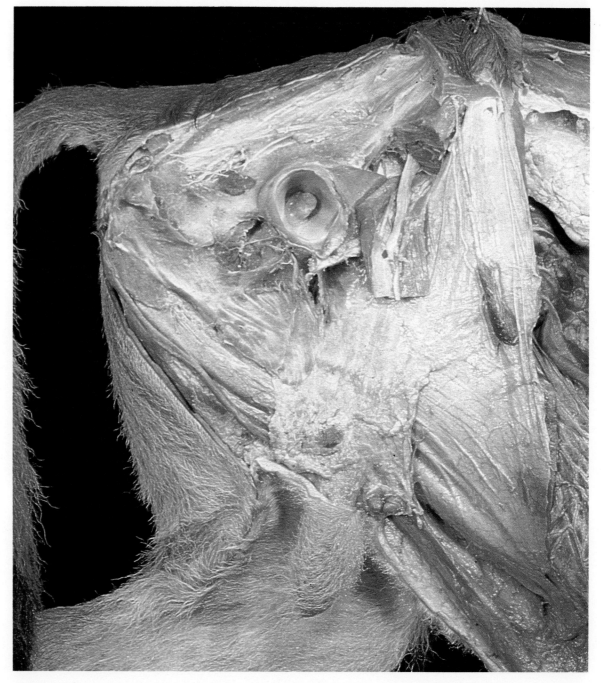

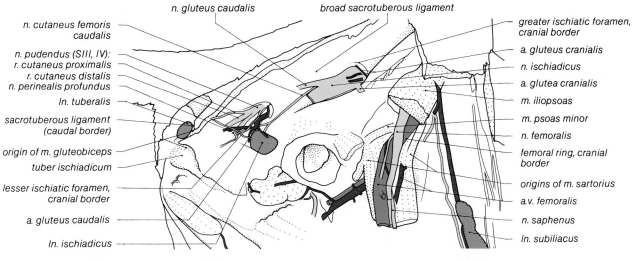

n. cutaneus femoris caudalis

n. gluteus caudalis

broad sacrotuberous ligament

n. pudendus (SIII, IV):
r. cutaneus proximalis
r. cutaneus distalis
n. perinealis profundus

ln. tuberalis

sacrotuberous ligament (caudal border)

origin of m. gluteobiceps

tuber ischiadicum

lesser ischiatic foramen, cranial border

a. gluteus caudalis

ln. ischiadicus

greater ischiatic foramen, cranial border

a. gluteus cranialis

n. ischiadicus

a. glutea cranialis

m. iliopsoas

m. psoas minor

n. femoralis

femoral ring, cranial border

origins of m. sartorius

a.v. femoralis

n. saphenus

ln. subiliacus

Fig. 9.20 The ischiatic foramina and femoral ring of the bull calf, in right lateral view.
This is a closer view of a part of the dissection shown in the previous figures, but the rectus femoris muscle has been shortened slightly.

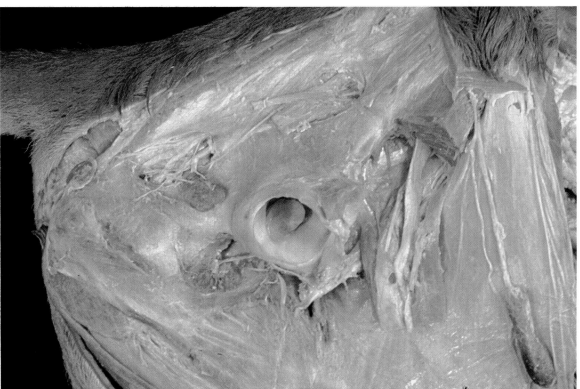

Fig. 9.21 Superficial inguinal structures of the bull calf, in right lateral view.

The structures traversing the inguinal canal are discernable through the thin lateral suspensory lamina immediately ventral to the superficial inguinal ring (see figs. 9.22 and 9.23).

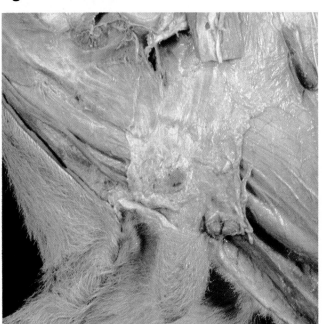

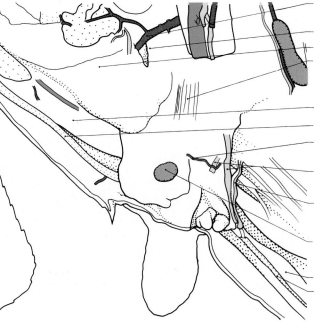

a. circumflexa femoris medialis

prepubic tendon

symphyseal tendon

lateral suspensory lamina (scrotal and mammary) covering inguinal structures

penile body

m. retractor penis

a. epigastrica caudalis superficialis

n. genitofemoralis (LIII, IV) r. cranialis

n. lumbalis II r. cutaneus medialis ventralis

ln. inguinale superficiale beneath lateral suspensory lamina

penile body

m. preputialis caudalis

Fig. 9.22 The superficial inguinal ring of the bull calf: right lateral view (1).

The lateral suspensory lamina has been partially removed to reveal the structures that traverse the inguinal canal, and those at the neck of the scrotum.

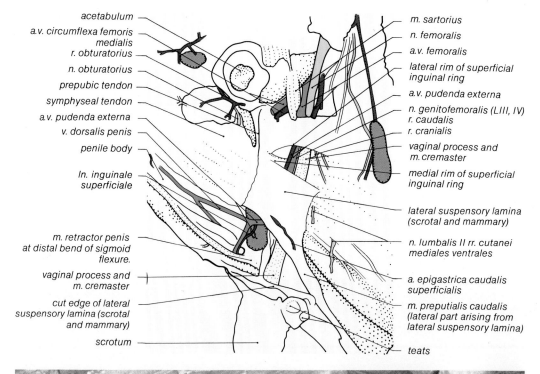

acetabulum
a.v. circumflexa femoris medialis
r. obturatorius
n. obturatorius
prepubic tendon
symphyseal tendon
a.v. pudenda externa
v. dorsalis penis
penile body
ln. inguinale superficiale
m. retractor penis at distal bend of sigmoid flexure.
vaginal process and m. cremaster
cut edge of lateral suspensory lamina (scrotal and mammary)
scrotum

m. sartorius
n. femoralis
a.v. femoralis
lateral rim of superficial inguinal ring
a.v. pudenda externa
n. genitofemoralis (LIII, IV) r. caudalis
r. cranialis
vaginal process and m. cremaster
medial rim of superficial inguinal ring
lateral suspensory lamina (scrotal and mammary)
n. lumbalis II rr. cutanei mediales ventrales
a. epigastrica caudalis superficialis
m. preputialis caudalis (lateral part arising from lateral suspensory lamina)
teats

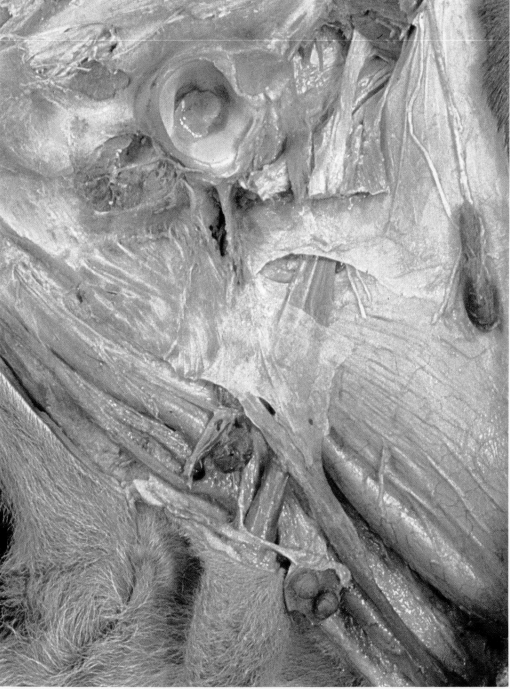

Fig. 9.23 The superficial inguinal ring of the bull calf: right lateral view (2).

The remaining part of the lateral suspensory lamina (see figs. 9.21 and 9.22) has been reflected to reveal the superficial ring and its traversing structures more clearly. It should be stressed that the clear-cut lateral rim of the superficial inguinal ring seen in figs. 9.22 – 9.27 is an artefact. It is merely the line along which the deep fascia of the lateral suspensory lamina has been cut. The ventral border of the 'pelvic tendon' of the external oblique abdominal muscle is the true lateral rim of the ring.

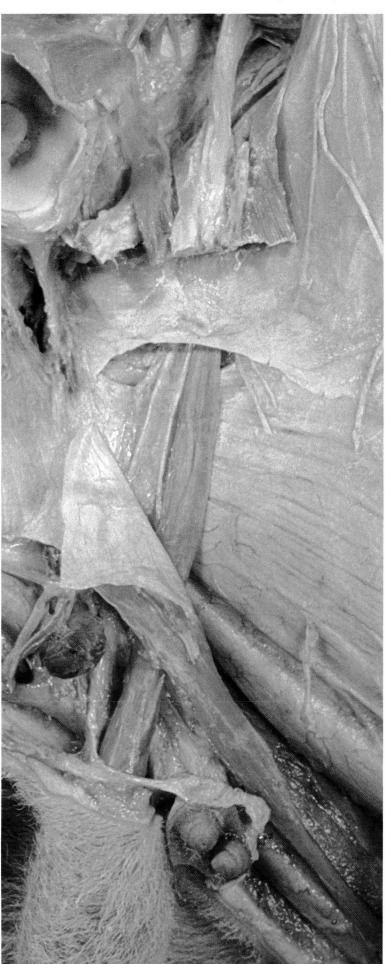

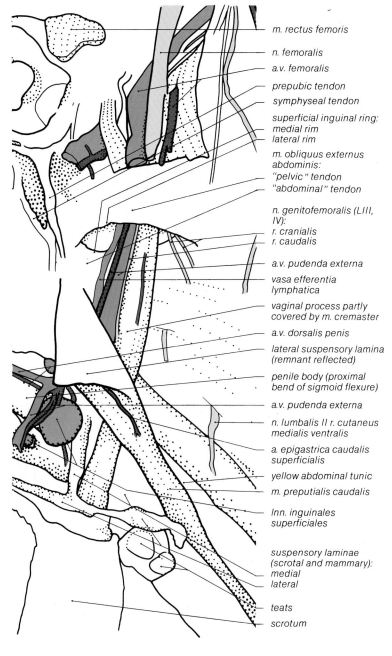

m. rectus femoris

n. femoralis

a.v. femoralis

prepubic tendon

symphyseal tendon

superficial inguinal ring:
medial rim
lateral rim

m. obliquus externus abdominis:
"pelvic" tendon
"abdominal" tendon

n. genitofemoralis (LIII, IV):
r. cranialis
r. caudalis

a.v. pudenda externa

vasa efferentia lymphatica

vaginal process partly covered by m. cremaster

a.v. dorsalis penis

lateral suspensory lamina (remnant reflected)

penile body (proximal bend of sigmoid flexure)

a.v. pudenda externa

n. lumbalis II r. cutaneus medialis ventralis

a. epigastrica caudalis superficialis

yellow abdominal tunic

m. preputialis caudalis

lnn. inguinales superficiales

suspensory laminae (scrotal and mammary):
medial
lateral

teats

scrotum

Fig. 9.24 Fasciae and vessels of the inguinal and scrotal regions in the bull calf: right lateral view.

Lateral and medial scrotal and mammary fasciae of the bull are readily comparable with the mammary suspensory laminae of the cow (see figs. 9.5 and 9.18). The dartos tunic is formed by adherence of the lateral lamina to the scrotal skin. The dartos septum is the direct continuation of the medial lamina into the scrotum.

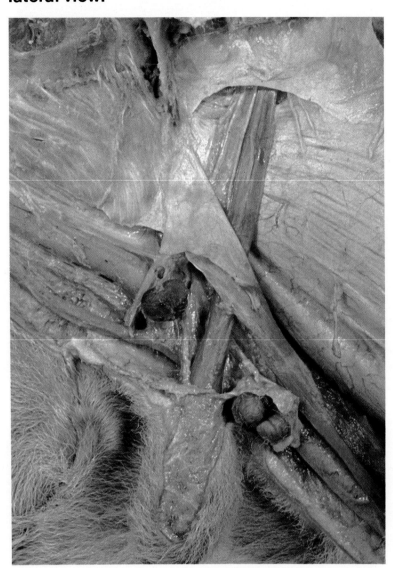

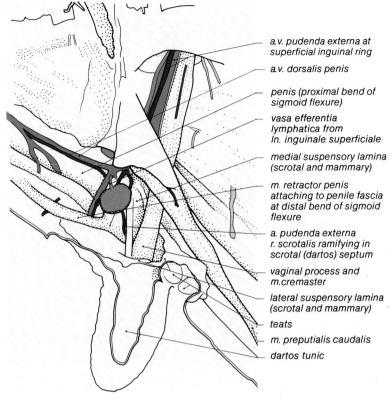

a.v. pudenda externa at superficial inguinal ring

a.v. dorsalis penis

penis (proximal bend of sigmoid flexure)

vasa efferentia lymphatica from ln. inguinale superficiale

medial suspensory lamina (scrotal and mammary)

m. retractor penis attaching to penile fascia at distal bend of sigmoid flexure

a. pudenda externa r. scrotalis ramifying in scrotal (dartos) septum

vaginal process and m.cremaster

lateral suspensory lamina (scrotal and mammary)

teats

m. preputialis caudalis

dartos tunic

Fig. 9.25 The prepuce and preputial orifice of the bull calf, in right lateral view.

A flap of skin has been reflected from the region immediately dorsal to the preputial orifice and the umbilicus. The specimen is at the stage of dissection shown in fig. 9.21.

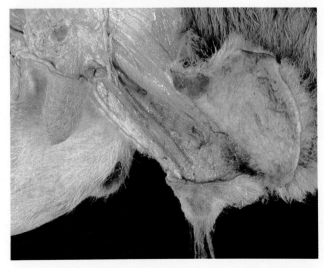

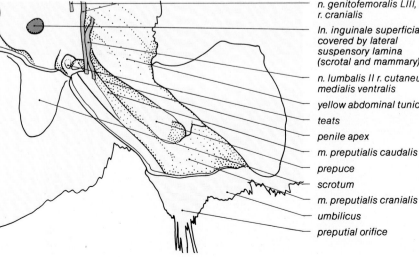

n. genitofemoralis LIII, IV r. cranialis

ln. inguinale superficiale covered by lateral suspensory lamina (scrotal and mammary)

n. lumbalis II r. cutaneus medialis ventralis

yellow abdominal tunic

teats

penile apex

m. preputialis caudalis

prepuce

scrotum

m. preputialis cranialis

umbilicus

preputial orifice

Fig. 9.26 The scrotum of the bull calf, in right lateral view.

The fascial layers of the scrotum can be subdivided in a more complex fashion, but for practical purposes the simple arrangement shown in this dissection and those preceding it is adequate.

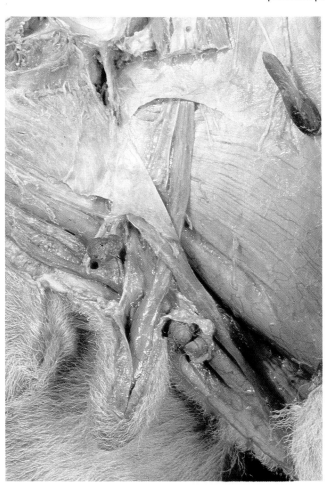

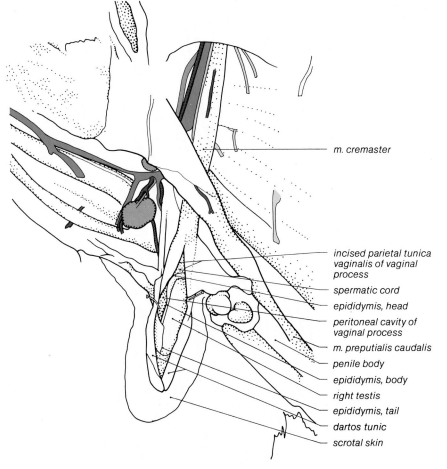

a. testicularis, within spermatic cord

n. genitofemoralis LIII, IV:
r. cranialis
r. caudalis

a.v. pudenda externa

vasa efferentia lymphatica

origin of medial suspensory lamina (scrotal and mammary) from yellow abdominal tunic

a. epigastrica caudalis superficialis

m. retractor penis (pars penina)

a. pudenda externa r. scrotalis (in dartos septum)

m. preputialis caudalis

m. cremaster

scrotal (dartos) septum

teats

parietal tunica vaginalis of vaginal process

dartos tunic (incised)

scrotal skin

Fig. 9.27 The scrotal contents of the bull calf, in right lateral view.

The wall of the vaginal process has been incised and pinned out to show the contents of the peritoneal vaginal cavity. In this specimen the body of the epididymis is not so medial in position as is usual because the testis has rotated on its long axis, (see fig. 8.38).

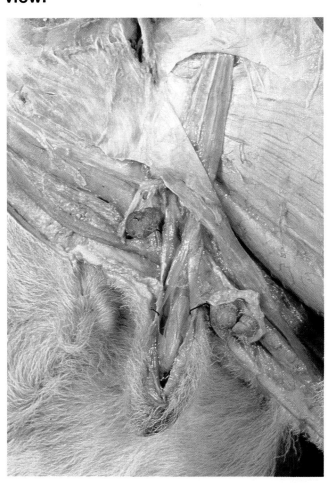

m. cremaster

incised parietal tunica vaginalis of vaginal process

spermatic cord

epididymis, head

peritoneal cavity of vaginal process

m. preputialis caudalis

penile body

epididymis, body

right testis

epididymis, tail

dartos tunic

scrotal skin

Index

References in this index are to page numbers, not to figures. The index lists the pages on which each structure has been labelled in the drawings that accompany the photographs.

In general, the names chosen for the labels to the drawings conform to the Anatomica Veterinaria (1973); the index lists these names as they appear in the labels.

Arteries, lymph nodes, muscles, nerves, veins, and their trunks are indexed under the usual abbreviations (a., ln., m., n., v., t.) as in the labels. For most other structures the anglicized names are used, but the classical name has been retained where it is much more familiar than the anglicized form (*e.g. corpus luteum, crista terminalis*).